Cardiovascular Outcomes of Treatments Available for Patients with Type 1 and 2 Diabetes

Editor

GUILLERMO E. UMPIERREZ

ENDOCRINOLOGY AND METABOLISM CLINICS OF NORTH AMERICA

www.endo.theclinics.com

Consulting Editor
ADRIANA G. IOACHIMESCU

March 2018 • Volume 47 • Number 1

ELSEVIER

1600 John F. Kennedy Boulevard • Suite 1800 • Philadelphia, Pennsylvania, 19103-2899

http://www.theclinics.com

ENDOCRINOLOGY AND METABOLISM CLINICS OF NORTH AMERICA Volume 47, Number 1
March 2018 ISSN 0889-8529, ISBN 13: 978-0-323-58397-8

Editor: Stacy Eastman
Developmental Editor: Meredith Madeira

Endocrinology and Metabolism Clinics of North America (ISSN 0889-8529) is published quarterly by Elsevier Inc., 360 Park Avenue South, New York, NY 10010-1710. Months of issue are March, June, September, and December. Periodicals postage paid at New York, NY and additional mailing offices. Subscription prices are USD 357.00 per year for US individuals, USD 721.00 per year for US institutions, USD 100.00 per year for US students and residents, USD 447.00 per year for Canadian individuals, USD 893.00 per year for Canadian institutions, USD 490.00 per year for international individuals, USD 893.00 per year for international institutions, and USD 245.00 per year for international and Canadian and foreign students/residents. To receive student/resident rate, orders must be accompanied by name of affiliated institution, date of term, and the signature of program/residency coordinator on institution letterhead. Orders will be billed at individual rate until proof of status is received. Foreign air speed delivery is included in all *Clinics* subscription prices. All prices are subject to change without notice. **POSTMASTER:** Send address changes to *Endocrinology and Metabolism Clinics of North America*, Elsevier Health Sciences Division, Subscription Customer Service, 3251 Riverport Lane, Maryland Heights, MO 63043. **Customer Service: Telephone: 1-800-654-2452** (U.S. and Canada); **1-314-447-8871** (outside U.S. and Canada). **Fax: 1-314-447-8029. E-mail: journalscustomerservice-usa@elsevier.com (for print support); journalsonlinesupport-usa@elsevier.com (for online support).**

Reprints. For copies of 100 or more, of articles in this publication, please contact the Commercial Rights Department, Elsevier Inc., 360 Park Avenue South, New York, NY 10010-1710; phone: +1-212-633-3874; fax: +1-212-633-3820; E-mail: reprints@elsevier.com.

Endocrinology and Metabolism Clinics of North America is covered in *MEDLINE/PubMed (Index Medicus), EMBASE/Excerpta Medica, Current Contents/Clinical Medicine, Current Contents/Life Sciences, Science Citation Index, ISI/BIOMED, BIOSIS,* and *Chemical Abstracts*.

Printed in the United States of America.

Contributors

CONSULTING EDITOR

ADRIANA G. IOACHIMESCU, MD, PhD, FACE
Associate Professor of Medicine and Neurosurgery, Co-Director, The Emory Pituitary Center, Emory University School of Medicine, Atlanta, Georgia, USA

EDITOR

GUILLERMO E. UMPIERREZ, MD, CDE, FACE, FACP
Professor of Medicine, Director Clinical Research, Center of Diabetes and Metabolism, Emory University, Director, Diabetes and Metabolism Section, Grady Health System, Atlanta, Georgia, USA

AUTHORS

MOHAMMED K. ALI, MD, MSc, MBA
Advisor, Division of Diabetes Translation, Centers for Disease Control and Prevention, Associate Professor, Hubert Department of Global Health, Rollins School of Public Health, Emory University, Department of Family and Preventive Medicine, Emory University School of Medicine, Atlanta, Georgia, USA

GEORGE L. BAKRIS, MD
Section of Endocrinology, Diabetes, and Metabolism, Department of Medicine, ASH Comprehensive Hypertension Center, The University of Chicago Medicine, Chicago, Illinois, USA

DEEPAK L. BHATT, MD, MPH
Executive Director, Interventional Cardiovascular Programs, Division of Cardiovascular Medicine, Brigham and Women's Hospital, Heart and Vascular Center, Professor of Medicine, Harvard Medical School, Boston, Massachusetts, USA

BEN BRANNICK, MD
Chief Clinical Endocrinology Fellow, Division of Endocrinology, Diabetes and Metabolism, The University of Tennessee Health Science Center, Memphis, Tennessee, USA

SAM DAGOGO-JACK, MD
Professor of Medicine and Director, Division of Endocrinology, Diabetes and Metabolism, The University of Tennessee Health Science Center, Memphis, Tennessee, USA

FARHEEN K. DOJKI, MD
Section of Endocrinology, Diabetes, and Metabolism, Department of Medicine, ASH Comprehensive Hypertension Center, The University of Chicago Medicine, Chicago, Illinois, USA

MAYA FAYFMAN, MD
Assistant Professor of Medicine, Division of Endocrinology, Metabolism and Lipids, Emory University School of Medicine, Atlanta, Georgia, USA

VIVIAN A. FONSECA, MD, FRCP
Professor of Medicine and Pharmacology, Tullis Tulane Alumni Chair in Diabetes, Chief, Section of Endocrinology, Tulane University Health Sciences Center, Southeast Louisiana Veterans Health Care System, New Orleans, Louisiana, USA

RODOLFO J. GALINDO, MD
Assistant Professor of Medicine, Division of Endocrinology, Metabolism and Lipids, Emory University School of Medicine, Atlanta, Georgia, USA

HERTZEL C. GERSTEIN, MD, MSc
Professor, Department of Medicine, Population Health Research Institute, McMaster University, Hamilton Health Sciences, Hamilton, Ontario, Canada

EDWARD W. GREGG, PhD
Chief, Epidemiology and Statistics Branch, Division of Diabetes Translation, Centers for Disease Control and Prevention, Atlanta, Georgia, USA

ANDREA V. HAAS, MD
Fellow, Division of Endocrinology, Diabetes, and Hypertension, Brigham and Women's Hospital, Harvard Medical School, Boston, Massachusetts, USA

IRL B. HIRSCH, MD
Professor, Division of Metabolism, Endocrinology and Nutrition, University of Washington, Seattle, Washington, USA

SILVIO E. INZUCCHI, MD
Professor of Medicine, Clinical Chief, Section of Endocrinology, Yale School of Medicine, Medical Director, Yale Diabetes Center, Yale-New Haven Hospital, New Haven, Connecticut, USA

ANDERS JORSAL, BSc, MD, PhD
Research Fellow, Resident Doctor, Department of Cardiology, Aarhus University Hospital, Department of Clinical Medicine, Faculty of Health, Aarhus University, Aarhus, Denmark

MARIAN SUE KIRKMAN, MD
Professor of Medicine, Division of Endocrinology, The University of North Carolina at Chapel Hill, Chapel Hill, North Carolina, USA

MARY T. KORYTKOWSKI, MD
Professor, Department of Medicine, Division of Endocrinology, University of Pittsburgh, Pittsburgh, Pennsylvania, USA

MIKHAIL KOSIBOROD, MD
Professor, Department of Medicine, University of Missouri-Kansas City, Department of Cardiology, Saint Luke's Mid America Heart Institute, Kansas City, Missouri, USA

DRAGANA LOVRE, MD
Assistant Professor of Medicine, Section of Endocrinology, Tulane University Health Sciences Center, Southeast Louisiana Veterans Health Care Systems, New Orleans, Louisiana, USA

HUSSAIN MAHMUD, MD
Clinical Assistant Professor of Medicine, Division of Endocrinology, UPMC, Pittsburgh, Pennsylvania, USA

ARJUN MAJITHIA, MD
Division of Cardiovascular Medicine, Lahey Hospital & Medical Center, Burlington, Massachusetts, USA

MARIE E. McDONNELL, MD
Chief, Diabetes Section, Division of Endocrinology, Diabetes, and Hypertension, Brigham and Women's Hospital, Harvard Medical School, Boston, Massachusetts, USA

JOHN J.V. McMURRAY, BSc (Hons), MB ChB (Hons), MD, FRCP, FESC, FACC, FAHA, FMedSci, FRSE
Professor of Medical Cardiology, Deputy Director (Clinical), Honorary Consultant Cardiologist, BHF Cardiovascular Research Centre, Institute of Cardiovascular & Medical Sciences, University of Glasgow, Queen Elizabeth University Hospital, Glasgow, United Kingdom

ADAM J. NELSON, BMedSc, MBBS
South Australian Health and Medical Research Institute, Adelaide, South Australia, Australia

STEPHEN J. NICHOLLS, MBBS, PhD, FRACP
South Australian Health and Medical Research Institute, Adelaide, South Australia, Australia

FRANCISCO J. PASQUEL, MD, MPH
Assistant Professor of Medicine, Division of Endocrinology, Emory University School of Medicine, Atlanta, Georgia, USA

SIMON K. ROCHELAU, BMBS
South Australian Health and Medical Research Institute, Adelaide, South Australia, Australia

REEMA SHAH, MD
Department of Medicine, Population Health Research Institute, McMaster University, Hamilton Health Sciences, Hamilton, Ontario, Canada

SULAY SHAH, MD
Endocrinology Fellow, Section of Endocrinology, Tulane University Health Sciences Center, New Orleans, Louisiana, USA

AANU SIHOTA, MD
Endocrinology Fellow, Section of Endocrinology, Tulane University Health Sciences Center, New Orleans, Louisiana, USA

SAVITHA SUBRAMANIAN, MD
Associate Professor, Division of Metabolism, Endocrinology and Nutrition, University of Washington, Seattle, Washington, USA

GUILLERMO E. UMPIERREZ, MD, CDE, FACE, FACP
Professor of Medicine, Director Clinical Research, Center of Diabetes and Metabolism, Emory University, Director, Diabetes and Metabolism Section, Grady Health System, Atlanta, Georgia, USA

HENRIK WIGGERS, BSc, MD, PhD, DMSc
Associate Professor of Medical Cardiology, Consultant Cardiologist, Department of Cardiology, Aarhus University Hospital, Department of Clinical Medicine, Faculty of Health, Aarhus University, Aarhus, Denmark

Contents

> Atherosclerotic cardiovascular disease (ASCVD) is a leading global cause of death and accounts for most deaths among individuals with diabetes. This article reviews the latest observational and trial data on changes in the relationship between diabetes and ASCVD risk, remaining gaps in how the role of each risk factor is understood, and current knowledge about specific interventions. Differences between high-income countries and low-income and middle-income countries are examined, barriers and facilitators are discussed, and a discussion around the concept of ideal cardiovascular health factors (Life's Simple 7) is focused on.

> Prediabetes is a state characterized by impaired fasting glucose or impaired glucose tolerance. This article discusses the pathophysiology and macrovascular complications of prediabetes. The pathophysiologic defects underlying prediabetes include insulin resistance, alpha- and beta-cell dysfunction, increased lipolysis, inflammation, and suboptimal incretin effect. Recent studies have revealed that the long-term complications of diabetes manifest in some people with prediabetes; these complications include microvascular and macrovascular disorders. Finally, the authors present an overview of randomized control trials aimed at preventing progression from prediabetes to type 2 diabetes and discuss their implications for macrovascular risk reduction.

> The most common cause of death among adults with diabetes is cardiovascular disease (CVD). In this concise review on pathogenesis of CVD in diabetes, the 4 common conditions, atherosclerosis, microangiopathy, diabetic cardiomyopathy, and cardiac autonomic neuropathy, are explored and illustrated to be caused by interrelated pathogenetic factors. Each of these diagnoses can present alone or, commonly, along with others owing to overlapping pathophysiology. Although the spectrum of

physiologic abnormalities that characterize the diabetes milieu is broad and goes beyond hyperglycemia, the authors highlight the most relevant evidence supporting the current knowledge of potent factors that contribute to CVD in diabetes.

Savitha Subramanian and Irl B. Hirsch

Type 1 diabetes mellitus, an autoimmune disorder characterized by beta-cell destruction and absolute insulin deficiency, is associated with significantly increased cardiovascular disease risk, but the mechanisms underlying this enhanced risk are unclear. Results of the pivotal Diabetes Control and Complications Trial/Epidemiology of Diabetes Interventions and Complications study have shown that compared with conventional therapy, intensive glycemic control results in decreased cardiovascular morbidity and mortality. Evidence from this study also revealed contributions of blood pressure, renal disease, body weight, and lipids to cardiovascular disease in type 1 diabetes mellitus. Extrapolating from existing evidence, this article addresses clinical strategies to mitigate cardiovascular risks.

Marian Sue Kirkman, Hussain Mahmud, and Mary T. Korytkowski

People with type 2 diabetes mellitus are at high risk of morbidity and mortality from cardiovascular disease (CVD). Based on observed relationships between hyperglycemia and CVD, several large clinical trials have investigated the ability of treatment strategies to achieve hemoglobin A_{1c} less than 7% (53 mmol/mol) as a way of reducing this risk. These studies demonstrate that intensified glycemic therapy may reduce CVD risk in younger patients with recent-onset type 2 diabetes mellitus but not in high-risk older individuals with established disease. Attention to blood pressure and lipid-lowering therapies with modified glycemic goals for older high-risk individuals is recommended.

Hertzel C. Gerstein and Reema Shah

As recently as 20 years ago there were no randomized controlled trials of potentially cardiovascular protective therapies in people with type 2 diabetes. The ongoing cardiovascular trials bring the needed evidence. Both primary and subsidiary analyses have transformed diabetes from a largely eminence-based specialty to one that is firmly evidence based. These studies have provided evidence supporting glucose-lowering drugs for patients with cardiovascular risk factors. Randomized controlled trials such as those described here will continue to challenge assumptions and create new approaches and paradigms that can be pursued to reduce and hopefully eliminate serious cardiovascular and other consequences of diabetes.

ENDOCRINOLOGY AND METABOLISM CLINICS OF NORTH AMERICA

VISIT THE CLINICS ONLINE!
Access your subscription at:
www.theclinics.com

Foreword

Diabetes and Atherosclerotic Cardiovascular Disease

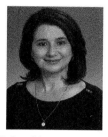

Adriana G. Ioachimescu, MD, PhD, FACE
Consulting Editor

The "Cardiovascular Outcomes of Treatments Available for Patients with Type 1 and 2 Diabetes" issue of the *Endocrinology and Metabolism Clinics of North America* is dedicated to a rapidly evolving field of great importance for physicians caring for patients with or at risk for diabetes mellitus. The guest editor is Dr Guillermo E. Umpierrez, a renowned diabetologist and prolific investigator at Emory University. Dr Umpierrez is an expert in management of inpatient hyperglycemia and senior author of the recent American Association of Clinical Endocrinologists consensus statement with regards to treatment of type 2 diabetes. Dr Umpierrez gathered an international group of experts to compile a thorough review of the growing body of evidence in this important field with relevance to the practice of endocrinologists, cardiologists, internists, and other specialists.

More than 400 million people worldwide have prediabetes and are at risk for microvascular and macrovascular complications even before the diagnosis of type 2 diabetes is made. Drs Brannick and Dagogo-Jack from University of Tennessee Health Science Center review the pathophysiology of prediabetes, the predicting factors of progression to type 2 diabetes, and the interventions to offset diabetes and its complications. Drs Pasquel and Gregg from Emory University in Atlanta explain the epidemiology trends with regards to atherosclerotic cardiovascular disease in diabetes and review the preventative strategies of cardiovascular and cerebrovascular events. Drs Haas and McDonnell from Harvard Medical School take us on a journey that unveils the pathogenesis of cardiovascular disease in diabetes. Dr Kirkman from University of North Carolina at Chapel Hill and Drs Mahmud and Korytkowski from University of Pittsburgh tackle the issue of intensive blood glucose control in relation to vascular outcomes in type 2 diabetes and underscore the risk of adverse cardiovascular risks of severe hypoglycemia. Drs Gerstein and Shah from McMaster University in Hamilton, Canada perform a thorough overview of cardiovascular outcome trials of glucose-lowering drugs in type 2 diabetes. Drs Jorsal and Wiggers from Aarhus University

Endocrinol Metab Clin N Am 47 (2018) xiii–xiv
https://doi.org/10.1016/j.ecl.2017.12.002
0889-8529/18/© 2017 Published by Elsevier Inc.

Hospital in Denmark and Dr McMurray from University of Glasgow in United Kingdom present the current evidence on the interaction between glucose-lowering drugs and heart failure. Dr Inzucchi from Yale University reviews the current evidence that allows physicians to practice personalized glucose management in patients with type 2 diabetes and cardiovascular disease. Dr Subramanian from University of Washington in Seattle targets specifically the relationship between intensive diabetes treatment and cardiovascular outcomes in patients with type 1 diabetes. Drs Galindo, Fayfman, and Umpierrez from Emory University in Atlanta provide a comprehensive review on management of hyperglycemia in hospitalized patients in several settings, including post–cardiac surgery. Dr Kosiborod from University of Missouri-Kansas City delivers a review on hyperglycemia in acute coronary syndromes from mechanisms to management strategies. Drs Dojki and Bakris from University of Chicago update us on blood pressure targets and modalities to achieve those in patients with diabetes according to clinical trials. Drs Nelson and Nicholls from South Australian Health and Medical Research Institute present a review of lipid-lowering strategies and lipid goals in type 2 diabetes. Dr Majithia from Lahey Medical Center and Dr Bhatt from Harvard Medical School tackle the controversial issue of preventative aspirin use, while also summarizing evidence for use of antiplatelet therapy in patients with cardiovascular complications. Drs Lovre, Shah, Sihota, and Fonseca from Tulane University in New Orleans perform a comprehensive review on the interaction between hyperglycemia, chronic kidney disease, and dyslipidemia.

We hope you will find this issue of the *Endocrinology and Metabolism Clinics of North America* informative and useful in your practice. This is an excellent issue for physicians who practice internal medicine, endocrinology, cardiology, nephrology, or surgery, and an essential collection for physicians in training. We thank Dr Umpierrez for guest-editing this extremely important issue, the team of authors for their contributions, and the Elsevier editorial staff for their continuous support.

Adriana G. Ioachimescu, MD, PhD, FACE
Emory University School of Medicine
The Emory Pituitary Center
1365 B Clifton Road, Northeast, B6209
Atlanta, GA 30322, USA

E-mail address:
aioachi@emory.edu

Preface

Diabetes and Atherosclerotic Cardiovascular Disease: Novel Insights and Therapeutic Strategies

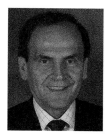

Guillermo E. Umpierrez, MD, CDE, FACE, FACP
Editor

Atherosclerotic cardiovascular disease (ASCVD), defined as coronary heart disease, cerebrovascular disease, or peripheral arterial disease, is the leading cause of morbidity and mortality for individuals with diabetes. Whether it is type 1 or type 2 diabetes, there is substantial evidence to support and that increasing hyperglycemia, uncontrolled blood pressure, and hyperlipidemia lead to an increase in cardiovascular disease risk. The death rate due to ASCVD in patients with diabetes is two to four times higher than those without diabetes, and large cross-sectional studies have reported that over two-thirds of the deaths in patients aged >65 years with diabetes are attributed to ASCVD.

Intensive glycemic control trials have clearly demonstrated a reduction in risk for microvascular complications in patients with type 1 and type 2 diabetes. The short-term impact on ASCVD, however, remains uncertain. Results of large randomized controlled trials and meta-analyses have shown that intensive glycemic control is associated with a relative reduction in CV events attributed primarily to a decrease in acute myocardial infarction rates; however, there was no effect of intensive glycemic control on rates of stroke, cardiovascular mortality, or all-cause mortality.

Common comorbidities in patients with diabetes, including hypertension and dyslipidemia, are well-established risk factors for ASCVD in patients with type 1 and type 2 diabetes. Numerous studies have shown the efficacy of controlling individual cardiovascular risk factors in preventing or slowing ASCVD in people with diabetes. In addition, large benefits are seen when multiple cardiovascular risk factors are addressed simultaneously. Risk factor modification in patients with diabetes during the past

Endocrinol Metab Clin N Am 47 (2018) xv–xvi
https://doi.org/10.1016/j.ecl.2017.12.001
0889-8529/18/© 2017 Published by Elsevier Inc.

two decades has improved the 10-year coronary heart disease risk ASCVD morbidity and mortality among US adults.

Since 2008, the US Food Drug Administration mandated that all new antidiabetic agents must undergo an adequately powered, glycemic-equipoised, cardiovascular outcome trial in high-risk type 2 diabetic patients, during the postmarketing phase, to demonstrate its safety by showing noninferiority against placebo. Most of these trials were conducted with drugs working through incretin pathway, dipeptidyl peptidase-4 inhibitors, and glucagon-like peptide-1 receptor agonists, and two trials with sodium-glucose–linked transporter-2 receptor inhibitors. The results of these trials suggest that ASCVD risk reduction may be driven more by drug strategy than the HbA1c level achieved in patients with type 2 diabetes.

In this issue, we discuss the epidemiology, pathophysiology, and management of ASCVD in patients with diabetes type 1 and type 2. We provide practical information on the diagnosis, prevention, and treatment of cardiovascular risk factors in patients with prediabetes and diabetes. In addition, we review recent recommendations on the treatment of hyperglycemia and diabetes during cardiovascular surgery, chronic kidney disease, and heart failure.

I would like to thank all the contributing authors for their diligent and scholarly reviews and for sharing their wisdom. I hope you will enjoy their perspectives and incorporate the information into your practice.

Guillermo E. Umpierrez, MD, CDE, FACE, FACP
Center of Diabetes and Metabolism
Emory University
Diabetes and Metabolism Section
Grady Health System
49 Jesse Hill Jr Drive
Atlanta, GA 30303, USA

E-mail address:
geumpie@emory.edu

The Evolving Epidemiology of Atherosclerotic Cardiovascular Disease in People with Diabetes

Francisco J. Pasquel, MD, MPH[a],*, Edward W. Gregg, PhD[b],
Mohammed K. Ali, MD, MSc, MBA[b,c,d]

KEYWORDS

- Cardiovascular • Diabetes • Epidemiology • Life's Simple 7
- Ideal cardiovascular health • Atherosclerosis

KEY POINTS

- Incidence rates of coronary artery disease and stroke in people with diabetes are declining in high-income countries; nevertheless, the absolute numbers are high and costs are expected to significantly increase in the next decades.
- The patterns of epidemiologic transitions in risk factors for diabetes and cardiovascular disease are different across the world and may be driven by changes in demographics, nutritional changes, sedentariness, tobacco use, and access to interventions.
- Achievement of hemoglobin c, blood pressure, and low-density lipoprotein cholesterol management goals has improved in the United States but remains suboptimal.
- Prevention strategies could simultaneously maintain or improve all cardiovascular health metrics, both behavioral (healthy weight, physical activity, healthy diet, and no smoking) and biological (glucose, blood pressure, and cholesterol).
- Atherosclerosis starts in childhood and primordial prevention in early life could have important benefits across the lifespan.

Disclosure Statement: No potential conflicts of interest relevant to this article. The findings and conclusions in this report are those of the authors and do not necessarily represent the official position of the Centers for Disease Control and Prevention.
[a] Division of Endocrinology, Emory University School of Medicine, 69 Jesse Hill Jr. Drive Southeast, Atlanta, GA 30303, USA; [b] Division of Diabetes Translation, Centers for Disease Control and Prevention, 4770 Buford Highway, Mailstop F-75, Atlanta, GA 30341, USA; [c] Hubert Department of Global Health, Rollins School of Public Health, Emory University, 1518 Clifton Road, Atlanta, GA 30322, USA; [d] Department of Family and Preventive Medicine, Emory University School of Medicine, 4500 North Shallowford Road, Suite B, Atlanta, GA 30338, USA
* Corresponding author.
E-mail address: fpasque@emory.edu

Endocrinol Metab Clin N Am 47 (2018) 1–32
https://doi.org/10.1016/j.ecl.2017.11.001
0889-8529/18/© 2017 Elsevier Inc. All rights reserved.

INTRODUCTION

Cardiovascular disease (CVD) is the leading global cause of death, accounting for 17.3 million deaths per year.[1] In 2015, 85% of all deaths due to CVD were related to atherosclerotic CVD (ASCVD), including coronary heart disease (CHD) and stroke (15.2 million deaths).[2] The burden of CVD is growing faster than the ability to combat it in large part due to the obesity and type 2 diabetes mellitus (T2D) epidemics.[3] Among patients with T2D older than 65 years, ASCVD accounts for up to 7 of 10 deaths.[4]

The relationship between diabetes and CVD is unique and evolving. First, part of this evolution is that other CVD risk factors are changing (eg, mean blood pressure, cholesterol levels, and smoking prevalence have declined since 1980, particularly in high-income countries),[5–7] likely affecting the excess risk of ASCVD in T2D. Second, changes in the incidence and prevalence trends and the health profile of newly diagnosed individuals with T2D in the past decades may have been influenced by changing diagnostic thresholds, screening practices, and higher number of younger individuals diagnosed with the disease.[8] Third, although incidence rates of myocardial infarction (MI) and of stroke are declining, the absolute numbers are still high and there is higher recognition of other cardiovascular comorbidities like nonischemic heart failure with reduced or preserved ejection fraction.[2,9] Fourth, the patterns of these evolutions vary across the world, partially driven by changes in demographics (aging populations), nutritional changes (higher-calorie diets), more sedentariness, and continued/growing tobacco use in low-income and middle-income countries (LMICs), compared with declines in high-income countries.[2,8,10]

Urgent measures to address ASCVD risk in people with diabetes could ameliorate health and economic impacts. Different primordial, primary, and secondary ASCVD prevention strategies are recommended by professional organizations and new large collaborative efforts are emerging. This article reviews results from the latest observational and trial data on changes in the relationship between diabetes and ASCVD risk, the remaining gaps in how the role of each major risk factor for ASCVD among people with diabetes is understood, interventions to address each specific risk factor, and what is (and is not) known about the use of those interventions in practice. Where possible, differences between high-income and LMIC settings are examined, barriers and facilitators are discussed, and a discussion around the concept of ideal cardiovascular health factors (ie, Life's Simple 7) is focused on.

US AND GLOBAL TRENDS IN ATHEROSCLEROTIC CARDIOVASCULAR DISEASE AMONG PEOPLE WITH DIABETES

Significant changes in mortality trends have been observed in the past 4 decades. In the United States and several other high-income countries worldwide, the CHD mortality rate peaked during the 1960s, then reversed direction and has steadily fallen since then.[11,12] Recent estimates, however, show that the decline in US CVD mortality rates have flattened to less than 1% per year since 2011 and that the death rate for 2015 actually increased by 1% for the first time since 1969.[3] Globally, the absolute number of CVD-related deaths continues to increase, largely driven by increased numbers of deaths in LMICs,[2,13] although age-standardized death rates have decreased, **Table 1**.

There are differences between high and LMICs in terms of the patterns of ASCVD in people with diabetes. Large reductions in the rates of classic complications of T2D have been observed in high-income countries over the past 20 years. Although there are few data, it is hypothesized that burden of CVD is growing in LMICs.[8,11]

In the United States, large reductions in the incidence of diabetes-related complications were observed between 1990 and 2010, with the greatest reduction observed for

Table 1
Global cause-specific mortality for cardiovascular disease and diabetes

Global Deaths	All-Age Deaths (Millions) 2005→2015	Percentage Change 2005→2015	Age-Standardized Rates of Death per 100,000
CVD	15.9→17.9	↑12.5% (10.6–14.4)	↓15.6% (14.2–16.9)
Ischemic heart disease	7.6→8.9	↑16.6% (14.6–18.6)	↓12.8% (11.4–14.2)
Ischemic stroke	2.8→3.0	↑7.9% (5.2–10.6)	↓20.2% (22.1–18.1)
Hemorrhagic stroke	3.3→3.3	← →2.7%(−0.6–6.4)	↓21.9% (24.3–19.0)
Peripheral vascular disease	0.04→0.05	↑37.7% (30.1–46.5)	← → 0.3% (−5.9–6.3)
Diabetes	1.2→1.5	↑ 32.1% (27.7–36.3)	← → 0.4% (−2.7–3.6)

← →, No significant change over time; →, absolute change over time; ↑↓, significant increase or decrease over time.

Data from GBD Mortality and Causes of Death Collaborators. Global, regional, and national life expectancy, all-cause mortality, and cause-specific mortality for 249 causes of death, 1980–2015: a systematic analysis for the Global Burden of Disease Study 2015. Lancet 2016;388(10053):1459–544.

MI, stroke, and limb amputation[14] (**Fig. 1**A). Similarly, other high-income countries have experienced a significant decline in the rate of ASCVD complications.[8] On the other hand, in LMICs, where most people with obesity and diabetes live[15,16] and where most of the global deaths (approximately 70%) related to CVD occur,[13] the trends of ASCVD-related mortality has decreased in a lower magnitude in the general population or in many countries a flat mortality or slight increases have been observed.[11] No data are available on ASCVD trends specifically among individuals with diabetes in LMICs.

Along with population growth and aging, there has been a worldwide increase in the age-standardized prevalence of diabetes since 1980.[17] In the United States, a potential decrease in the incidence of diabetes was suggested in 2014 based on self-report data from the National Health Interview Survey[18]; however, it has been suggested that the observed decline was likely an artifact of nonbiological factors, especially related to changes in diagnostic criteria[19] Recent reports show that the prevalence of diabetes among adults increased in the US from 8.4% (1988–1994 period)[20] to 12.2% in 2015,[21] with the highest prevalence among those aged 46 to 65 years. It is possible that changes in the incidence/prevalence of diabetes has changed its relationship with ASCVD, as lower glycemic diagnostic thresholds and higher screening rates could have resulted in a larger and healthier population of individuals with diabetes; however there are no objective data to support this.

Over the past several decades, subjects with and without diabetes have benefited similarly from the decline in CVD rates.[22] It is not clear, however, why the magnitude of the drop in the rate of macrovascular complications in the United States in recent years has been significantly higher among people with diabetes versus the general public[14] (**Fig. 1**). One explanation could be the simultaneous impact of the results of the United Kingdom Prospective Diabetes Study (UKPDS) with an emphasis on blood pressure control by professional associations along with the publication of Adult Treatment Panel III guidelines for statin use in patients with diabetes.[23,24] Trends have shown a decline in blood pressure that seem similar among individuals with and without diabetes but of lower magnitude in recent years.[25,26] Simultaneously, there has been a higher use of statins among people with diabetes along with an

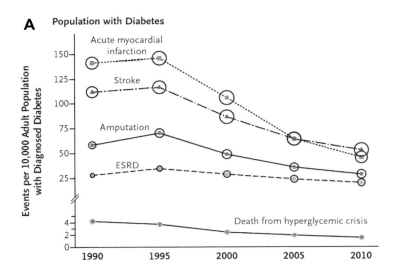

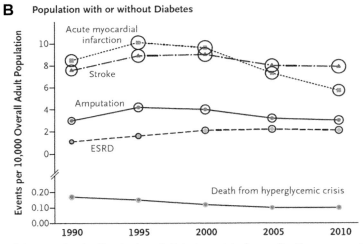

Fig. 1. Trends in age-standardized rates of diabetes-related complications among US adults with diagnosed diabetes, 1990 to 2010. Denominators are from the National Health Interview Survey (*A*) and the U.S. Census Bureau (*B*). ESRD, end-stage renal disease. (*From* Gregg EW, Li Y, Wang J, et al. Changes in diabetes-related complications in the United States, 1990–2010. N Engl J Med 2014;370(16):1514–23; with permission.)

apparent higher decline in cholesterol levels compared with individuals without diabetes.[27,28] The use of statins has also been lower among individuals without diabetes with dyslipidemia who would qualify for statin use.[21,28–30] In addition, compared with individuals without diabetes, statins seem to benefit people with diabetes in higher magnitude.[31–33] It is also possible that simultaneous management of multiple risk factors in patients with diabetes could have led to a substantial decline in cardiovascular events and mortality.[34,35] In addition, the nationwide adoption and meaningful use of electronic health records potentially could have had an impact on prevention efforts in patients with diabetes in the past few years.[36,37]

IDEAL CARDIOVASCULAR HEALTH (LIFE'S SIMPLE 7)

According to the World Health Organization (WHO), hypertension, tobacco use, high blood glucose, physical inactivity, overweight and obesity, and high cholesterol levels are among the top risk factors for death globally.[38] Most of these factors are associated with incident CVD and diabetes, and patients with diabetes have a high prevalence of most risk factors.[10,21,38,39]

For people without preexisting CVD, the American Heart Association created a set of central goals that together reflect ideal cardiovascular health. The concept is useful from public health and individual clinical levels and allows decision makers and health care providers to track how people do with regard to achievement of optimal levels of 7 metrics (Life's Simple 7).[40] These cardiovascular health metrics include ideal health behaviors (no smoking, healthy weight, physical activity at goal levels, and pursuit of a diet consistent with current guideline recommendations) and ideal biological factors (untreated total cholesterol <200 mg/dL, untreated blood pressure <120/<80 mm Hg, and fasting blood glucose <100 mg/dL).[4,41] Results of a recent meta-analysis show that greater achievement of ideal cardiovascular health metrics is associated with an impressively lower risk of CVD (relative risk [RR] 0.20; 95% CI, 0.11–0.37), cardiovascular mortality (RR 0.25; 95% CI, 0.10–0.63), and all-cause mortality (RR 0.55; 95% CI, 0.37–0.80).[42] Over recent years, blood pressure, low-density lipoprotein cholesterol (LDL-C), and glycemic control in patients with diabetes have improved in the United States; however, only a minority of individuals are at control for all these factors[43–45] (**Fig. 2**). In addition to these 3 metrics, achieving behavioral goals (no smoking, maintaining a healthy weight, physical activity, and healthy diet) is challenging for patients with diabetes. Combined data from the Atherosclerosis Risk in Communities Study (ARIC),[46] the Multi-Ethnic Study of Atherosclerosis (MESA),[47] and the Jackson Heart Study (JHS)[48] showed that individuals with diabetes who achieved individual or combined goals of hemoglobin A_{1c} (A_{1c}), blood pressure, and LDL-C (ABCs) control had a substantially lower risk of CHD and CVD[49] (**Fig. 3**).

In patients with diabetes it is presumed that most cardiovascular benefits are achieved from improving blood pressure and cholesterol levels; however, the impact of glycemic control on ASCVD in high-risk patients is less clear.[50–55] Interventions on smoking cessation, lifestyle changes, the introduction of a Mediterranean diet or the Dietary Approach to Stop Hypertension (DASH), and the use of newer antidiabetic agents with proved cardiovascular benefits could add further benefits to patients with diabetes. Analyses and interventions addressing simultaneously these 3 biological (ABCs) metrics and all 4 behavioral factors in patients with diabetes are limited. Areas for future research include the cumulative effect of addressing all cardiovascular health metrics among subjects with diabetes.

IDEAL BIOLOGICAL FACTORS (GLYCEMIC CONTROL, BLOOD PRESSURE, AND CHOLESTEROL)

In the United States, significant improvements have been observed in the prevalence of patients with diabetes that meet ABC management goals.[43,45] Large declines in the rates of vascular complications have also been observed in other high-income countries.[8,14] Despite this progress, achievement of ABC goals remains suboptimal, particularly among minority groups, and the absolute number of complications continues to increase.[2,43,45,56]

Glycemic Control and Diabetes as Coronary Heart Disease Equivalent

A causal relationship between hyperglycemia and microvascular complications is well established and the rate of microvascular complications in people with diabetes is

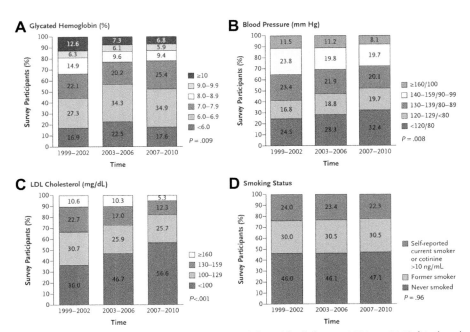

Fig. 2. Distribution of risk factors among US adults with diabetes, 1999 to 2010 (National Health and Nutrition Examination Survey). During the last period (2007–2010), 52.2% met A_{1C} goal less than 7%, 56.8% met LDL-C goal less than 100 mg/dL (primary prevention), 23.2% met LDL-C less than 70 mg/dL (secondary prevention), and 51% met blood pressure goal less than 130/80. Tobacco use was reported in 22.3%. Only 14.3% met ABC and tobacco use targets. The distributions for glycated hemoglobin level (*A*), blood pressure (*B*), low-density lipoprotein (LDL) cholesterol level (*C*), and smoking status (*D*) are shown according to time periods designated in the National Health and Nutrition Examination Survey. Data are weighted percentages. (*From* Ali MK, Bullard KM, Saaddine JB, et al. Achievement of goals in U.S. diabetes care, 1999-2010. N Engl J Med 2013;368(17):1613–24; with permission.)

thought to be at least 10 times to 20 times that of the nondiabetic population.[8] The high prevalence of ASCVD in individuals with diabetes has been recognized for more than a century[57]; however, a causal relationship between diabetes and macrovascular complications is less well understood given the overlap with multiple comorbidities and risk factors.

For several years, diabetes has been considered a CHD risk equivalent[58] and more recently as a CHD risk equivalent for peripheral arterial disease and carotid artery stenosis[59]; nevertheless other reports suggest that the risk is considerably lower.[60,61] The duration and severity of diabetes could explain this discrepancy. Recently, in the REasons for Geographic and Racial Differences in Stroke Study, participants with diabetes only (no CHD or albuminuria) had lower risk of CHD events than did those with prevalent CHD; however, those with severe diabetes (defined by insulin use and/or with albuminuria) had similar risk to those with prevalent CHD (hazard ratio [HR] 0.88 [95% CI, 0.72–1.09]), whereas individuals with diabetes and CHD had the highest risk of additional events (**Fig. 4**).

Glycated hemoglobin and fasting blood glucose seem reliable screening tools in patients with CVD[62] and are closely linked to incident cardiovascular events.[63–67] Among individuals 55 years to 64 years of age, it is estimated that for every 1 mmol/L (18 mg/

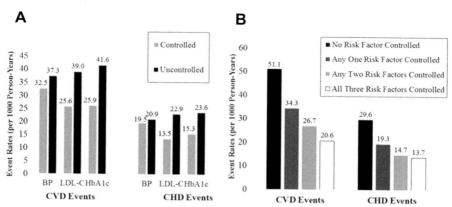

Fig. 3. Unadjusted CVD and CHD event rates per 1000 person-years for subjects with diabetes, by status of being at target level for individual risk factors BP, LDL-C, and A₁c (A) and by the number of risk factors at target levels (B). BP target, 130/80 mm Hg; LDL-C target, 2.6 mmol/L (100 mg/dL); and A₁c target, 53.0 mmol/mol (7%). Data from 3 cohorts (MESA, ARIC, and JHS). BP, blood pressure; HbA1c, glycated hemoglobin. (*From* Wong ND, Zhao Y, Patel R, et al. Cardiovascular risk factor targets and cardiovascular disease event risk in diabetes: a pooling project of the atherosclerosis risk in communities study, multi-ethnic study of atherosclerosis, and Jackson Heart Study. Diabetes Care 2016;39(5):668–76; with permission.)

dL) higher fasting plasma glucose, the RRs are 1.18 (1.08–1.29) for ischemic heart disease and 1.14 (1.01–1.29) for total stroke.[68] The potential benefit of intensive glucose-lowering treatment, however, may be offset by the potential harm associated with severe hypoglycemia.[69]

National US estimates suggest a modest improvement in glycemic control over time. Between the 1999 to 2002 period and the 2007 to 2010 period, the proportion of patients with poor glycemic control decreased approximately 6% (95% CI, −10.5 to −1.1) and the proportions of patients who met the recommended targets for glycated hemoglobin level increased by 8% (95% CI, 0.8–15.0). Nevertheless, approximately half of patients still had a glycated hemoglobin greater than 7% in the 2007 to 2010 period.[43] Follow-up results from 2 landmark trials (Diabetes Control and Complications Trial and UKPDS) in patients with type 1 diabetes mellitus and T2D showed that better glycemic control early during the disease process is associated with lower cardiovascular risk, suggesting a long-term benefit of initial good glycemic control, termed *legacy* effect or *metabolic memory*, by some investigators.[57,70]

The Action to Control Cardiovascular Risk in Diabetes (ACCORD) trial,[51] the Action in Diabetes and Vascular Disease: PreterAx and Diamicron Modified-Release Controlled Evaluation (ADVANCE) trial,[50] and Veterans Affairs Diabetes Trial (VADT)[52] were 3 landmark randomized controlled trials (RCTs) of shorter duration, aiming to examine the effect of intensively lowering glycated hemoglobin and other cardiovascular risk levels on cardiovascular events in older, poorly controlled patients, with ACCORD aiming at the lowest A₁c target (<6%). Intensive therapy in this trial was associated with a decreased number of MIs on follow-up, yet there was a significantly higher mortality observed in the intensive arm.[51,71] This study was stopped prematurely due to the unexpected increase in all-cause mortality after approximately 3.7 years of follow-up. The risk of cardiovascular mortality noted during the active phase of ACCORD (HR 1.49; 95% CI, 1.19, 1.87) decreased after 8.8 years but

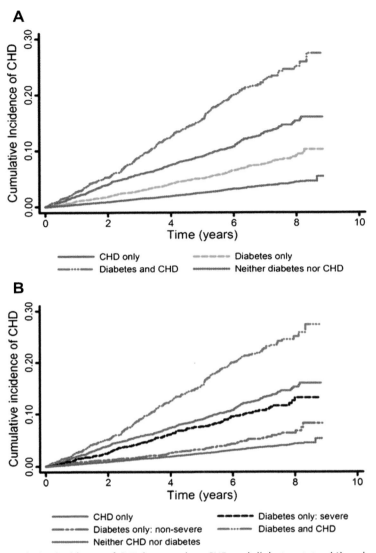

Fig. 4. Cumulative incidence of CHD by prevalent CHD and diabetes status (*A*) and prevalent CHD and diabetes (insulin use and/or albuminuria) status (*B*). Severe diabetes is defined as insulin use and/or albuminuria. (*From* Mondesir FL, Brown TM, Muntner P. Diabetes, diabetes severity, and coronary heart disease risk equivalence: REasons for Geographic and Racial Differences in Stroke (REGARDS). Am Heart J 2016;181:43–51; with permission.)

remained significantly higher (HR 1.20; 95% CI, 1.03, 1.39).[53] Similarly, intensive therapy in ADVANCE and VADT was not associated with decreased cardiovascular mortality.[50,52]

Among patients with diabetes using insulin therapy, a long-standing debate has been the association of insulin use and increased risk of death observed in observational studies, particularly based on a dose-dependent fashion. A recent observational study that accounted for time-dependent factors did not find major cardiovascular harms associated with insulin therapy.[72] These findings are consistent with results from randomized clinical trials, such as those suggesting that different basal insulins do not seem to increase cardiovascular mortality.[73–75]

Recently, 2 classes of antidiabetes medications (glucagon-like peptide-1 receptor analogs[76,77] and sodium-glucose cotransporter-2 [SGLT-2] inhibitors[78,79]) have shown decreased numbers of cardiovascular events in patients with high baseline risk. SGLT-2 inhibitors (canagliflozin and empagliflozin) showed not only a reduction in cardiovascular death but also a markedly significant decrease in hospitalization for heart failure that seems largely independent from a potential modification of the natural history of atherosclerosis. These findings have been reproduced in real-world practice.[80] The impact at large scale of these costly medications on population health is unknown.

Blood Pressure, Clear Benefits—Moving Targets

In 2010, high blood pressure was the leading risk factor for deaths due to CVD, chronic kidney disease, and diabetes worldwide, accounting for more than 40% of deaths from these diseases.[81] In the United States, hypertension is highly prevalent among patients with diabetes (74%; 95% CI, 70%–77%).[21]

Large randomized trials have clearly shown that controlling blood pressure with antihypertensive agents reduces cardiovascular events in patients with diabetes.[23,82,83] Based on estimates derived from US data, even modest changes in blood pressure (such as 5 mm Hg, the mean reduction in DASH) could significantly reduce more than 600,000 CHD events over a 10-year period.[84]

Current guidelines suggest a blood pressure target of 140/90 mm Hg for most patients, yet the blood pressure target has been a matter of intense debate in recent years.[85–87] The ACCORD BP study[88] evaluated the potential benefits of targeting a systolic blood pressure (SBP) level below 120 mm Hg versus a level below 140 mm Hg in patients with T2D. The lower target did not reduce the rate of a composite outcome of fatal and nonfatal major cardiovascular events after 4.7 years. Even though there was a reduction in the secondary endpoint of total stroke, the number of events in this study was lower than expected.[88,89] Serious adverse events that were attributed to antihypertensive drugs (ie, hypotension, bradycardia or arrhythmia, and hyperkalemia) were significantly higher in the intensive-therapy group.[88] Two meta-analyses evaluating SBP targets in patients with diabetes suggested that a target of 140/90 mm Hg is preferable in this population.[90,91] These 2 analyses found conflicting results for lower blood pressure targets (more harm was observed if pretreatment SBP was <140 mm Hg[91] vs a potential lower risk for stroke for SBP <130 mm Hg[90]).

The Systolic Blood Pressure Intervention Trial[92] compared the same targets (120 mm Hg vs 140 mm Hg) and found that the intensive target significantly reduced the primary endpoint (composite outcome: MI, other acute coronary syndrome, stroke, heart failure, or death from cardiovascular causes) by 25% (HR 0.75; 95% CI, 0.64–0.89). This study did not include patients with diabetes, and the results cannot be extrapolated to this population. A more recent meta-analysis of 42 RCTs, including 30 trials that enrolled patients with diabetes, showed that reducing SBP to levels below currently recommended targets significantly reduces the risk of CVD and all-cause mortality (with the lowest risk at 120–124 mm Hg). A subanalysis of subjects with diabetes was not feasible due to insufficient data.[86] Outcomes of intensive blood pressure reduction for patients with diabetes warrant further investigation.[86,90–92]

Multiple antihypertensive agents, including angiotensin-converting enzyme (ACE) inhibitors, angiotensin receptor blockers (ARBs), diuretics, and calcium channel blockers, have been shown effective in reducing cardiovascular events in patients with diabetes.[93] Agents that target the renin-angiotensin system (RAS) (ACE inhibitors and ARBs) have been for several years the agents of choice for patients with diabetes and hypertension. Nevertheless, the superiority of these agents for the prevention of CVD outcomes in patients with diabetes has not been consistent. A recent meta-analysis[94] showed that RAS blockers were of similar efficacy compared with thiazides, calcium channel blockers, and β-blockers. These findings are consistent with the recommendations from the Eighth Joint National Committee on prevention, detection, evaluation, and treatment of high blood pressure and led to recent changes in the recommendations by the American Diabetes Association.[93] RAS blockers, however, remain as the agents of choice for patients with diabetes and albuminuria.[93]

Dyslipidemia, Still Based on Low-Density Lipoprotein Cholesterol

A causal relationship between blood cholesterol levels and atherosclerosis is well established.[95,96] Large-scale clinical trials have clearly demonstrated the safety and remarkable effectiveness of statins to reduce cardiovascular morbidity and mortality.[95] LDL-C management is a major goal to reduce cardiovascular complications in patients with diabetes.

In addition to statins, a reduction in saturated fat, cholesterol, and trans-fat intake and increasing plant stanols/sterols, omega-3 fatty acids, and viscous fiber (such as in oats, legumes, and citrus) are recommended to improve the lipid profile of patients with diabetes.[93] Furthermore, glycemic control can have a substantial effect in patients with hypertriglyceridemia and poor glucose control.

The ideal LDL-C goal has been a matter of debate in recent years. Results of clinical trials with nonstatin lipid-lowering agents have demonstrated that lowering LDL-C levels beyond current goals in patients with high cardiovascular risk can further decrease the risk of cardiovascular events.[32,97]

A meta-analysis, including 14 randomized clinical trials showed that there was a 9% proportional reduction in all-cause mortality per millimore per liter (39 mg/dL) reduction in LDL-C among individuals with diabetes (rate ratio [RR] 0.91; 99% CI, 0.82–1.01), which was similar to the 13% reduction among those without diabetes (RR 0.87; 99% CI, 0.82–0.92).[98] After 5 years, it was estimated that about 40 fewer people with diabetes had major vascular events per 1000 persons assigned to statin therapy.[98]

Despite the clear evidence of lipid-lowering therapies on cardiovascular risk reduction, major gaps still exist. In the United States, for the period of 2011 to 2014, 3 of 4 adults (75.2%; 95% CI, 68.7–80.8) were eligible for primary prevention of ASCVD with statin therapy, however, only 58.2% (95% CI, 49.7–66.3) of those eligible were on lipid-lowering therapy.[21] For secondary prevention, approximately 1 of 5 people (23.3%; 95% CI, 18.9–28.3) was eligible for statin therapy; however, only 2 of 3 eligible individuals were on lipid-lowering therapy during that period.[8]

The role of therapies targeting high triglycerides in patients with diabetes is less well established. Results from a prespecified subgroup analysis from ACCORD suggested a benefit of combination therapy of statin and fibrates in male participants with both a high baseline triglyceride level and a low baseline high-density lipoprotein cholesterol (HDL-C) level.[99] The heterogeneity of treatment response by baseline lipids was sustained after 9.7 years of follow-up in this cohort.[100] Given inconclusive findings of large prospective studies and variable use in clinical practice, targeting triglycerides and HDL-C is currently not an intervention well studied at the population health level.

IDEAL HEALTH BEHAVIORS (HEALTHY WEIGHT, PHYSICAL ACTIVITY, HEALTHY DIET, AND NO SMOKING)

Maintaining a Healthy Weight; Are More Aggressive Interventions Needed?

Obesity may be a bigger health crisis than hunger and is a leading risk factor for death and disabilities globally.[101] The mortality burden of high body mass index (BMI) approximately doubled from 1980 to 2010 worldwide and is expected to increase further in coming years.[81,101] In 2014, more than 1.9 billion adults were overweight and of these more than 600 million had obesity. In addition, it is estimated that approximately 41 million children under 5 years old had overweight or obesity in 2014.[102] Recent estimates show that more than two-thirds of deaths related to high BMI were due to CVD globally.[103] Obesity is independently associated with both CVD[104] and T2D.[105] In the United States approximately 9 of 10 individuals with T2D have overweight or obesity (88%; 95% CI, 85%–90%).[8]

The amount and distribution of adiposity play important roles in influencing multiple cardiometabolic traits and the development of cardiometabolic diseases. Central adiposity, however, may pose higher risk for stroke and CHD.[106] According to National Health and Nutrition Examination Survey data, abdominal adiposity based on waist circumference has increased progressively in the United States since the 1960s,[107] including an upward trend from 1999 to 2012.[108]

Insulin resistance, a condition linked to central adiposity, has been considered a major factor driving the increased risk of diabetes and CVD.[109] Results from the Bogalusa Heart Study showed that hyperinsulinism during early life (5 years to 23 years) is associated with worse cardiovascular risk years later.[110,111] A recent report showed that BMI levels precede hyperinsulinemia during childhood and that this 1-directional relationship plays a role in the development of hypertension.[112] It is known that the metabolic syndrome, a constellation of factors that include central adiposity, insulin resistance, dyslipidemia, and hypertension as defined either by the National Cholesterol Education Program or WHO criteria, is associated with increased CVD mortality.[113]

According to the degree of insulin sensitivity, prevalence of the metabolic syndrome, cardiorespiratory fitness, or the number of cardiometabolic abnormalities, a highly prevalent subgroup of individuals with obesity but without apparent atherosclerosis has been characterized as "metabolically healthy."[114–116] Nevertheless, meta-analyses of prospective cohorts suggest that individuals with obesity considered metabolically healthy are still at an increased risk of diabetes and cardiovascular events compared with metabolically healthy normal-weight individuals and that there is no healthy pattern of increased weight.[117–119]

Sustained weight loss of 3% to 5% can result in clinically meaningful reductions in triglycerides, blood glucose, A_{1C}, and risk of T2D. Greater amounts of weight loss can reduce blood pressure, improve LDL-C and HDL-C, and reduce the need for diabetes and cardiovascular medications.[120]

Major challenges exist to achieve significant weight loss with medical therapy among patients with diabetes or to implement lifestyle interventions, particularly among patients with marked obesity. Bariatric surgery procedures have evolved significantly in the past 2 decades and are now considered a safe and effective alternative for the management of obesity.[121] Five-year outcome data from the Surgical Treatment and Medications Potentially Eradicate Diabetes Efficiently trial showed that bariatric surgery achieving marked weight loss, significantly improved the cardiometabolic profile of patients with diabetes, and decreased use of diabetes and cardiovascular medications.[122] Similar benefits on cardiometabolic risk factors have been observed in adolescents undergoing bariatric surgery, including remission of T2D in up to 95% of participants with diabetes at baseline.[123] After approximately 11 years of follow-up, bariatric surgery for severe obesity was associated with long-term weight loss and decreased overall mortality in the Swedish Obese Subjects study, a prospective but nonrandomized intervention. Mortality was related mostly to MI and cancer in this study.[124]

Bariatric surgery also seems cost effective and has the potential to reduce lifetime health care costs by 30%.[121,125] It has, for many years, been recommended as a therapeutic option for individuals with obesity and T2D; however, widespread bariatric surgery is limited because of multiple socioeconomic barriers, limited numbers of bariatric surgeons and specialized centers, and uncertain public health support.[121,125]

Lifestyle Changes, Look AHEAD, and Beyond

It is known that low levels of fitness are associated with increased risk of CVD mortality among patients with diabetes independently of weight.[126] Furthermore, the addition of cardiorespiratory fitness to traditional risk factors significantly improves the reclassification of risk for adverse cardiovascular outcomes.[127] Lifestyle interventions can reduce cardiovascular risk in patients both with and without diabetes.[39] It is also known that the amount of exercise among patients with diabetes is a major determinant of glycemic control.[128]

Randomized interventions have confirmed improvements in cardiometabolic risk with lifestyle interventions that include exercise in patients with short-term and long-term diabetes duration.[129–133] The impact of short-term lifestyle interventions, however, on hard cardiovascular outcomes later in life is not clear.[134,135]

Results from the American Cancer Society Cancer Prevention Study[136] showed that in overweight people with diabetes (N = 4970), intentional weight loss was associated with approximately 25% reduction in mortality (RR 0.75; 95% CI, 0.67–0.84) and 28% reduction in CVD and diabetes mortality (RR 0.72; 95% CI, 0.63–0.82) during a 12-year follow-up.

The Look AHEAD (Action for Health in Diabetes) trial was a landmark study that randomized 5145 patients with overweight or obesity and T2D to an intensive lifestyle intervention that promoted weight loss (decreased caloric intake and increased physical activity) or to receive diabetes support and education (control group). In this study, modest weight loss of 5% to less than 10% was associated with significant improvements in CVD risk factors at 1 year[131]; nevertheless, at 10 years of follow-up, the trial was stopped early based on futility analysis. The primary CVD outcome occurred in 403 patients in the intervention group and in 418 in the control group (1.83 and 1.92 events per 100 person-years, respectively; HR in the intervention group, 0.95; and 95% CI, 0.83–1.09).[135] Similarly, lifestyle modification programs based on the Diabetes Prevention Program study have shown clinically meaningful weight and cardiometabolic health improvements over a short period of observation.[133]

A recent intervention with intense physical activity that exceeded some of the limitations of Look AHEAD (different levels of supervised exercise and total exercise volume [duration, frequency, and intensity]) showed a 74% reduction in the use of glucose-lowering medication after 12 months; however, the durability and impact of this findings on CVD are not known. Mild hypoglycemia was reported in 13% of participants on the intensive intervention.[137] Similarly, in an exploratory analysis of Look AHEAD, intensive lifestyle intervention was associated with a greater likelihood of partial remission of T2D.[138]

The length of observation and magnitude of weight loss might be important factors to determine the impact of lifestyle interventions. In the Da Qing Diabetes Prevention Study, a 6-year program for Chinese people with impaired glucose tolerance, lifestyle intervention reduced cardiovascular and all-cause mortality after 23 years of follow-up.[139] An analysis of individuals who lost at least 10% of their bodyweight in the first year of Look AHEAD had a 21% lower risk of the primary composite outcome, including death from cardiovascular causes, nonfatal acute MI, nonfatal stroke, or admission to hospital for angina (adjusted HR 0.79; 95% CI, 0.64–0.98) compared with individuals with stable weight or weight gain.[140] A recent analysis evaluating the heterogeneity in response to lifestyle intervention in Look AHEAD showed that baseline A_{1C} and health status distinguished people who would benefit from the intervention and identified 3 relevant groups. Participants who had both low starting A_{1C} (<6·8%) and good health status (>48 on the 36-Item Short Form Health Survey) had an impressive 45% reduction in incidence of the composite primary outcome.[141] On the other hand, those with low starting A_{1C} but poor health status had twice the risk. Areas for future research include improving our understanding of heterogeneity in response to interventions to design diverse menus of individualized lifestyle interventions to improve population health.[141]

Mediterranean and Dietary Approach to Stop Hypertension Diets

Global dietary patterns have shifted in nearly every nation in the world. In the United States, suboptimal diet is a leading risk factor for death and disability.[10] Specifically, diets that are high in calories, saturated fats, salt, and sugars but low in fruits and vegetables have been implicated in the development of cardiometabolic risk factors and CVD[10,142] (**Fig. 5**). At the global level, for example, 1.65 million annual deaths from cardiovascular causes were attributed to excess sodium intake.[143] In the United States, dietary factors were estimated associated with a substantial proportion of deaths from heart disease, stroke, and T2D. The largest numbers of estimated diet-related cardiometabolic deaths were related to high sodium (66,508 deaths in 2012; 9.5% of all cardiometabolic deaths), low nuts/seeds (59,374; 8.5%), high processed meats (57,766; 8.2%), low seafood omega-3 fats (54,626; 7.8%), low

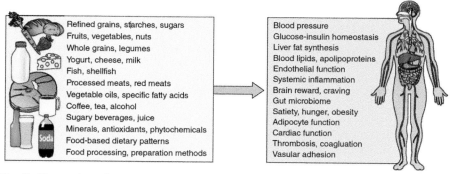

Fig. 5. Diet and cardiovascular and metabolic risk — pathways and mechanisms. Each of these dietary factors influences many or even all of these pathways, which could also be modified in some cases by underlying individual characteristics. (*From* Mozaffarian D. Dietary and policy priorities for cardiovascular disease, diabetes, and obesity: a comprehensive review. Circulation 2016;133(2):187–225; with permission.)

vegetables (53,410; 7.6%), low fruits (52,547; 7.5%), and high sugar-sweetened beverages (51,694; 7.4%).[144]

Current US federal agricultural subsidies focus on financing the production of corn, soybeans, wheat, rice, sorghum, dairy, and livestock.[145] In a recent study, higher consumption of calories from subsidized food commodities was associated with a greater probability of cardiometabolic risks, including obesity, dysglycemia, dyslipidemia, and higher C-reactive protein level.[142]

Data from RCTs show that lower intake of dietary saturated fat and replaced with polyunsaturated vegetable oil reduced CVD by approximately 30%, a reduction similar to that observed with statin treatment.[146] The Prevención con Dieta Mediterránea trial enrolled patients with T2D or at least 3 of the following major risk factors: smoking, hypertension, elevated LDL-C levels, low HDL-C levels, overweight or obesity, and a family history of premature CHD. The 2 Mediterranean diet groups received either extravirgin olive oil (approximately 1 L per week) or 30 g of mixed nuts per day (15 g of walnuts, 7.5 g of hazelnuts, and 7.5 g of almonds) at no cost. The control group received small nonfood gifts. This landmark study showed that assignment to a Mediterranean diet significantly reduced the incidence of major cardiovascular events. The HRs were 0.70 (95% 0.54–0.92) for the group receiving extravirgin olive oil and 0.72 (95% CI, 0.54–0.96) for the diet with nuts group.[147] Similarly, results of a meta-analysis showed also that the use of the Mediterranean diet is associated with lower A_{1C} levels and improved cardiovascular risk factors in patients with diabetes.[148]

The DASH is recommended to lower blood pressure.[149] The DASH can also affect other cardiometabolic parameters and has been associated with a reduction of approximately 13% in the 10-year Framingham risk score for CVD.[150] A modified DASH higher in vegetable fats and lower in carbohydrates compared with the conventional DASH results in larger cardiometabolic benefits.[10] In particular, replacing carbohydrates with unsaturated fat may improve insulin sensitivity and might be more beneficial for patients with diabetes.[151]

Recent studies have challenged the diet-heart hypothesis.[152–154] In a recent analysis of dietary intake in 18 countries, a diet high in carbohydrates was associated with increased all-cause mortality whereas saturated fat consumption was surprisingly associated with lower all-cause mortality.[153] Although further clarification is awaited, eating more fish, fruits, vegetables, and whole grains is recommended as well as avoiding salt, sugar, industrial trans fats, and overeating.[155–158]

Tobacco Use Is Still Prevalent

Reducing the prevalence of smoking in the US has been a public health priority since the landmark Surgeon General's report on smoking in 1964 and has been a notable achievement in public health.[12,159] Heavy taxes on tobacco products, placing warning labels on cigarette packs, imposing advertising restrictions, prohibiting minors from purchasing tobacco products, advertising campaigns, and banning smoking in public places are among the policy initiatives that contributed to this reduction[12] (**Fig. 6**). According to results from the Bogalusa Heart Study, cigarette smoking in young adults significantly exacerbates the adverse effects of age and metabolic syndrome on subclinical atherosclerosis, which underscores the importance of prevention and cessation of tobacco use in the young.[160] In patients with CHD, quitting smoking is associated with a substantial reduction (RR 0.64; 95% CI, 0.58–0.71) in risk of all-cause mortality.[161] The impact of smoking cessation can be observed after a short period of time. An RCT showed a 77% RR reduction (95% CI, 27%–93%) in all-cause mortality among hospitalized smokers with acute CVD assigned to an intensive

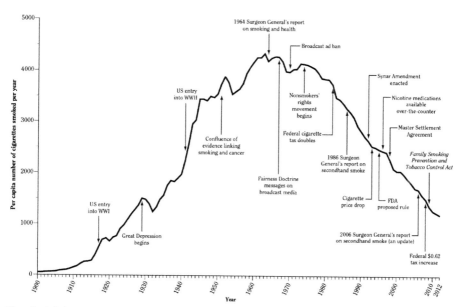

Fig. 6. Adult per capita cigarette consumption and major smoking and health events, United States, 1900 to 2012. FDA, Food and Drug Administration; WW, World War. (*From* US Department of Health Human Services. The health consequences of smoking—50 years of progress: a report of the Surgeon General. Atlanta (GA): US Department of Health and Human Services, Centers for Disease Control and Prevention, National Center for Chronic Disease Prevention and Health Promotion, Office on Smoking and Health; 2014. p. 17; with permission.)

smoking cessation program and followed for 24 months.[162] Only sparse data are available regarding the efficacy of smoking cessation interventions in people with diabetes.[163]

During the past decade, however, US data show that the prevalence of tobacco use remains high among patients with diabetes and has not changed significantly between 1999 and 2010.[43] Further research may help identify best strategies to combat tobacco use among individuals with diabetes.

ADDITIONAL RISK FACTORS
Age, Gender, and Duration of Diabetes

Globally, life expectancy increased from 61.7 years in 1980 to 71.8 years in 2015.[2] In the United States, an increase in the prevalence of CVD is largely attributable to the aging of the population, increasing numbers of members of higher-risk minority groups in the population, and people with diabetes living longer.[3,164] Increasing numbers of individuals younger than 40 years are being diagnosed with diabetes,[165,166] and they are less likely to have good glycemic control and receive organ-protective medications.[43,166]

Patients with early-onset T2D seem to have a more aggressive disease, with increased risk of cardiovascular complications compared with those with late-onset diabetes[167,168] that seems mostly attributable to the duration of disease.[169] Patients with early-onset T2D also have higher risk of cardiovascular death compared with those with type 1 diabetes mellitus with similar age of onset.[168] Similarly, earlier onset of diabetes among older adults is also associated with worse diabetes-related complications.[170,171]

Women with diabetes have more than a 40% increased risk of incident CHD compared with men with diabetes (RR 1.44; 95% CI, 1.27, 1.63).[172] The excess risk of stroke associated with diabetes is also significantly higher in women compared with men (RR 2.28; 95% CI, 1.93–2.69).[173] Similar gender disparities have been reported among patients with type 1 diabetes.[174] A meta-analysis, including more than 200,000 people with type 1 diabetes mellitus and more than 15,000 events, showed that compared with men, women had a 40% greater excess risk of all-cause mortality and more than twice the risk of incident CHD (standardized mortality ratio 2.54 [95% CI, 1.80–3.60]).[174] Despite this increased risk, it has been reported that CVD risk factors are managed less aggressively in women with diabetes compared with men.[175]

Areas for future research include efforts to understand the mechanisms responsible for the substantial gender difference in diabetes-related risk of ASCVD events.[172,173]

Hypercoagulability and Antiplatelet Therapy

Patients with diabetes have increased risk for thrombogenesis[176]; however, the response to aspirin in patients with diabetes seems different from the response among people without diabetes, particularly for primary prevention. The results of meta-analyses suggest that low-dose aspirin therapy in patients with diabetes may be associated with a decrease in stroke among women and a decrease in MI in men.[177] But in general, the benefits of aspirin for primary prevention are considered of lower magnitude compared with the effect on nondiabetic populations.[178] Recent follow-up results from the Japanese Primary Prevention of Atherosclerosis With Aspirin for Diabetes trial showed that low-dose aspirin therapy did not decrease the risk for cardiovascular events in patients with diabetes but increased risk for gastrointestinal bleeding.[179] Current recommendations suggest that low-dose aspirin should be considered in patients with high cardiovascular risk (10-year risk >10%) and for those at intermediate risk but not for those at low risk for ASCVD (10-year risk <5%).[57]

The role of aspirin therapy for secondary prevention in patients with diabetes has been recognized and is broadly recommended. Between 1999 to 2000 and 2011 to 2012, the use of aspirin increased from 4% to 28% among US adults with CHD, showing an increasing but persistently low use of aspirin for secondary prevention in high risk individuals.[180]

WHAT IS ON THE HORIZON?

The underlying mechanisms that lead to ASCVD in patients with diabetes are largely unknown. Systems epidemiology approaches using tools, such as high-resolution metabolomics and integrative *omics* approaches, provide an unprecedented opportunity to study underlying biological pathways in diabetes and ASCVD in large populations.[181–187] Metabolomics also offers a unique opportunity to explore the interactions between the genome and the environment (eg, modification of risk factors) and better understand future disease risk and new targets for disease prevention.[188–190] Metabolomics has also recently emerged as a potential tool for objective dietary assessment.[190,191]

Targeting multiple risk factors associated with highly complex diseases is a major challenge in the management of chronic conditions, such as CVD and diabetes, and large gaps exist in the achievement of care goals in actual practice,[192] despite evidence from clinical trials.[35,193] National US programs aiming to improve diabetes care have encountered significant barriers in the implementation process and achievement of goals,[194] and the long-term effects on diabetes-related complications and cost-efficiency of such programs are unknown.[194]

Recently, a multicomponent quality improvement strategy comprising nonphysician care coordinators and decision-support electronic health records in South Asia showed that over a median of 28 months, a greater percentage of intervention participants achieved the primary outcome (18.2% vs 8.1%; RR 2.24 [95% CI, 1.71–2.92]) defined as achieving A_{1C} level less than 7% plus blood pressure less than 130/80 mm Hg and/or LDL-C level less than 100 mg/dL.[192] The findings of this study are encouraging and were of larger magnitude compared with smaller quality-improvement interventions.[195] Additional studies in other settings might help clarify the role of such interventions.

In 2016, the WHO and the US Centers for Disease Control and Prevention launched the Global Hearts Initiative, a new program to support governments in strengthening the prevention and control of CVD through programs focusing on tobacco control (MPOWER), salt reduction (SHAKE), and management of CVD in primary health care (HEARTS) (http://www.who.int/cardiovascular_diseases/global-hearts/en/). The initiative aims to accelerate progress toward achieving the United Nations Sustainable Development Goal (Goal 3.4)[196] of reducing premature deaths from heart attacks and stroke by one-third by 2030.

SUMMARY AND POTENTIAL PUBLIC HEALTH IMPLICATIONS

Noncommunicable diseases, including CVD and diabetes, are responsible for 63% of all deaths worldwide.[197] These diseases have been largely attributed to poor diet, a leading risk factor for death and disability that is closely linked to the obesity and T2D epidemics.[3,4,10] It is estimated that if the major risk factors for NCDs were eliminated, approximately three-quarters of heart disease, stroke, and T2D would be prevented.[197]

Diabetes is one of the most important public health challenges of the twenty-first century.[198] Globally, the prevalence of diabetes has nearly quadrupled in the past 35 years, with a greater rate increase in LMICs.[17] The estimated global cost of diabetes for 2015 was $1.31 trillion (95% CI, 1.28–1.36) or 1.8% (95% CI, 1.8–1.9) of global gross domestic product.[199] In the United States alone, approximately 30.2 million people (22.4% of total global estimates) have diabetes,[17,21] and the prevalence is expected to increase as a consequence of the progressive obesity epidemic and increased life expectancy.[19,200] The burden of CVD is growing in the United States and it is estimated that the cost ($ 555 billion in 2016) will double to $1.1 trillion by 2035.[3] These epidemics are leading to a dramatic increase in the absolute number of cardiovascular events, despite the marked decrease in the rate of diabetes complications in the past decades.[8] In addition to premature death and high cost of medical care, ASCVD and diabetes lead to a decrease in quality of life, high individual and economic burdens of associated morbidities, and decreased work productivity.[57,201]

T2D and CVD share many common risk factors, including central adiposity, insulin resistance/dysglycemia, dyslipidemia, and high blood pressure. These traits cluster together in an identifiable pattern linked by obesity and insulin resistance.[202] That said, the traditional approach to treatment is to address each factor individually; a more holistic, preventive approach that centers around ideal health behaviors may actually have larger impacts than piecemeal and individual risk factor-focused interventions.

To reduce CVD incidence and mortality, both prevention and treatment are essential: primary prevention to reduce incidence and mortality and secondary prevention and treatment to improve quality of life, reduce recurrences, and reduce mortality.[12]

Results from prospective studies show that early number of ideal cardiovascular health metrics present in childhood predict subsequent cardiometabolic health.[203,204] In recent years, more emphasis has been placed on the prevention of risk factor development (primordial prevention) along with a focus on the promotion of ideal cardiovascular health in children and the improvement in cardiovascular health metric scores in those with poor or intermediate cardiovascular health metrics.[205,206] These constructs address simultaneously the risk of obesity, CVD and T2D, and would benefit from more research to delineate ideal interventions early in life.

Atherosclerosis starts early in life, and risk factors during childhood are known to be predictive.[207,208] Even moderate cholesterol level elevations in early adulthood predict risk for future CHD.[209] Critical to achievement of ideal cardiovascular health and disease prevention is maintenance of ideal metrics from birth through childhood to young adulthood and beyond.[206] Of concern, younger adults with diabetes are less likely than older adults to meet goals for treatment and preventive practices,[43,166,210] and it is unclear whether physician inattentiveness, poor access to health care, or other factors account for these gaps.[43] Important areas for future research include examination of the gap among younger adults with diabetes to avoid an impending epidemic of young-onset diabetic complications,[43,168] as well as studies assessing intensive risk factor control in early-onset diabetes.[211]

In the United States, millions of patients are treated with statins for primary and secondary prevention of ASCVD events, and the costs are decreasing as medications become generic.[212] It is estimated that the cost for statins decreased from $17.2 billion (out-of-pocket cost, $6.9 billion) in 2002 to 2003 to $16.9 billion (out-of-pocket cost, $3.3 billion) in 2012 to 2013.[28] Despite these advances, a large proportion of patients still remains untreated.[21,28–30] In addition, major health care disparities have been observed, with lower use of statins among women, racial/ethnic minorities, and uninsured individuals.[28]

Areas for future research include more emphasis on lifestyle interventions in older patients with diabetes. Recent analyses of Look AHEAD show that the magnitude of weight loss and the heterogeneity in the response to a lifestyle intervention can determine who will benefit the most from such intervention.[140,141,213] Interventions in at-risk populations have also shown the long-term impact on cardiovascular mortality.[139]

Even though the Life's Simple 7 concept was designed to prevent CVD in the general nondiabetic population, outcomes research suggests that improving each factor[214] could add additional benefits beyond control of ABCs alone and that multidisciplinary approaches could improve the risk profile and reduce ASCVD events in patients with cardiometabolic disease. Professional organizations could consider a stronger emphasis and more comprehensive approach targeting all cardiovascular health measures (such as Life's Simple 7) beyond the use of blood pressure, cholesterol, and antiplatelet medications to reduce cardiovascular risk.[93]

Social and environmental factors are important in shaping dietary habits and population-based approaches to improve global dietary quality.[10] Several approaches may be effective in shaping dietary habits, including media and education campaigns, food labeling, economic incentives, changes of local food environment, comprehensive school- and work-based interventions, restrictions on advertising and marketing, and direct regulation, providing flexibility to policy-makers and allowing for synergistic multicomponent campaigns.[215] Models such as Shape Up Somerville have shown that increasing opportunities for healthy food and physical activity through a child-targeted, community-based environmental change intervention has a significant impact in decreasing childhood obesity with a potential to change parental BMI.[216,217]

Intersectoral collaborations that implement cost-effective multicomponent interventions for the management of diabetes and cardiometabolic risk factors are potential solutions at the local and population levels.[192] These include community-based programs that address the social determinants of health, environmental, and policy-level interventions. To develop such approaches, public health professionals could engage the research community, community-based organizations, schools and workplaces, agriculture and food industry, local and national governments, and international organizations, especially in LMIC.[158,215]

Given that atherosclerosis starts in childhood, future prevention efforts will benefit from acting upon the vast evidence from observational studies and available randomized controlled trials to prioritize action against modifiable risk factors.[218,219] The National Children's Study was a planned large-scale, long-term study of US children and their parents designed to study environmental influences on child health and development.[219] Based on the advice of an expert group, however, the study was closed in 2014 during its planning phase due to feasibility concerns. A new initiative, the Environmental influences on Child Health Outcomes Program,[220] will leverage existing cohorts totaling 50,000 children and help understanding of how environmental factors in early development influence the risk of obesity and cardiometabolic risk in children.

Optimizing health behaviors in early life has the potential to combat the diabetes and CVD epidemics. On the other hand, the results of the Three-City Study[214] in elderly individuals (mean age 74 years) also suggest that it is never too late to improve cardiovascular health to limit the time spent with illness and disability.[214,221]

REFERENCES

1. World Health Organization. Cardiovascular Disease (CVDs). Available at: http://www.who.int/cardiovascular_diseases/en. Accessed August 22, 2017.
2. GBD Mortality and Causes of Death Collaborators. Global, regional, and national life expectancy, all-cause mortality, and cause-specific mortality for 249 causes of death, 1980-2015: a systematic analysis for the Global Burden of Disease Study 2015. Lancet 2016;388(10053):1459–544.
3. American Heart Association & American Stroke Association. Cardiovascular Disease: A Costly Burden for America. Projections through 2035. Available at: http://www.heart.org/idc/groups/heart-public/@wcm/@adv/documents/downloadable/ucm_491543.pdf. Accessed August 22, 2017.
4. Benjamin EJ, Blaha MJ, Chiuve SE, et al. Heart disease and stroke statistics-2017 update: a report from the American Heart Association. Circulation 2017;135(10):e146–603.
5. Danaei G, Finucane MM, Lin JK, et al. National, regional, and global trends in systolic blood pressure since 1980: systematic analysis of health examination surveys and epidemiological studies with 786 country-years and 5.4 million participants. Lancet 2011;377(9765):568–77.
6. Farzadfar F, Finucane MM, Danaei G, et al. National, regional, and global trends in serum total cholesterol since 1980: systematic analysis of health examination surveys and epidemiological studies with 321 country-years and 3.0 million participants. Lancet 2011;377(9765):578–86.
7. Guo F, Garvey WT. Trends in Cardiovascular Health Metrics in Obese Adults: National Health and Nutrition Examination Survey (NHANES), 1988-2014. J Am Heart Assoc 2016;5(7) [pii:e003619].
8. Gregg EW, Sattar N, Ali MK. The changing face of diabetes complications. Lancet Diabetes Endocrinol 2016;4(6):537–47.

9. Dinesh Shah A, Langenberg C, Rapsomaniki E, et al. Type 2 diabetes and incidence of a wide range of cardiovascular diseases: a cohort study in 1.9 million people. Lancet 2015;385(Suppl 1):S86.
10. Mozaffarian D. Dietary and policy priorities for cardiovascular disease, diabetes, and obesity: a comprehensive review. Circulation 2016;133(2):187–225.
11. Ali MK, Jaacks LM, Kowalski AJ, et al. Noncommunicable diseases: three decades of global data show a mixture of increases and decreases in mortality rates. Health Aff 2015;34(9):1444–55.
12. Ford ES, Capewell S. Proportion of the decline in cardiovascular mortality disease due to prevention versus treatment: public health versus clinical care. Annu Rev Public Health 2011;32:5–22.
13. Roth GA, Huffman MD, Moran AE, et al. Global and regional patterns in cardiovascular mortality from 1990 to 2013. Circulation 2015;132(17):1667–78.
14. Gregg EW, Li Y, Wang J, et al. Changes in diabetes-related complications in the United States, 1990-2010. N Engl J Med 2014;370(16):1514–23.
15. Guariguata L, Whiting DR, Hambleton I, et al. Global estimates of diabetes prevalence for 2013 and projections for 2035. Diabetes Res Clin Pract 2014;103(2): 137–49.
16. Dagenais GR, Gerstein HC, Zhang X, et al. Variations in diabetes prevalence in low-, middle-, and high-income countries: results from the prospective urban and rural epidemiological study. Diabetes Care 2016;39(5):780–7.
17. NCD Risk Factor Collaboration. Worldwide trends in diabetes since 1980: a pooled analysis of 751 population-based studies with 4.4 million participants. Lancet 2016;387(10027):1513–30.
18. Geiss LS, Wang J, Cheng YJ, et al. Prevalence and incidence trends for diagnosed diabetes among adults aged 20 to 79 years, United States, 1980-2012. JAMA 2014;312(12):1218–26.
19. Selvin E, Ali MK. Declines in the incidence of diabetes in the U.S.-real progress or artifact? Diabetes Care 2017;40(9):1139–43.
20. Cheng YJ, Imperatore G, Geiss LS, et al. Secular changes in the age-specific prevalence of diabetes among U.S. adults: 1988-2010. Diabetes Care 2013; 36(9):2690–6.
21. Centers for Disease Control and Prevention. National diabetes statistics report, 2017. Atlanta (GA): Centers for Disease Control and Prevention, U.S. Dept of Health and Human Services; 2017.
22. Fox CS, Coady S, Sorlie PD, et al. Trends in cardiovascular complications of diabetes. JAMA 2004;292(20):2495–9.
23. Tight blood pressure control and risk of macrovascular and microvascular complications in type 2 diabetes: UKPDS 38. UK Prospective Diabetes Study Group. BMJ 1998;317(7160):703–13.
24. Mann D, Reynolds K, Smith D, et al. Trends in statin use and low-density lipoprotein cholesterol levels among US adults: impact of the 2001 National Cholesterol Education Program guidelines. Ann Pharmacother 2008;42(9):1208–15.
25. Yoon SS, Gu Q, Nwankwo T, et al. Trends in blood pressure among adults with hypertension: United States, 2003 to 2012. Hypertension 2015;65(1):54–61.
26. Egan BM, Zhao Y, Axon RN. US trends in prevalence, awareness, treatment, and control of hypertension, 1988-2008. JAMA 2010;303(20):2043–50.
27. Preis SR, Pencina MJ, Hwang SJ, et al. Trends in cardiovascular disease risk factors in individuals with and without diabetes mellitus in the Framingham Heart Study. Circulation 2009;120(3):212–20.

28. Salami JA, Warraich H, Valero-Elizondo J, et al. National trends in statin use and expenditures in the US adult population from 2002 to 2013: insights from the Medical Expenditure Panel Survey. JAMA Cardiol 2017;2(1):56–65.

29. Harrington RA. Statins-almost 30 years of use in the United States and still not quite there. JAMA Cardiol 2017;2(1):66.

30. Johansen ME, Green LA, Sen A, et al. Cardiovascular risk and statin use in the United States. Ann Fam Med 2014;12(3):215–23.

31. Pyorala K, Pedersen TR, Kjekshus J, et al. Cholesterol lowering with simvastatin improves prognosis of diabetic patients with coronary heart disease. A subgroup analysis of the Scandinavian Simvastatin Survival Study (4S). Diabetes Care 1997;20(4):614–20.

32. Cannon CP, Blazing MA, Giugliano RP, et al. Ezetimibe added to statin therapy after acute coronary syndromes. N Engl J Med 2015;372(25):2387–97.

33. Goldberg RB, Mellies MJ, Sacks FM, et al. Cardiovascular events and their reduction with pravastatin in diabetic and glucose-intolerant myocardial infarction survivors with average cholesterol levels: subgroup analyses in the cholesterol and recurrent events (CARE) trial. The Care Investigators. Circulation 1998; 98(23):2513–9.

34. Gaede P, Lund-Andersen H, Parving HH, et al. Effect of a multifactorial intervention on mortality in type 2 diabetes. N Engl J Med 2008;358(6):580–91.

35. Gaede P, Vedel P, Larsen N, et al. Multifactorial intervention and cardiovascular disease in patients with type 2 diabetes. N Engl J Med 2003;348(5):383–93.

36. Reed M, Huang J, Graetz I, et al. Outpatient electronic health records and the clinical care and outcomes of patients with diabetes mellitus. Ann Intern Med 2012;157(7):482–9.

37. Charles D, Gabriel M, Furukawa MF. Adoption of electronic health record systems among US non-federal acute care hospitals: 2008–2013. ONC data brief 2013;9:1–9.

38. Narayan KM, Ali MK, Koplan JP. Global noncommunicable diseases–where worlds meet. N Engl J Med 2010;363(13):1196–8.

39. Zhang X, Devlin HM, Smith B, et al. Effect of lifestyle interventions on cardiovascular risk factors among adults without impaired glucose tolerance or diabetes: a systematic review and meta-analysis. PLoS One 2017;12(5):e0176436.

40. American Heart Association. My Life Check: Life's Simple 7. American Heart Association Web site. Available at: http://mylifecheck.heart.org/. Accessed August 22, 2017.

41. Lloyd-Jones DM, Hong Y, Labarthe D, et al. Defining and setting national goals for cardiovascular health promotion and disease reduction: the American Heart Association's strategic Impact Goal through 2020 and beyond. Circulation 2010; 121(4):586–613.

42. Fang N, Jiang M, Fan Y. Ideal cardiovascular health metrics and risk of cardiovascular disease or mortality: a meta-analysis. Int J Cardiol 2016;214:279–83.

43. Ali MK, Bullard KM, Saaddine JB, et al. Achievement of goals in U.S. diabetes care, 1999-2010. N Engl J Med 2013;368(17):1613–24.

44. Wong ND, Patao C, Wong K, et al. Trends in control of cardiovascular risk factors among US adults with type 2 diabetes from 1999 to 2010: comparison by prevalent cardiovascular disease status. Diab Vasc Dis Res 2013;10(6):505–13.

45. Stark Casagrande S, Fradkin JE, Saydah SH, et al. The prevalence of meeting A1C, blood pressure, and LDL goals among people with diabetes, 1988-2010. Diabetes Care 2013;36(8):2271–9.

46. The Atherosclerosis Risk in Communities (ARIC) Study: design and objectives. The ARIC investigators. Am J Epidemiol 1989;129(4):687–702.

47. Bild DE, Bluemke DA, Burke GL, et al. Multi-ethnic study of atherosclerosis: objectives and design. Am J Epidemiol 2002;156(9):871–81.

48. Carpenter MA, Crow R, Steffes M, et al. Laboratory, reading center, and coordinating center data management methods in the Jackson Heart Study. Am J Med Sci 2004;328(3):131–44.

49. Wong ND, Zhao Y, Patel R, et al. Cardiovascular risk factor targets and cardiovascular disease event risk in diabetes: a pooling project of the atherosclerosis risk in communities study, Multi-Ethnic Study of Atherosclerosis, and Jackson Heart Study. Diabetes Care 2016;39(5):668–76.

50. Advance Collaborative Group, Patel A, MacMahon S, Chalmers J, et al. Intensive blood glucose control and vascular outcomes in patients with type 2 diabetes. N Engl J Med 2008;358(24):2560–72.

51. Action to Control Cardiovascular Risk in Diabetes Study Group, Gerstein HC, Miller ME, Byington RP, et al. Effects of intensive glucose lowering in type 2 diabetes. N Engl J Med 2008;358(24):2545–59.

52. Duckworth W, Abraira C, Moritz T, et al. Glucose control and vascular complications in veterans with type 2 diabetes. N Engl J Med 2009;360(2):129–39.

53. ACCORD Study Group. Nine-year effects of 3.7 years of intensive glycemic control on cardiovascular outcomes. Diabetes Care 2016;39(5):701–8.

54. Hayward RA, Reaven PD, Wiitala WL, et al. Follow-up of glycemic control and cardiovascular outcomes in type 2 diabetes. N Engl J Med 2015;372(23):2197–206.

55. Zoungas S, Chalmers J, Neal B, et al. Follow-up of blood-pressure lowering and glucose control in type 2 diabetes. N Engl J Med 2014;371(15):1392–406.

56. Aviles-Santa L, Colon-Ramos U, Lindberg NM, et al. From sea to shining sea, and the great plains to patagonia: a review on current knowledge of diabetes mellitus in hispanics/latinos in the U.S. and Latin America. Front Endocrinol, in press.

57. Low Wang CC, Hess CN, Hiatt WR, et al. Clinical update: cardiovascular disease in diabetes mellitus: atherosclerotic cardiovascular disease and heart failure in type 2 diabetes mellitus - mechanisms, management, and clinical considerations. Circulation 2016;133(24):2459–502.

58. Haffner SM, Lehto S, Ronnemaa T, et al. Mortality from coronary heart disease in subjects with type 2 diabetes and in nondiabetic subjects with and without prior myocardial infarction. N Engl J Med 1998;339(4):229–34.

59. Newman JD, Rockman CB, Kosiborod M, et al. Diabetes mellitus is a coronary heart disease risk equivalent for peripheral vascular disease. Am Heart J 2017;184:114–20.

60. Bulugahapitiya U, Siyambalapitiya S, Sithole J, et al. Is diabetes a coronary risk equivalent? Systematic review and meta-analysis. Diabet Med 2009;26(2):142–8.

61. Rana JS, Liu JY, Moffet HH, et al. Diabetes and prior coronary heart disease are not necessarily risk equivalent for future coronary heart disease events. J Gen Intern Med 2016;31(4):387–93.

62. Sattar N, Preiss D. Screening for diabetes in patients with cardiovascular disease: HbA1c trumps oral glucose tolerance testing. Lancet Diabetes Endocrinol 2016;4(7):560–2.

63. Selvin E, Steffes MW, Zhu H, et al. Glycated hemoglobin, diabetes, and cardiovascular risk in nondiabetic adults. N Engl J Med 2010;362(9):800–11.

64. Santos-Oliveira R, Purdy C, da Silva MP, et al. Haemoglobin A1c levels and subsequent cardiovascular disease in persons without diabetes: a meta-analysis of prospective cohorts. Diabetologia 2011;54(6):1327–34.
65. Emerging Risk Factors Collaboration, Sarwar N, Gao P, Seshasai SR, et al. Diabetes mellitus, fasting blood glucose concentration, and risk of vascular disease: a collaborative meta-analysis of 102 prospective studies. Lancet 2010; 375(9733):2215–22.
66. Gerstein HC, Pogue J, Mann JF, et al. The relationship between dysglycaemia and cardiovascular and renal risk in diabetic and non-diabetic participants in the HOPE study: a prospective epidemiological analysis. Diabetologia 2005; 48(9):1749–55.
67. Rao Kondapally Seshasai S, Kaptoge S, Thompson A, et al. Diabetes mellitus, fasting glucose, and risk of cause-specific death. N Engl J Med 2011;364(9): 829–41.
68. Singh GM, Danaei G, Farzadfar F, et al. The age-specific quantitative effects of metabolic risk factors on cardiovascular diseases and diabetes: a pooled analysis. PLoS One 2013;8(7):e65174.
69. Boussageon R, Bejan-Angoulvant T, Saadatian-Elahi M, et al. Effect of intensive glucose lowering treatment on all cause mortality, cardiovascular death, and microvascular events in type 2 diabetes: meta-analysis of randomised controlled trials. BMJ 2011;343:d4169.
70. Murray P, Chune GW, Raghavan VA. Legacy effects from DCCT and UKPDS: what they mean and implications for future diabetes trials. Curr Atheroscler Rep 2010;12(6):432–9.
71. Group AS, Gerstein HC, Miller ME, et al. Long-term effects of intensive glucose lowering on cardiovascular outcomes. N Engl J Med 2011;364(9):818–28.
72. Gamble JM, Chibrikov E, Twells LK, et al. Association of insulin dosage with mortality or major adverse cardiovascular events: a retrospective cohort study. Lancet Diabetes Endocrinol 2017;5(1):43–52.
73. Holman RR, Paul SK, Bethel MA, et al. 10-year follow-up of intensive glucose control in type 2 diabetes. N Engl J Med 2008;359(15):1577–89.
74. Origin Trial Investigators, Gerstein HC, Bosch J, Dagenais GR, et al. Basal insulin and cardiovascular and other outcomes in dysglycemia. N Engl J Med 2012; 367(4):319–28.
75. Marso SP, McGuire DK, Zinman B, et al. efficacy and safety of degludec versus glargine in type 2 diabetes. N Engl J Med 2017;377(8):723–32.
76. Marso SP, Daniels GH, Brown-Frandsen K, et al. Liraglutide and cardiovascular outcomes in type 2 diabetes. N Engl J Med 2016;375(4):311–22.
77. Marso SP, Bain SC, Consoli A, et al. Semaglutide and cardiovascular outcomes in patients with type 2 diabetes. N Engl J Med 2016;375(19):1834–44.
78. Zinman B, Wanner C, Lachin JM, et al. Empagliflozin, cardiovascular outcomes, and mortality in type 2 diabetes. N Engl J Med 2015;373(22):2117–28.
79. Neal B, Perkovic V, Mahaffey KW, et al. Canagliflozin and cardiovascular and renal events in type 2 diabetes. N Engl J Med 2017;377(7):644–57.
80. Kosiborod M, Cavender MA, Fu AZ, et al. Lower risk of heart failure and death in patients initiated on sodium-glucose cotransporter-2 inhibitors versus other glucose-lowering drugs: The CVD-REAL Study (Comparative Effectiveness of Cardiovascular Outcomes in New Users of Sodium-Glucose Cotransporter-2 Inhibitors). Circulation 2017;136(3):249–59.
81. Global Burden of Metabolic Risk Factors for Chronic Diseases Collaboration. Cardiovascular disease, chronic kidney disease, and diabetes mortality burden

of cardiometabolic risk factors from 1980 to 2010: a comparative risk assessment. Lancet Diabetes Endocrinol 2014;2(8):634–47.

82. Hansson L, Zanchetti A, Carruthers SG, et al. Effects of intensive blood-pressure lowering and low-dose aspirin in patients with hypertension: principal results of the Hypertension Optimal Treatment (HOT) randomised trial. HOT Study Group. Lancet 1998;351(9118):1755–62.

83. Patel A, Advance Collaborative Group, MacMahon S, et al. Effects of a fixed combination of perindopril and indapamide on macrovascular and microvascular outcomes in patients with type 2 diabetes mellitus (the ADVANCE trial): a randomised controlled trial. Lancet 2007;370(9590):829–40.

84. Erlinger TP, Vollmer WM, Svetkey LP, et al. The potential impact of nonpharmacologic population-wide blood pressure reduction on coronary heart disease events: pronounced benefits in African-Americans and hypertensives. Prev Med 2003;37(4):327–33.

85. Yancy CW, Bonow RO. New blood pressure-lowering targets-finding clarity. JAMA Cardiol 2017;2(7):719–20.

86. Bundy JD, Li C, Stuchlik P, et al. Systolic blood pressure reduction and risk of cardiovascular disease and mortality: a systematic review and network meta-analysis. JAMA Cardiol 2017;2(7):775–81.

87. James PA, Oparil S, Carter BL, et al. 2014 evidence-based guideline for the management of high blood pressure in adults: report from the panel members appointed to the Eighth Joint National Committee (JNC 8). JAMA 2014;311(5): 507–20.

88. Group AS, Cushman WC, Evans GW, et al. Effects of intensive blood-pressure control in type 2 diabetes mellitus. N Engl J Med 2010;362(17):1575–85.

89. Nilsson PM. ACCORD and risk-factor control in type 2 diabetes. N Engl J Med 2010;362(17):1628–30.

90. Emdin CA, Rahimi K, Neal B, et al. Blood pressure lowering in type 2 diabetes: a systematic review and meta-analysis. JAMA 2015;313(6):603–15.

91. Brunstrom M, Carlberg B. Effect of antihypertensive treatment at different blood pressure levels in patients with diabetes mellitus: systematic review and meta-analyses. BMJ 2016;352:i717.

92. Sprint Research Group, Wright JT Jr, Williamson JD, Whelton PK, et al. A randomized trial of intensive versus standard blood-pressure control. N Engl J Med 2015;373(22):2103–16.

93. American Diabetes Association. 9. Cardiovascular disease and risk management. Diabetes Care 2017;40(Suppl 1):S75–87.

94. Bangalore S, Fakheri R, Toklu B, et al. Diabetes mellitus as a compelling indication for use of renin angiotensin system blockers: systematic review and meta-analysis of randomized trials. BMJ 2016;352:i438.

95. Steinberg D. Thematic review series: the pathogenesis of atherosclerosis. An interpretive history of the cholesterol controversy, part V: the discovery of the statins and the end of the controversy. J Lipid Res 2006;47(7):1339–51.

96. Endo A. A historical perspective on the discovery of statins. Proc Jpn Acad Ser B Phys Biol Sci 2010;86(5):484–93.

97. Ridker PM, Revkin J, Amarenco P, et al. Cardiovascular efficacy and safety of bococizumab in high-risk patients. N Engl J Med 2017;376(16):1527–39.

98. Cholesterol Treatment Trialists (CTT) Collaborators, Kearney PM, Blackwell L, Collins R, et al. Efficacy of cholesterol-lowering therapy in 18,686 people with diabetes in 14 randomised trials of statins: a meta-analysis. Lancet 2008; 371(9607):117–25.

99. Accord Study Group, Ginsberg HN, Elam MB, Lovato LC, et al. Effects of combination lipid therapy in type 2 diabetes mellitus. N Engl J Med 2010;362(17): 1563–74.
100. Elam MB, Ginsberg HN, Lovato LC, et al. Association of fenofibrate therapy with long-term cardiovascular risk in statin-treated patients with type 2 diabetes. JAMA Cardiol 2017;2(4):370–80.
101. Bhupathiraju SN, Hu FB. Epidemiology of obesity and diabetes and their cardiovascular complications. Circ Res 2016;118(11):1723–35.
102. World Health Organization. Obesity and overweight. Available at: http://www.who.int/mediacentre/factsheets/fs311/en/. Accessed August 22, 2017.
103. G. B. D. Obesity Collaborators, Afshin A, Forouzanfar MH, Reitsma MB, et al. Health effects of overweight and obesity in 195 countries over 25 years. N Engl J Med 2017;377(1):13–27.
104. Hubert HB, Feinleib M, McNamara PM, et al. Obesity as an independent risk factor for cardiovascular disease: a 26-year follow-up of participants in the Framingham Heart Study. Circulation 1983;67(5):968–77.
105. Cassano PA, Rosner B, Vokonas PS, et al. Obesity and body fat distribution in relation to the incidence of non-insulin-dependent diabetes mellitus. A prospective cohort study of men in the normative aging study. Am J Epidemiol 1992; 136(12):1474–86.
106. Dale CE, Fatemifar G, Palmer TM, et al. Causal Associations of Adiposity and Body Fat Distribution With Coronary Heart Disease, Stroke Subtypes, and Type 2 Diabetes Mellitus: A Mendelian Randomization Analysis. Circulation 2017;135(24):2373–88.
107. Okosun IS, Chandra KM, Boev A, et al. Abdominal adiposity in U.S. adults: prevalence and trends, 1960-2000. Prev Med 2004;39(1):197–206.
108. Ford ES, Maynard LM, Li C. Trends in mean waist circumference and abdominal obesity among US adults, 1999-2012. JAMA 2014;312(11):1151–3.
109. Reaven GM. Banting lecture 1988. Role of insulin resistance in human disease. Diabetes 1988;37(12):1595–607.
110. Bao W, Srinivasan SR, Berenson GS. Persistent elevation of plasma insulin levels is associated with increased cardiovascular risk in children and young adults. The Bogalusa Heart Study. Circulation 1996;93(1):54–9.
111. Zhang H, Zhang T, Li S, et al. Long-term impact of childhood adiposity on adult metabolic syndrome is modified by insulin resistance: the Bogalusa Heart Study. Sci Rep 2015;5:17885.
112. Zhang T, Zhang H, Li Y, et al. Temporal relationship between childhood body mass index and insulin and its impact on adult hypertension: The Bogalusa Heart Study. Hypertension 2016;68(3):818–23.
113. Lakka HM, Laaksonen DE, Lakka TA, et al. The metabolic syndrome and total and cardiovascular disease mortality in middle-aged men. JAMA 2002; 288(21):2709–16.
114. Stefan N, Kantartzis K, Machann J, et al. Identification and characterization of metabolically benign obesity in humans. Arch Intern Med 2008;168(15): 1609–16.
115. Wildman RP, Muntner P, Reynolds K, et al. The obese without cardiometabolic risk factor clustering and the normal weight with cardiometabolic risk factor clustering: prevalence and correlates of 2 phenotypes among the US population (NHANES 1999-2004). Arch Intern Med 2008;168(15):1617–24.

116. Ortega FB, Lee DC, Katzmarzyk PT, et al. The intriguing metabolically healthy but obese phenotype: cardiovascular prognosis and role of fitness. Eur Heart J 2013;34(5):389–97.

117. Kramer CK, Zinman B, Retnakaran R. Are metabolically healthy overweight and obesity benign conditions?: A systematic review and meta-analysis. Ann Intern Med 2013;159(11):758–69.

118. Eckel N, Meidtner K, Kalle-Uhlmann T, et al. Metabolically healthy obesity and cardiovascular events: a systematic review and meta-analysis. Eur J Prev Cardiol 2016;23(9):956–66.

119. Bell JA, Kivimaki M, Hamer M. Metabolically healthy obesity and risk of incident type 2 diabetes: a meta-analysis of prospective cohort studies. Obes Rev 2014; 15(6):504–15.

120. Jensen MD, Ryan DH, Apovian CM, et al. 2013 AHA/ACC/TOS guideline for the management of overweight and obesity in adults: a report of the American College of Cardiology/American Heart Association Task Force on Practice Guidelines and The Obesity Society. Circulation 2014;129(25 Suppl 2):S102–38.

121. Bariatric surgery: why only a last resort? Lancet Diabetes Endocrinol 2014;2(2):91.

122. Schauer PR, Bhatt DL, Kirwan JP, et al. Bariatric surgery versus intensive medical therapy for diabetes - 5-year outcomes. N Engl J Med 2017;376(7):641–51.

123. Inge TH, Courcoulas AP, Jenkins TM, et al. Weight loss and health status 3 years after bariatric surgery in adolescents. N Engl J Med 2016;374(2):113–23.

124. Sjostrom L, Narbro K, Sjostrom CD, et al. Effects of bariatric surgery on mortality in Swedish obese subjects. N Engl J Med 2007;357(8):741–52.

125. Laiteerapong N, Huang ES. The public health implications of the cost-effectiveness of bariatric surgery for diabetes. Diabetes Care 2010;33(9): 2126–8.

126. Church TS, LaMonte MJ, Barlow CE, et al. Cardiorespiratory fitness and body mass index as predictors of cardiovascular disease mortality among men with diabetes. Arch Intern Med 2005;165(18):2114–20.

127. Ross R, Blair SN, Arena R, et al. Importance of assessing cardiorespiratory fitness in clinical practice: a case for fitness as a clinical vital sign: a scientific statement from the American Heart Association. Circulation 2016;134(24): e653–99.

128. Umpierre D, Ribeiro PA, Schaan BD, et al. Volume of supervised exercise training impacts glycaemic control in patients with type 2 diabetes: a systematic review with meta-regression analysis. Diabetologia 2013;56(2):242–51.

129. Ornish D, Scherwitz LW, Billings JH, et al. Intensive lifestyle changes for reversal of coronary heart disease. JAMA 1998;280(23):2001–7.

130. Balducci S, Zanuso S, Nicolucci A, et al. Effect of an intensive exercise intervention strategy on modifiable cardiovascular risk factors in subjects with type 2 diabetes mellitus: a randomized controlled trial: the Italian Diabetes and Exercise Study (IDES). Arch Intern Med 2010;170(20):1794–803.

131. Wing RR, Lang W, Wadden TA, et al. Benefits of modest weight loss in improving cardiovascular risk factors in overweight and obese individuals with type 2 diabetes. Diabetes Care 2011;34(7):1481–6.

132. Andrews RC, Cooper AR, Montgomery AA, et al. Diet or diet plus physical activity versus usual care in patients with newly diagnosed type 2 diabetes: the Early ACTID randomised controlled trial. Lancet 2011;378(9786):129–39.

133. Mudaliar U, Zabetian A, Goodman M, et al. Cardiometabolic risk factor changes observed in diabetes prevention programs in us settings: a systematic review and meta-analysis. PLoS Med 2016;13(7):e1002095.

134. Deijle IA, Van Schaik SM, Van Wegen EE, et al. Lifestyle interventions to prevent cardiovascular events after stroke and transient ischemic attack: systematic review and meta-analysis. Stroke 2017;48(1):174–9.
135. Look Ahead Research Group, Wing RR, Bolin P, Brancati FL, et al. Cardiovascular effects of intensive lifestyle intervention in type 2 diabetes. N Engl J Med 2013;369(2):145–54.
136. Williamson DF, Thompson TJ, Thun M, et al. Intentional weight loss and mortality among overweight individuals with diabetes. Diabetes Care 2000;23(10): 1499–504.
137. Johansen MY, MacDonald CS, Hansen KB, et al. Effect of an intensive lifestyle intervention on glycemic control in patients with type 2 diabetes: a randomized clinical trial. JAMA 2017;318(7):637–46.
138. Gregg EW, Chen H, Wagenknecht LE, et al. Association of an intensive lifestyle intervention with remission of type 2 diabetes. JAMA 2012;308(23):2489–96.
139. Li G, Zhang P, Wang J, et al. Cardiovascular mortality, all-cause mortality, and diabetes incidence after lifestyle intervention for people with impaired glucose tolerance in the Da Qing Diabetes Prevention Study: a 23-year follow-up study. Lancet Diabetes Endocrinol 2014;2(6):474–80.
140. Look Ahead Research Group, Gregg EW, Jakicic JM, Blackburn G, et al. Association of the magnitude of weight loss and changes in physical fitness with long-term cardiovascular disease outcomes in overweight or obese people with type 2 diabetes: a post-hoc analysis of the Look AHEAD randomised clinical trial. Lancet Diabetes Endocrinol 2016;4(11):913–21.
141. Baum A, Scarpa J, Bruzelius E, et al. Targeting weight loss interventions to reduce cardiovascular complications of type 2 diabetes: a machine learning-based post-hoc analysis of heterogeneous treatment effects in the Look AHEAD trial. Lancet Diabetes Endocrinol 2017;5(10):808–15.
142. Siegel KR, McKeever Bullard K, Imperatore G, et al. Association of higher consumption of foods derived from subsidized commodities with adverse cardiometabolic risk among US Adults. JAMA Intern Med 2016;176(8):1124–32.
143. Mozaffarian D, Fahimi S, Singh GM, et al. Global sodium consumption and death from cardiovascular causes. N Engl J Med 2014;371(7):624–34.
144. Micha R, Penalvo JL, Cudhea F, et al. Association between dietary factors and mortality from heart disease, stroke, and type 2 diabetes in the United States. JAMA 2017;317(9):912–24.
145. Franck C, Grandi SM, Eisenberg MJ. Agricultural subsidies and the American obesity epidemic. Am J Prev Med 2013;45(3):327–33.
146. Sacks FM, Lichtenstein AH, Wu JHY, et al. Dietary fats and cardiovascular disease: a presidential advisory from the American Heart Association. Circulation 2017;136(3):e1–23.
147. Estruch R, Ros E, Salas-Salvado J, et al. Primary prevention of cardiovascular disease with a Mediterranean diet. N Engl J Med 2013;368(14):1279–90.
148. Esposito K, Maiorino MI, Bellastella G, et al. A journey into a Mediterranean diet and type 2 diabetes: a systematic review with meta-analyses. BMJ Open 2015; 5(8):e008222.
149. Appel LJ, Moore TJ, Obarzanek E, et al. A clinical trial of the effects of dietary patterns on blood pressure. DASH Collaborative Research Group. N Engl J Med 1997;336(16):1117–24.
150. Siervo M, Lara J, Chowdhury S, et al. Effects of the Dietary Approach to Stop Hypertension (DASH) diet on cardiovascular risk factors: a systematic review and meta-analysis. Br J Nutr 2015;113(1):1–15.

151. Gadgil MD, Appel LJ, Yeung E, et al. The effects of carbohydrate, unsaturated fat, and protein intake on measures of insulin sensitivity: results from the Omni-Heart trial. Diabetes Care 2013;36(5):1132–7.

152. Ramsden CE, Zamora D, Majchrzak-Hong S, et al. Re-evaluation of the traditional diet-heart hypothesis: analysis of recovered data from Minnesota Coronary Experiment (1968-73). BMJ 2016;353:i1246.

153. Dehghan M, Mente A, Zhang X, et al. Associations of fats and carbohydrate intake with cardiovascular disease and mortality in 18 countries from five continents (PURE): a prospective cohort study. Lancet 2017;390(10107):2050–62.

154. de Souza RJ, Mente A, Maroleanu A, et al. Intake of saturated and trans unsaturated fatty acids and risk of all cause mortality, cardiovascular disease, and type 2 diabetes: systematic review and meta-analysis of observational studies. BMJ 2015;351:h3978.

155. Veerman JL. Dietary fats: a new look at old data challenges established wisdom. BMJ 2016;353:i1512.

156. Miller V, Mente A, Dehghan M, et al. Fruit, vegetable, and legume intake, and cardiovascular disease and deaths in 18 countries (PURE): a prospective cohort study. Lancet 2017;390(10107):2037–49.

157. Satija A, Bhupathiraju SN, Spiegelman D, et al. Healthful and unhealthful plant-based diets and the risk of coronary heart disease in U.S. Adults. J Am Coll Cardiol 2017;70(4):411–22.

158. Toledo E, Martinez-Gonzalez MA. Fruits, vegetables, and legumes: sound prevention tools. Lancet 2017;390(10107):2017–8.

159. US Department of Health Human Services. The health consequences of smoking—50 years of progress: a report of the Surgeon General. Atlanta (GA): US Department of Health and Human Services, Centers for Disease Control and Prevention, National Center for Chronic Disease Prevention and Health Promotion, Office on Smoking and Health; 2014. p. 17.

160. Li S, Yun M, Fernandez C, et al. Cigarette smoking exacerbates the adverse effects of age and metabolic syndrome on subclinical atherosclerosis: the Bogalusa Heart Study. PLoS One 2014;9(5):e96368.

161. Critchley JA, Capewell S. Mortality risk reduction associated with smoking cessation in patients with coronary heart disease: a systematic review. JAMA 2003;290(1):86–97.

162. Mohiuddin SM, Mooss AN, Hunter CB, et al. Intensive smoking cessation intervention reduces mortality in high-risk smokers with cardiovascular disease. Chest 2007;131(2):446–52.

163. Tonstad S, Lawrence D. Varenicline in smokers with diabetes: A pooled analysis of 15 randomized, placebo-controlled studies of varenicline. J Diabetes Investig 2017;8(1):93–100.

164. Boyle JP, Thompson TJ, Gregg EW, et al. Projection of the year 2050 burden of diabetes in the US adult population: dynamic modeling of incidence, mortality, and prediabetes prevalence. Popul Health Metr 2010;8:29.

165. Harron KL, Feltbower RG, McKinney PA, et al. Rising rates of all types of diabetes in south Asian and non-south Asian children and young people aged 0-29 years in West Yorkshire, U.K., 1991-2006. Diabetes Care 2011;34(3):652–4.

166. Yeung RO, Zhang Y, Luk A, et al. Metabolic profiles and treatment gaps in young-onset type 2 diabetes in Asia (the JADE programme): a cross-sectional study of a prospective cohort. Lancet Diabetes Endocrinol 2014;2(12):935–43.

167. Hillier TA, Pedula KL. Complications in young adults with early-onset type 2 diabetes: losing the relative protection of youth. Diabetes Care 2003;26(11): 2999–3005.

168. Constantino MI, Molyneaux L, Limacher-Gisler F, et al. Long-term complications and mortality in young-onset diabetes: type 2 diabetes is more hazardous and lethal than type 1 diabetes. Diabetes Care 2013;36(12):3863–9.

169. Huo X, Gao L, Guo L, et al. Risk of non-fatal cardiovascular diseases in early-onset versus late-onset type 2 diabetes in China: a cross-sectional study. Lancet Diabetes Endocrinol 2016;4(2):115–24.

170. Selvin E, Coresh J, Brancati FL. The burden and treatment of diabetes in elderly individuals in the u.s. Diabetes Care 2006;29(11):2415–9.

171. Huang ES, Laiteerapong N, Liu JY, et al. Rates of complications and mortality in older patients with diabetes mellitus: the diabetes and aging study. JAMA Intern Med 2014;174(2):251–8.

172. Peters SA, Huxley RR, Woodward M. Diabetes as risk factor for incident coronary heart disease in women compared with men: a systematic review and meta-analysis of 64 cohorts including 858,507 individuals and 28,203 coronary events. Diabetologia 2014;57(8):1542–51.

173. Peters SA, Huxley RR, Woodward M. Diabetes as a risk factor for stroke in women compared with men: a systematic review and meta-analysis of 64 cohorts, including 775,385 individuals and 12,539 strokes. Lancet 2014; 383(9933):1973–80.

174. Huxley RR, Peters SA, Mishra GD, et al. Risk of all-cause mortality and vascular events in women versus men with type 1 diabetes: a systematic review and meta-analysis. Lancet Diabetes Endocrinol 2015;3(3):198–206.

175. Wexler DJ, Grant RW, Meigs JB, et al. Sex disparities in treatment of cardiac risk factors in patients with type 2 diabetes. Diabetes Care 2005;28(3):514–20.

176. Osende JI, Badimon JJ, Fuster V, et al. Blood thrombogenicity in type 2 diabetes mellitus patients is associated with glycemic control. J Am Coll Cardiol 2001; 38(5):1307–12.

177. Xie M, Shan Z, Zhang Y, et al. Aspirin for primary prevention of cardiovascular events: meta-analysis of randomized controlled trials and subgroup analysis by sex and diabetes status. PLoS One 2014;9(10):e90286.

178. Antithrombotic Trialists' Collaboration. Collaborative meta-analysis of randomised trials of antiplatelet therapy for prevention of death, myocardial infarction, and stroke in high risk patients. BMJ 2002;324(7329):71–86.

179. Saito Y, Okada S, Ogawa H, et al. Low-dose aspirin for primary prevention of cardiovascular events in patients with type 2 diabetes mellitus: 10-year follow-up of a randomized controlled trial. Circulation 2017;135(7):659–70.

180. Shah NS, Huffman MD, Ning H, et al. Trends in myocardial infarction secondary prevention: the National Health and Nutrition Examination Surveys (NHANES), 1999-2012. J Am Heart Assoc 2015;4(4) [pii:e001709].

181. Cornelis MC, Hu FB. Systems epidemiology: a new direction in nutrition and metabolic disease research. Curr Nutr Rep 2013;2(4):225–35.

182. Guasch-Ferre M, Hruby A, Toledo E, et al. Metabolomics in prediabetes and diabetes: a systematic review and meta-analysis. Diabetes Care 2016;39(5): 833–46.

183. Lee S, Zhang C, Kilicarslan M, et al. Integrated network analysis reveals an association between plasma mannose levels and insulin resistance. Cell Metab 2016;24(1):172–84.

184. Lawler PR, Akinkuolie AO, Chu AY, et al. Atherogenic lipoprotein determinants of cardiovascular disease and residual risk among individuals with low low-density lipoprotein cholesterol. J Am Heart Assoc 2017;6(7) [pii:e005549].

185. Liu J, Semiz S, van der Lee SJ, et al. Metabolomics based markers predict type 2 diabetes in a 14-year follow-up study. Metabolomics 2017;13(9):104.

186. Mardinoglu A, Stancakova A, Lotta LA, et al. Plasma mannose levels are associated with incident type 2 diabetes and cardiovascular disease. Cell Metab 2017;26(2):281–3.

187. Perrino C, Barabasi AL, Condorelli G, et al. Epigenomic and transcriptomic approaches in the post-genomic era: path to novel targets for diagnosis and therapy of the ischaemic heart? Position paper of the European Society of Cardiology Working Group on Cellular Biology of the Heart. Cardiovasc Res 2017;113(7):725–36.

188. Ruiz-Canela M, Toledo E, Clish CB, et al. Plasma branched-chain amino acids and incident cardiovascular disease in the PREDIMED Trial. Clin Chem 2016; 62(4):582–92.

189. Guasch-Ferre M, Zheng Y, Ruiz-Canela M, et al. Plasma acylcarnitines and risk of cardiovascular disease: effect of Mediterranean diet interventions. Am J Clin Nutr 2016;103(6):1408–16.

190. Garcia-Perez I, Posma JM, Gibson R, et al. Objective assessment of dietary patterns by use of metabolic phenotyping: a randomised, controlled, crossover trial. Lancet Diabetes Endocrinol 2017;5(3):184–95.

191. Bhupathiraju SN, Hu FB. One (small) step towards precision nutrition by use of metabolomics. Lancet Diabetes Endocrinol 2017;5(3):154–5.

192. Ali MK, Singh K, Kondal D, et al. Effectiveness of a multicomponent quality improvement strategy to improve achievement of diabetes care goals: a randomized, controlled trial. Ann Intern Med 2016;165(6):399–408.

193. Bittner V, Bertolet M, Barraza Felix R, et al. Comprehensive cardiovascular risk factor control improves survival: the BARI 2D trial. J Am Coll Cardiol 2015;66(7): 765–73.

194. Haw JS, Tantry S, Vellanki P, et al. National strategies to decrease the burden of diabetes and its complications. Curr Diab Rep 2015;15(9):65.

195. Tricco AC, Ivers NM, Grimshaw JM, et al. Effectiveness of quality improvement strategies on the management of diabetes: a systematic review and meta-analysis. Lancet 2012;379(9833):2252–61.

196. United Nations. Transforming our world: the 2030 Agenda for Sustainable Development. Available at: https://sustainabledevelopment.un.org/post2015/transformingourworld. Accessed November 2, 2017.

197. World Health Organization. Noncommunicable diseases (NCDs). Available at: http://www.who.int/features/factfiles/noncommunicable_diseases/en/. Accessed August 22, 2017.

198. Zimmet P, Alberti KG, Magliano DJ, et al. Diabetes mellitus statistics on prevalence and mortality: facts and fallacies. Nat Rev Endocrinol 2016;12(10):616–22.

199. Bommer C, Heesemann E, Sagalova V, et al. The global economic burden of diabetes in adults aged 20-79 years: a cost-of-illness study. Lancet Diabetes Endocrinol 2017;5(6):423–30.

200. Fryar CD, Carroll MD, Ogden CL. Prevalence of overweight, obesity, and extreme obesity among adults aged 20 and over: United States, 1960-1962 through 2013-2014. National Center for Health Statistics. Division of Health and Nutrition Examination Surveys; 2016. Available at: https://www.cdc.gov/nchs/data/hestat/obesity_adult_13_14/obesity_adult_13_14.pdf. Accessed August 22, 2017.

201. American Diabetes Association. Economic costs of diabetes in the U.S. in 2012. Diabetes Care 2013;36(4):1033–46.
202. Meigs JB. Epidemiology of type 2 diabetes and cardiovascular disease: translation from population to prevention: the Kelly West award lecture 2009. Diabetes Care 2010;33(8):1865–71.
203. Laitinen TT, Pahkala K, Magnussen CG, et al. Ideal cardiovascular health in childhood and cardiometabolic outcomes in adulthood: the Cardiovascular Risk in Young Finns Study. Circulation 2012;125(16):1971–8.
204. McGill HC Jr, McMahan CA, Zieske AW, et al. Effects of nonlipid risk factors on atherosclerosis in youth with a favorable lipoprotein profile. Circulation 2001; 103(11):1546–50.
205. Weintraub WS, Daniels SR, Burke LE, et al. Value of primordial and primary prevention for cardiovascular disease: a policy statement from the American Heart Association. Circulation 2011;124(8):967–90.
206. Steinberger J, Daniels SR, Hagberg N, et al. Cardiovascular health promotion in children: challenges and opportunities for 2020 and beyond: a scientific statement from the American Heart Association. Circulation 2016;134(12):e236–255.
207. McMahan CA, Gidding SS, Viikari JS, et al. Association of Pathobiologic Determinants of Atherosclerosis in Youth risk score and 15-year change in risk score with carotid artery intima-media thickness in young adults (from the Cardiovascular Risk in Young Finns Study). Am J Cardiol 2007;100(7):1124–9.
208. Berenson GS, Srinivasan SR, Bao W, et al. Association between multiple cardiovascular risk factors and atherosclerosis in children and young adults. The Bogalusa Heart Study. N Engl J Med 1998;338(23):1650–6.
209. Navar-Boggan AM, Peterson ED, D'Agostino RB Sr, et al. Hyperlipidemia in early adulthood increases long-term risk of coronary heart disease. Circulation 2015; 131(5):451–8.
210. Song SH, Gray TA. Early intensive cardiovascular risk management in young people with type 2 diabetes. Diabetes Res Clin Pract 2011;92(3):e70–72.
211. Song SH. Early-onset type 2 diabetes: high lifetime risk for cardiovascular disease. Lancet Diabetes Endocrinol 2016;4(2):87–8.
212. Weintraub WS. Perspective on trends in statin use. JAMA Cardiol 2017;2(1): 11–2.
213. Gregg EW, Wing R. Looking again at the Look AHEAD study. Lancet Diabetes Endocrinol 2017;5(10):763–4.
214. Gaye B, Canonico M, Perier MC, et al. Ideal cardiovascular health, mortality, and vascular events in elderly subjects: the three-city study. J Am Coll Cardiol 2017; 69(25):3015–26.
215. Afshin A, Micha R, Khatibzadeh S, et al. Dietary policies to reduce noncommunicable diseases. The handbook of global health policy. Chichester (United Kingdom): Wiley; 2014. p. 175–93.
216. Economos CD, Hyatt RR, Must A, et al. Shape Up Somerville two-year results: a community-based environmental change intervention sustains weight reduction in children. Prev Med 2013;57(4):322–7.
217. Coffield E, Nihiser AJ, Sherry B, et al. Shape Up Somerville: change in parent body mass indexes during a child-targeted, community-based environmental change intervention. Am J Public Health 2015;105(2):e83–89.
218. Smith GC, Pell JP. Parachute use to prevent death and major trauma related to gravitational challenge: systematic review of randomised controlled trials. BMJ 2003;327(7429):1459–61.

219. National Children's Study (NCS). NICHD. Available at: http://www.nichd.nih.gov/research/NCS/Pages/default.aspx. Accessed August 27, 2017.

220. Environmental influences on Child Health Outcomes (ECHO) program. NIH. Available at: http://www.nih.gov/echo. Accessed August 27, 2017.

221. Alexander KP. Low-hanging fruit for a healthy old age. J Am Coll Cardiol 2017; 69(25):3027–8.

Prediabetes and Cardiovascular Disease
Pathophysiology and Interventions for Prevention and Risk Reduction

Ben Brannick, MD, Sam Dagogo-Jack, MD*

KEYWORDS

- Impaired fasting glucose • Impaired glucose tolerance • Prediabetes complications
- Cardiovascular disease • Macrovascular

KEY POINTS

- Prediabetes carries an increased risk in cardiovascular disease.
- Significant physiologic, metabolic, and biochemical features are dysregulated in prediabetes.
- Extensive randomized, controlled trials have demonstrated that lifestyle modification can decrease the rate of progression from prediabetes to diabetes.
- Early detection and intervention is vitally important for the prevention of prediabetes progression to diabetes.

INTRODUCTION

Type 2 diabetes mellitus (T2DM) is one of the major causes of premature morbidity and mortality worldwide with the World Health Organization reporting that 1 in 10 adults worldwide had T2DM in 2014.[1] In the United States, 1 of every 5 health care dollars is spent on diabetes-related health care.[2] Diabetes mellitus also imposes a huge drain in developing countries on national health budgets comprising on average at least 5% of their total health expenditures on diabetes in 2010.[3] Of these, macrovascular complications are the greatest contributor to the direct and indirect costs of diabetes.[4] The

Disclosure Statement: Dr B. Brannick has nothing to disclose. Dr S. Dagogo-Jack is supported, in part, by Grant R01 DK067269 from the National Institutes of Health.
Authors' Contributions: S. Dagogo-Jack, as senior author, created the design and content of this article. Both S. Dagogo-Jack and B. Brannick drafted, revised and produced the final version of the article.
Division of Endocrinology, Diabetes and Metabolism, University of Tennessee Health Science Center, 920 Madison Avenue, Suite 300A, Memphis, TN 38163, USA
* Corresponding author.
E-mail address: sdj@uthsc.edu

Endocrinol Metab Clin N Am 47 (2018) 33–50
https://doi.org/10.1016/j.ecl.2017.10.001
0889-8529/18/© 2017 Elsevier Inc. All rights reserved.

endo.theclinics.com

development of T2DM is punctuated by an interlude of prediabetes, itself a toxic state that is associated with the development of macrovascular complications.

DIAGNOSIS AND THE BURDEN OF PREDIABETES

The prelude to diabetes is prediabetes in what can be described as a continuum from normoglycemia through worsening dysglycemia. Prediabetes is defined specifically as impaired glucose tolerance (IGT) and/or impaired fasting glucose.[5] According to the American Diabetes Association, IGT is defined as a 2-hour plasma glucose value in the 75-g oral glucose tolerance test (OGTT) of 140 to 199 mg/dL (7.8 to 11.0 mmol/L).[6] Impaired fasting glucose is defined as a fasting plasma glucose of 100 to 125 mg/dL (5.6 to 6.9 mmol/L).[6] Finally prediabetes can also be defined as a hemoglobin A1c (HbA1c) of 5.7% to 6.4% (39–46 mmol/mol).[6,7] It bears stressing that the American Diabetes Association criteria stipulate normal glucose tolerance (NGT) as a fasting glucose level less of than 100 mg/dL and a 2-hour postload OGTT plasma glucose level of less than 140 mg/dL. With regard to using HbA1c as a diagnosis of prediabetes, it must be stressed that there are many well characterized "pitfalls" such as anemia, chronic kidney disease, and other systemic illness and hematologic disorders that disrupt the reliability of HbA1c as an integrated measure of mean plasma glucose.[8–12] In particular, racial and ethnic differences in the relationship between blood glucose values and HbA1c call for caution when using HbA1c levels for the diagnosis of prediabetes.[8–14] It is always prudent to confirm diagnosis with actual blood glucose measurement before instituting therapeutic measures.[8] Estimates by the Centers for Disease Control and Prevention in the United States indicated that there were approximately 29 million adults with diabetes and 86 million with prediabetes in 2014.[15,16] Worldwide, there are more than 400 million people with prediabetes and projections indicate that more than 470 million people will have prediabetes by 2030.[17] In addition, many studies from across the globe have pointed out that the risk of many comorbidities are the same in diabetes and prediabetes and affect all age groups.[18–23]

PATHOPHYSIOLOGIC DEFECTS IN PREDIABETES

The known pathophysiologic defects that underlie T2DM are being increasingly recognized in the prediabetic state.[24–28] The natural progression of dysglycemia involves increasing insulin resistance and loss of pancreatic beta-cell function.[29] Significant defects in insulin action and secretion are consistently demonstrable in the prediabetic state of IGT.[30–32] Several cross-sectional studies and a few longitudinal studies have carefully documented the various defects leading to prediabetes and T2DM.[33–35]

FINDINGS FROM LONGITUDINAL ASSESSMENT OF INSULIN ACTION AND SECRETION

A landmark longitudinal study that tracked high-risk subjects from the stage of NGT to prediabetes reported that the transition to prediabetes was associated with an increase in body weight, increase in insulin resistance, and a decrease in endogenous insulin secretion (beta-cell dysfunction).[29] The study further demonstrated that progression from prediabetes to T2DM was accompanied by a worsening of weight gain, insulin resistance, and beta-cell dysfunction.[29] Thus, the salient finding from the longitudinal observation was that insulin resistance and beta-cell failure coevolve simultaneously rather than sequentially, as was previously believed. Individuals who maintained NGT status, despite weight gain and associated insulin resistance, were those who mounted a robust endogenous insulin secretory response.[29] Thus, if beta-cells cannot overcome insulin resistance, dysglycemia ensues. A supportive post mortem study reported approximately 40% deficit in relative beta-cell volume among individuals with prediabetes compared with those with normal fasting glucose concentrations.[35]

LIPOLYSIS, INCRETIN, ALPHA CELL, AND INFLAMMATION IN PREDIABETES

Further defects in the prediabetic state include increased lipolysis, decreased endogenous levels of glucagonlike peptide 1, and impaired postprandial suppression of glucagon secretion by the alpha-cells of the pancreas.[33,36–39] Additionally, as listed in **Table 1**, aberrant expression of proinflammatory cytokines adds to the toxic milieu of prediabetes. For instance, low adiponectin levels have been demonstrated to be predictive of progression from NGT to prediabetes, and from prediabetes to T2DM.[39,40] Increased levels of molecular markers such as intercellular adhesion molecule-1 and tumor necrosis factor-α have been reported.[41] **Fig. 1** shows the recognized pathophysiologic defects in T2DM, highlighting those that have also been described in prediabetes.[42,43]

Emerging insights regarding the gut microbiome and its association with cardiometabolic disorders, such as obesity, diabetes, dyslipidemia, and so on, have relevance to prediabetes. Recently, a disturbed gut microbiota expressed as gut dysbiosis (an intestinal physical barrier abnormality) has been associated with the progression and maintenance of obesity, T2DM, cardiovascular disease (CVD) and the metabolic syndrome.[44–49] Future research into this area will help to shed light onto the proximal chronology of the associated between gut dysbiosis and early dysglycemia and prediabetes.

PREDICTORS OF GLYCEMIC PROGRESSION TO PREDIABETES AND TYPE 2 DIABETES MELLITUS
Conversion from Prediabetes to Type 2 Diabetes Mellitus

An analysis of 6 prospective studies on progression from prediabetes to T2DM revealed the following features: (1) baseline fasting plasma glucose and the 2-hour OGTT glucose values were positively associated with diabetes risk, (2) the rate of progression from prediabetes to T2DM was exponential among subjects in the top quartile of baseline fasting plasma glucose but increased linearly with increasing 2-hour OGTT glucose levels, (3) incident diabetes occurred at higher rates in Hispanic, Mexican-Americans, Pima, and Nauruan populations than among other ethnicities

Table 1	
Pathophysiologic defects in prediabetes	
Defect	**References**
Loss of beta-cell volume	35
Defects in insulin action and secretion	24,26,29–31,33,50,51
Endothelial dysfunction	26,51
Arterial stiffness	69–71
Increased lipolysis	25,36
Reduced incretin levels	36,38
Increased hepatic glucose production	26,32,33
Impaired glucagon levels	33
Dysregulated cytokines	40,41,95

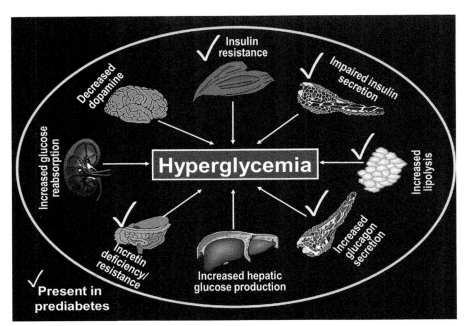

Fig. 1. Recognized pathophysiologic defects in type 2 diabetes mellitus and prediabetes. (*From* Dagogo-Jack S. Diabetes risks from prescription and nonprescription drugs. ADA press, Alexandria, VA, 2016. © 2016 by the American Diabetes Association. *Reprinted with permission from* American Diabetes Association.)

such as Caucasians, and (4) an increased body mass index predicted T2DM risk in low-risk populations but not in populations with the highest incidence of T2DM.[50,51] Of note, weight gain significantly predicted the risk of incident T2DM in African Americans in the Atherosclerosis Risk in Communities study.[52]

Normoglycemia to Prediabetes Transition

Longitudinal studies in subjects from a high-risk population (PIMA Indians) with baseline NGT indicated that weight gain, insulin resistance, and progressive loss of insulin secretory response to glucose predicted transition from NGT to IGT (prediabetes).[29,52] The longitudinal mean weight change in NGT → NGT subjects (nonprogressors) versus NGT → IGT progressors was 2.6 kg versus 5.2 kg during a 6-year follow-up period.[24]

In the BLSA (Baltimore Longitudinal Study of Aging), 62% of the initially NGT participants progressed to prediabetes during 10 years of follow-up, yielding an annualized rate of prediabetes 6.2% in the BLSA.[53] In the POP-ABC (Pathobiology of Prediabetes in a Biracial Cohort) study, initially normoglycemic African American and European American offspring of parents with T2DM were followed longitudinally for the primary outcome of incident prediabetes (impaired fasting glucose or IGT). During a mean 2.62 years of follow-up, 101 of 343 POP-ABC participants developed incident prediabetes, yielding an annualized rate of approximately 11%.[54] Compared with nonprogressors, POP-ABC participants who developed incident prediabetes were older, more likely to be male, had higher baseline body mass index and fat mass, had lower levels of physical activity (adjusted for food habits), lower measures of insulin sensitivity, disposition index, serum adiponectin, and high-density lipoprotein (HDL) cholesterol levels; and higher triglyceride levels.[40,54–56]

MACROVASCULAR COMPLICATIONS OF PREDIABETES

The macrovascular disorders associated with prediabetes include CVD, stroke, and peripheral vascular disease. As **Fig. 2** depicts, these disorders are established in patients with T2DM, but their initiation and progression are well-recognized to occur during the prediabetes stage.[57–60] In fact, the traditional CVD risk factors (dyslipidemia, obesity, hypertension) are quite prevalent among individuals with prediabetes.[61–66]

Cardiovascular Disease

A recent metaanalysis based on 35 studies reported data for the association between myocardial infarction and congestive heart failure as well as coronary artery disease and atherosclerosis have all been reported in individuals with prediabetes.[66–68] In the EPIC-Norfolk study, a 1% increase in HbA1c within the normal range was associated with increased 10-year cardiovascular mortality.[27] The EPIC-Norfolk findings are in accord with data from the Paris Prospective Study cohort, which showed a doubling of CVD mortality in IGT subjects compared with NGT subjects.[58] The finding of increased mortality is underscored by the fact that most patients with prediabetes harbor features of insulin resistance (metabolic) syndrome, including upper-body obesity, hypertriglyceridemia, decreased HDL cholesterol levels, and hypertension, among others. Components of the metabolic syndrome often can be identified in prediabetic subjects several years before the diagnosis of T2DM.[59,69] These features translate into advanced atherosclerotic vascular changes, which are often preceded by impairment of endothelium-dependent vasodilation, vascular smooth muscle dysfunction, and increased arterial stiffness.[70]

A recent cross-sectional study reported a positive association between prediabetes and the prevalence of arterial stiffness, suggesting that early intervention on prediabetes control might prevent arterial stiffness.[71] Remarkably, the prediabetes state is associated a nearly 3-fold higher prevalence of unrecognized myocardial infarction

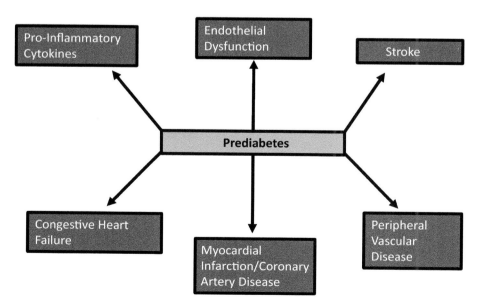

Fig. 2. Recognized macrovascular complications associated with prediabetes. (*Data from* Refs.[56–71])

compared with NGT status, as was demonstrated in the MESA (Multi-Ethnic Study of Atherosclerosis) study.[61]

More recently, a randomized controlled trial of 6522 patients with coronary artery disease and prediabetes found that although acarbose did not reduce the risk of major adverse cardiovascular events, it did reduce the incidence of diabetes.[72]

Stroke

Compared with NGT subjects, individuals with prediabetes have an increased risk of cerebrovascular diseases, including transient ischemic attack, stroke, and recurrent stroke.[64,73–76] A recent study by Tanaka and colleagues[77] demonstrated that both diabetes and prediabetes were associated with poor early prognosis 30 days after acute ischemic stroke. A study by Qiao and colleagues[78] indicates that the 2-hour postload OGTT glucose level is a strong predictor of stroke and future CVD. In the recently published KORA-MRI study (Cooperative Health Research in the Region of Augsburg-MRI), among 400 subjects who underwent MRI, 103 subjects had prediabetes and 54 had established diabetes. Subjects with prediabetes had an increased risk for carotid plaque and adverse functional cardiac parameters.[79]

In the IRIS trial (Insulin Resistance Intervention after Stroke) involving patients without diabetes who had insulin resistance along with a recent history of ischemic stroke or transient ischemic attack, treatment with pioglitazone significantly decreased the risks of stroke, myocardial infarction, or the development of T2DM as compared with placebo treament.[80,81]

Peripheral Vascular Disease

Prediabetes is common in patients with peripheral vascular disease; however, the exact mechanisms remain to be fully elucidated. The development of diabetes is independently associated with mortality in PVD patients in some but not all studies.[82,83]

Interactions Among Prediabetes and Cardiovascular Disease Risk Factors

Epidemiologic studies have shown that prediabetes is a strong predictor of CVD.[5,81–85] The studies include DECODE (Diabetes Epidemiology: Collaborative analysis Of Diagnostic criteria in Europe) and Funagata Diabetes Study, among others.[84–87] In the San Antonio Heart Study, there was evidence that the risk for CVD starts to increase long before the onset of clinical diabetes.[88–90] Obesity and overweight, known risk factors for T2DM and prediabetes, have also been associated with CVD risk.[91–94] Overweight and obesity have been frequently associated with low-grade, chronic, systemic inflammation characterized by increased levels of proinflammatory markers including tumor necrosis factor-alpha, interleukin-6, interleukin-8, and C-reactive protein.[95] Also, overweight people with prediabetes often present with dyslipidemia (higher triglycerides and lower HDL cholesterol)[95–100] Hypertension is another CVD risk factor that has been examined in prediabetes.[101–105] The DREAM (Diabetes REduction Assessment with ramipril and rosiglitazone Medication)[101] and NAVIGATOR (Long-term Study of Nateglinide+Valsartan to Prevent or Delay Type II Diabetes Mellitus and Cardiovascular Complications)[102] studies assessed the effect of blood pressure control on the progression from prediabetes to T2DM. Similarly, the Diabetes Prevention Program investigators reported lower rates of incident hypertension among prediabetic individuals randomized to the intensive lifestyle arm as compared with the placebo arm.[103]

INTERVENTION STUDIES TO PREVENT PROGRESSION FROM PREDIABETES TO TYPE 2 DIABETES MELLITUS AND DEVELOPMENT OF CARDIOVASCULAR DISEASE
Prevention of type 2 diabetes mellitus

Table 2 lists lifestyle and pharmacologic intervention studies to prevent T2DM among individuals enrolled with prediabetes. Lifestyle intervention has clearly been demonstrated to decrease progression to T2DM.[102–107] The results of the DPP (Diabetes Prevention Program), FDPS (Finnish Diabetes Prevention Study), and other pertinent studies showed approximately 60% risk reduction for incident T2DM in the lifestyle arm compared with placebo.[108–112] In both the DPP and FDPS, every 1 kg decrease in weight in the lifestyle arm was associated with 15% to 16% in future T2DM risk.[23,111,113–117]

There are also studies showing potential benefits from a variety of different pharmacotherapies.[23] Pioglitazone was found to decrease the risk of diabetes by approximately 70% in obese subjects with prediabetes in the ACT NOW (Actos Now for Prevention of Diabetes) study.[118] **Table 2** lists pertinent randomized controlled trials from around the world that demonstrated significant decrease in progression of prediabetes to diabetes. These include the STOP-NIDDM (Study to Prevent NIDDM; 25% risk reduction), XENDOS (XENical in the prevention of diabetes in obese subjects; 45% risk reduction), DREAM (62% risk reduction), CANOE (Low-dose combination therapy with rosiglitazone and metformin to prevent type 2 diabetes mellitus; 26% risk reduction), and the valsartan arm of the NAVIGATOR trial (14% risk reduction).[119–123] It must be noted, however, that in both the IDPP1 (Indian Diabetes Prevention Programme) and the follow-up study IDPP2, pharmacologic intervention provided no additional benefit beyond lifestyle modification in subjects randomized to lifestyle plus metformin or lifestyle plus pioglitazone arms.[124,125] Furthermore, all the medications tested for diabetes prevention have had untoward adverse effects (sometimes severe), and attempts to withdraw the medications have resulted in glycemic rebound.[126,127] Given these limitations of pharmacotherapy, the current guidelines from the American Diabetes Association recommend lifestyle modifications as the first-line approach for diabetes prevention.[6] Indications for possible use of metformin include women with a history of gestational diabetes and high-risk individuals unresponsive to optimal lifestyle modification.[6]

Prevention of Cardiovascular Disease in Prediabetes

Long-term follow-up of the Da Qing study demonstrated that diabetes prevention through lifestyle modification was associated with decreased cardiovascular and all-cause mortality after 23 years.[128] In the DPP, intensive lifestyle intervention that significantly decreased the risk of T2DM also reduced the need for antihypertensive medications.[103] The prevalence of hypertension in the DPP cohort at baseline was approximately 30% in the 3 comparison groups (placebo, metformin, lifestyle).[103] After 3 years of follow-up, the prevalence of hypertension was observed to have increased to approximately 40% in the placebo and metformin arms.[103] Surprisingly, the hypertension prevalence remained at the baseline rate of 30% in the intensive lifestyle group 3 years later.[103] Thus, lifestyle interventions designed to prevent T2DM also seems to have prevented incident hypertension in this initially prediabetic cohort.[103] The DPP investigators also reported that subjects assigned to intensive lifestyle intervention showed decreased blood pressure, increased HDL cholesterol levels, and lower triglyceride levels, as well as a reduction in the more atherogenic small, dense low-density lipoprotein particles during approximately 3 years of follow-up.[103] Consonant with these findings, there was a reduced need for

Table 2
Pertinent prediabetes intervention studies

Study	Intervention	Number of Subjects	Study Population	Risk Reduction	Years
Da Qing[117]	Diet and exercise	577	Chinese IGT adults, mean age 46, BMI 26	31%–46% after 6 y	1986–1992
Finnish DPS[115]	Diet and exercise	522	IGT adults, mean age 55, BMI 31	58% after 3.2 y	1993–1998
STOP-NIDDM[119]	Acarbose	1428	IGT adults, mean age 55, BMI 31	25% after 3.3 y	1995–1998
DPP[116]	Diet and exercise	3234	IGT adults, mean age 54 y, BMI 34	Metformin 31%, lifestyle 58% after 2 y	1996–1999
XENDOS[120]	Orlistat and diet and exercise	3305	Swedish, BMI >30, mean age 43, 21% with IGT	Entire group 37%, IGT 45% after 4 y	1997–2002
DREAM[121]	Rosiglitazone	5269	IGT and/or IFG subjects mean age 54.7 y, BMI 30.9	62% after approximately 3 y	2001–2003
IDDP-1[124]	Lifestyle modifications and metformin or lifestyle modifications	531	Indian, IGT mean age 46 y, BMI 25.8	Diet and exercise 28.5%, metformin 26.4%, diet and exercise and metformin 28.2% after 30 mo	2001–2004
ACT-NOW[127]	Pioglitazone	602	IGT, mean age 53, BMI 33	72% with pioglitazone over 2.4 y	2004–2006
CANOE[122]	Combination rosiglitazone and metformin vs placebo	207	IGT, mean age 50, BMI 31.3	26% in the combination group after 3.9 y	2004–2006
IDDP-2[125]	Lifestyle modifications or pioglitazone and lifestyle modifications	407	Indian IGT, mean age 45.3, BMI 25.9	28% though pioglitazone not additive to lifestyle modification	2006–2009
NAVIGATOR[123]	Nataglinide and lifestyle modifications or Valsartan and lifestyle modifications	9306	IGT, mean age 63.7, BMI 30.5	Nataglinide none, Valsartan 14%	2005–2010

Abbreviations: BMI, body mass index; IGT, impaired glucose tolerance.

lipid lowering medications in the DPP,[103,105,106] as has been observed by others.[107–109,118,129]

The Mediterranean diet is appealing as a specific nutritional recommendation, based on convincing reports of its benefits on cardiometabolic endpoints. For example, results from the PREDIMED (PREvención con DIeta MEDiterránea) randomized nutrition intervention trial for the primary prevention of CVD showed a 40% reduction in the incidence of T2DM in participants assigned to a Mediterranean diet supplemented with extra virgin olive oil compared with those assigned to a low-fat control diet.[130,131] Other reports on the Mediterranean diet showed concordant findings on cardiometabolic profile. Mediterranean-style diet has been shown to result in greater weight loss along with improvement in inflammatory markers compared with general lifestyle counseling (14 kg vs 3 kg; $P<.001$).[132–135]

Beside the impact of lifestyle intervention on CVD risk factors, there is considerable interest in knowing whether prevention of diabetes also prevents related CVD. This has been a question under investigation by the DPPOS (Diabetes Prevention Program Outcome Study) research group. Analysis of regression patterns in the DPPOS showed that individuals whose blood glucose returned to normal experienced a 56% long-term reduction in diabetes incidence compared with those who remained dysglycemic.[105] Although CVD outcomes data collection is still in progress, additional inference from the DPPOS study would suggest that regression from prediabetes to normal may also be associated with decreased risk for CVD.[107,136]

CLINICAL TRANSLATION AND SUMMARY

Prediabetes is a toxic cardiometabolic state associated with increased risk for microvascular and macrovascular complications.[137] Physicians and health care providers should screen patients routinely for prediabetes and refer those with the condition for intensive lifestyle counseling. The goal is to achieve and maintain greater than 5% weight loss through caloric restriction and increased physical activity, similar to the DPP and kindred studies (see **Table 2**).[6,34,62,63] Health care providers should endeavor to build strong ties within health care systems, communities, and payers, to increase the availability of evidence-based structured lifestyle programs.

In a recent survey, 33.6% of outpatients (out of 1.16 million outpatient visits analyzed) had prediabetes, based on HbA1c results. Amazingly, less than 1% of those patients whose HbA1c tests showed prediabetes were recognized and diagnosed as such by clinicians. Of the abysmally low numbers whose prediabetes status was properly captured in the clinical records, only 23% had documentation of treatment (lifestyle modification and/or metformin) in the medical record.[138] The prediabetes period presents an opportunity to intervene during the disease process. Primary care physicians, specialists, health systems, and patients themselves all have an obligation to ensure that the opportunity for prevention is not missed.[139–143]

Although it has long been known that diabetes confers significant cardiovascular risks, it is now becoming established that CVD risks precede diabetes and are evident in people with prediabetes. Given the millions of people with prediabetes around the globe, the impact on cardiovascular health is staggering. However, identifying and intervening in the at-risk prediabetic populations requires education, increased awareness, care coordination, organization, and novel reimbursement mechanisms at multiple levels (health systems, society, and individual).

REFERENCES

1. World Health Organization. Global status report on noncommunicable diseases 2016. Geneva (Switzerland): World Health Organization; 2016.
2. Dall TM, Yang W, Halder P, et al. The economic burden of elevated blood glucose levels in 2012. Diabetes Care 2014;37:3172–9.
3. Zhang P, Zhang X, Brown J, et al. Global healthcare expenditure on diabetes for 2010 and 2030. Diabetes Res Clin Pract 2010;87:293–301.
4. American Diabetes Association. Economic costs of diabetes in the U.S. in 2012. Diabetes Care 2013;36(4):1033–46.
5. DeFronzo RA, Abdul-Ghani M. Assessment and treatment of cardiovascular risk in prediabetes: impaired glucose tolerance and impaired fasting glucose. Am J Cardiol 2011;108:3B–24B.
6. American Diabetes Association. Standards of medical care in diabetes-2017. Diabetes Care 2017;40:S11–24.
7. World Health Organization (WHO) Consultation. Definition and diagnosis of diabetes and intermediate hyperglycaemia. Geneva (Switzerland): World Health Organization; 2006. Available at: http://www.who.int/diabetes/publications/Definition%20and%20diagnosis%20of%20diabetes_new.pdf. Accessed March 10, 2017.
8. Dagogo-Jack S. Pitfalls in the use of HbA1(c) as a diagnostic test: the ethnic conundrum. Nat Rev Endocrinol 2010;6:589–93.
9. Chapp-Jumbo E, Edeoga C, Wan J, et al. Ethnic disparity in hemoglobin A1c levels among normoglycemic offspring of parents with type 2 diabetes. Endocr Pract 2012;18:356–62.
10. Ebenibo S, Edeoga C, Wan J, et al. Glucoregulatory function among African Americans and European Americans with normal or pre-diabetic hemoglobin A1c levels. Metabolism 2014;63:767–72.
11. Herman WH, Dungan KM, Wolffenbuttel BH, et al. Racial and ethnic differences in mean plasma glucose, hemoglobin A1c, and 1,5-anhydroglucitol in over 2000 patients with type 2 diabetes. J Clin Endocrinol Metab 2009;94(5):1689–94.
12. Soranzo N. Genetic determinants of variability in glycated hemoglobin (HbA(1c)) in humans: review of recent progress and prospects for use in diabetes care. Curr Diab Rep 2011;11(6):562–9.
13. Herman WH. Are there clinical implications of racial differences in HbA1c? Yes, to not consider can do great harm! Diabetes Care 2016;39(8):1458–61.
14. Wolffenbuttel BH, Herman WH, Gross JL, et al. Ethnic differences in glycemic markers in patients with type 2 diabetes. Diabetes Care 2013;36(10):2931–6.
15. Centers for Disease Control and Prevention. National diabetes statistics report: estimates of diabetes and its burden in the United States, 2014. Atlanta (GA): US Department of Health and Human Services; 2014.
16. International Diabetes Federation. IDF diabetes atlas 2015. 7th edition. Brussels (Belgium): International Diabetes Federation; 2015.
17. Middelbeek RJW, Abrahamson MJ. Diabetes, prediabetes, and glycemic control in the United States: challenges and opportunities. Ann Intern Med 2014; 160:572–3.
18. Hu D, Fu P, Xie J, et al, MS for the InterASIA Collaborative Group. Increasing prevalence and low awareness, treatment and control of diabetes mellitus among Chinese adults: the InterASIA study. Diabetes Res Clin Pract 2008;81: 250–7.

19. Faeh D, William J, Tappy L, et al. Prevalence, awareness and control of diabetes in the Seychelles and relationship with excess body weight. BMC Public Health 2007;7:163.
20. Saadi H, Carruthers SG, Nagelkerke N, et al. Prevalence of diabetes mellitus and its complications in a population-based sample in Al Ain, United Arab Emirates. Diabetes Res Clin Pract 2007;78(3):369–77.
21. Echouffo-Tcheugui JB, Dagogo-Jack S. Preventing diabetes mellitus in developing countries. Nat Rev Endocrinol 2012;8:557–62.
22. Dagogo-Jack S. Predicting diabetes: our relentless quest for genomic nuggets. Diabetes Care 2012;35:193–5.
23. Tabák AG, Herder C, Rathmann W, et al. Prediabetes: a high-risk state for diabetes development. Lancet 2012;379:2279–90.
24. Defronzo RA. Banting lecture. From the triumvirate to the ominous octet: a new paradigm for the treatment of type 2 diabetes mellitus. Diabetes 2009;58:773–95.
25. Cerasi E, Luft R. The prediabetic state, its nature and consequences—a look toward the future. Diabetes 1972;21:685–94.
26. Halban PA, Polonsky KS, Bowden DW, et al. Beta-cell failure in type 2 diabetes: postulated mechanisms and prospects for prevention and treatment. Diabetes Care 2014;37:1751–8.
27. Khaw KT, Wareham N, Bingham S, et al. Association of hemoglobin A1c with cardiovascular disease and mortality in adults: the European Prospective Investigation. Ann Intern Med 2004;141:413–20.
28. Ford ES, Zhao G, Li C. Pre-diabetes and the risk for cardiovascular disease: a systematic review of the evidence. J Am Coll Cardiol 2010;55:1310–7.
29. Weyer C, Bogardus C, Mott DM, et al. The natural history of insulin secretory dysfunction and insulin resistance in the pathogenesis of type 2 diabetes mellitus. J Clin Invest 1999;104:787–94.
30. Kitabchi AE, Temprosa M, Knowler WC, et al, The Diabetes Prevention Program Research Group. Role of insulin secretion and sensitivity in the evolution of type 2 diabetes in the diabetes prevention program: effects of lifestyle intervention and metformin. Diabetes 2005;54:2404–14.
31. Eschwege E, Richard JL, Thibult N, et al. Coronary heart disease mortality in relation with diabetes, blood glucose and plasma insulin levels. The Paris prospective study, ten years later. Horm Metab Res Suppl 1985;15:41–6.
32. DeFronzo RA, Bonadonna RC, Ferrannini E. Pathogenesis of NIDDM. A balanced overview. Diabetes Care 1992;15:318–68.
33. Mitrakou A, Kelley D, Mokan M, et al. Role of reduced suppression of glucose production and diminished early insulin release in impaired glucose tolerance. N Engl J Med 1992;326:22–9.
34. Meigs JB, D'Agostino RB Sr, Nathan DM, et al. Longitudinal association of glycemia and microalbuminuria: the Framingham Offspring Study. Diabetes Care 2002;25:977–83.
35. Butler AE, Janson J, Bonner-Weir S, et al. Beta-cell deficit and increased beta-cell apoptosis in humans with type 2 diabetes. Diabetes 2003;52:102–10.
36. Dagogo-Jack S, Askari H, Tykodi G. Glucoregulatory physiology in subjects with low-normal, high-normal, or impaired fasting glucose. J Clin Endocrinol Metab 2009;94:2031–6.
37. DeFronzo R, Kanat M, Abdul-Ghani M. Treatment of prediabetes. World J Diabetes 2015;6:1207–22.

38. Toft-Nielsen MB, Damholt MB, Madsbad S, et al. Determinants of the impaired secretion of glucagon-like peptide-1 in type 2 diabetic patients. J Clin Endocrinol Metab 2001;86:3717–23.
39. Mather KJ, Funahashi T, Matsuzawa Y, et al. Diabetes prevention program. adiponectin, change in adiponectin, and progression to diabetes in the diabetes prevention program. Diabetes 2008;57:980–6.
40. Jiang Y, Owei I, Wan J, et al. Adiponectin levels predict prediabetes risk: the pathobiology of prediabetes in A biracial cohort (POP-ABC) study. BMJ Open Diabetes Res Care 2016;4(1):e000194.
41. Huang Z, Chen C, Li S, et al. Serum markers of endothelial dysfunction and inflammation increase in hypertension with prediabetes mellitus. Genet Test Mol Biomarkers 2016;20:322–7.
42. Dagogo-Jack S. Diabetes risks from prescription and nonprescription drugs. Alexandria (VA): ADA Press; 2016.
43. Lefèbvre PJ, Scheen AJ. The postprandial state and risk of cardiovascular disease. Diabet Med 1998;4:S63–8.
44. von Toerne C, Huth C, de Las Heras Gala T, et al. MASP1, THBS1, GPLD1 and ApoA-IV are novel biomarkers associated with prediabetes: the KORA F4 study. Diabetologia 2016;9:1882–92.
45. Turnbaugh PJ, Ley RE, Mahowald MA, et al. An obesity-associated gut microbiome with increased capacity for energy harvest. Nature 2006;444:1027–31.
46. Cani PD, Neyrinck AM, Fava F, et al. Selective increases of bifidobacteria in gut microflora improve high-fat-diet-induced diabetes in mice through a mechanism associated with endotoxaemia. Diabetologia 2007;50:2374–83.
47. Ridaura VK, Faith JJ, Rey FE, et al. Gut microbiota from twins discordant for obesity modulate metabolism in mice. Science 2013;341:1241214.
48. Koeth RA, Wang Z, Levison BS, et al. Intestinal microbiota metabolism of L-carnitine, a nutrient in red meat, promotes atherosclerosis. Nat Med 2013; 19:576–85.
49. Vrieze A, Van Nood E, Holleman F, et al. Transfer of intestinal microbiota from lean donors increases insulin sensitivity in individuals with metabolic syndrome. Gastroenterology 2012;143:913–6.
50. Edelstein SL, Knowler WC, Bain RP, et al. Predictors of progression from impaired glucose tolerance to NIDDM: an analysis of six prospective studies. Diabetes 1997;46:701–10.
51. Knowler WC, Bennett PH, Hamman RF, et al. Diabetes incidence and prevalence in Pima Indians: a 19-fold greater incidence than in Rochester, Minnesota. Am J Epidemiol 1978;108:497–505.
52. Brancati FL, Kao WH, Folsom AR, et al. Incident type 2 diabetes mellitus in African American and white adults: the atherosclerosis risk in communities study. JAMA 2000;283:2253–9.
53. Meigs JB, Muller DC, Nathan DM, et al. Baltimore longitudinal study of aging. The natural history of progression from normal glucose tolerance to type 2 diabetes in the Baltimore longitudinal study of aging. Diabetes 2003;52:1475–84.
54. Dagogo-Jack S, Edeoga C, Ebenibo S, et al, Pathobiology of Prediabetes in a Biracial Cohort (POP-ABC) Research Group. Lack of racial disparity in incident prediabetes and glycemic progression among black and white offspring of parents with type 2 diabetes: the pathobiology of prediabetes in a biracial cohort (POP-ABC) study. J Clin Endocrinol Metab 2014;99:E1078–87.
55. Boucher AB, Adesanya EA, Owei I, et al. Dietary habits and leisure-time physical activity in relation to adiposity, dyslipidemia, and incident dysglycemia in the

pathobiology of prediabetes in a biracial cohort study. Metabolism 2015;64:
1060–7.

56. Owei I, Umekwe N, Wan J, et al. Plasma lipid levels predict dysglycemia in a
biracial cohort of nondiabetic subjects: potential mechanisms. Exp Biol Med
(Maywood) 2016;241:1961–7.

57. Selvin E, Lazo M, Chen Y, et al. Diabetes mellitus, prediabetes, and incidence of
subclinical myocardial damage. Circulation 2014;130:1374–82.

58. Balkau B, Eschwège E, Papoz L, et al. Risk factors for early death in non-insulin
dependent diabetes and men with known glucose tolerance status. BMJ 1993;
307:295–9.

59. Dagogo-Jack S, Egbuonu N, Edeoga C. Principles and practice on non-
pharmacological interventions to reduce cardiometabolic risk. Med Princ Pract
2010;19:167–75.

60. Nyenwe EA, Dagogo-Jack S. Metabolic syndrome, prediabetes and the science
of primary prevention. Minerva Endocrinol 2011;36:129–45.

61. Stacey RB, Leaverton PE, Schocken DD, et al. Prediabetes and the association
with unrecognized myocardial infarction in the multi-ethnic study of atherosclerosis. Am Heart J 2015;170:923–8.

62. Hu FB, Stampfer MJ, Haffner SM, et al. Elevated risk of cardiovascular disease
prior to clinical diagnosis of type 2 diabetes. Diabetes Care 2002;25:1129–34.

63. Coutinho M, Gerstein HC, Wang Y, et al. Analysis of published data from 20
studies of 95,783 individuals followed for 12.4 years. Diabetes Care 1999;22:
233–40.

64. Smith NL, Barzilay JI, Shaffer D, et al. Fasting and 2-hour post challenge serum
glucose measures and risk of incident cardiovascular events in the elderly: the
cardiovascular health study. Arch Intern Med 2002;162:209–16.

65. Huang Y, Cai X, Mai W, et al. Association between prediabetes and risk of cardiovascular disease and all-cause mortality: systematic review and meta-analysis. BMJ 2016;355:i5953.

66. Bonora E, Kiechl S, Willeit J, et al. Carotid atherosclerosis and coronary heart
disease in the metabolic syndrome: prospective data from the Bruneck study.
Diabetes Care 2003;26:1251–7.

67. Tai ES, Goh SY, Lee JJ, et al. Lowering the criterion for impaired fasting glucose:
impact on disease prevalence and associated risk of diabetes and ischemic
heart disease. Diabetes Care 2004;27:1728–34.

68. Rijkelijkhuizen J, Nijpels J, Heine R, et al. High risk of cardiovascular mortality in
individuals with impaired fasting glucose is explained by conversion to diabetes: the Hoorn study. Diabetes Care 2007;30:332–6.

69. Dagogo-Jack S. Endocrinology & metabolism: complications of diabetes mellitus. In: Singh AK, editor. Scientific American medicine. Hamilton (Canada):
Decker Intellectual Properties; 2015.

70. Papa G, Degano C, Iurato MP, et al. Macrovascular complication phenotypes in
type 2 diabetic patients. Cardiovasc Diabetol 2013;12:20.

71. Wang J, Liu L, Zhou Y, et al. Increased fasting glucose and the prevalence of
arterial stiffness: a cross-sectional study in Chinese adults. Neurol Res 2014;
5:427–33.

72. Holman RR, Coleman RL, Chan JCN, et al, ACE Study Group. Effects of
acarbose on cardiovascular and diabetes outcomes in patients with coronary heart disease and impaired glucose tolerance (ACE): a randomised,
double-blind, placebo-controlled trial. Lancet Diabetes Endocrinol 2017;5
[pii:S2213-8587(17) 30309-1].

73. Roquer J, Rodríguez-Campello A, Cuadrado-Godia E, et al. Ischemic stroke in prediabetic patients. J Neurol 2014;261:1866–70.

74. Urabe T, Watada H, Okuma Y, et al. Prevalence of abnormal glucose metabolism and insulin resistance among subtypes of ischemic stroke in Japanese patients. Stroke 2009;40:1289–95.

75. Kernan WN, Viscoli CM, Inzucchi SE, et al. Prevalence of abnormal glucose tolerance following a transient ischemic attack or ischemic stroke. Arch Intern Med 2005;165:227–33.

76. Matz K, Keresztes K, Tatschl C, et al. Disorders of glucose metabolism in acute stroke patients: an underrecognized problem. Diabetes Care 2006;29:792–7.

77. Tanaka R, Ueno Y, Miyamoto N, et al. Impact of diabetes and prediabetes on the short-term prognosis in patients with acute ischemic stroke. J Neurol Sci 2013; 332:45–50.

78. Qiao Q, Pyörälä K, Pyörälä M, et al. Two hour glucose is a better risk predictor for incident coronary heart disease and cardiovascular mortality than fasting glucose. Eur Heart J 2002;23:1267–75.

79. Bamberg F, Hetterich H, Rospleszcz S, et al. Subclinical disease burden as assessed by whole-body MRI in subjects with prediabetes, subjects with diabetes, and normal control subjects from the general population: the KORA-MRI study. Diabetes 2017;1:158–69.

80. Holman RR, Coleman RL, Chan JCN, et al. IRIS trial investigators. Pioglitazone after ischemic stroke or transient ischemic attack. N Engl J Med 2016;374(14): 1321–31.

81. Inzucchi SE, Viscoli CM, Young LH, et al. IRIS trial investigators. Pioglitazone prevents diabetes in insulin-resistant patients with cerebrovascular disease. Diabetes Care 2016;39:1684–92.

82. Golledge J, Quigley F, Velu R, et al. Association of impaired fasting glucose, diabetes and their management with the presentation and outcome of peripheral artery disease: a cohort study. Cardiovasc Diabetol 2014;13:147.

83. Kamalesh M, Shen J. Diabetes and peripheral arterial disease in men: trends in prevalence, mortality, and effect of concomitant coronary disease. Clin Cardiol 2009;32:442–6.

84. The DECODE study group. Consequence of the new diagnostic criteria for diabetes in older men and women. Diabetes Care 1999;22:1667–71.

85. Zhang L, Qiao Q, Tuomilehto J, et al, DECODE Study Group. The impact of dyslipidaemia on cardiovascular mortality in individuals without a prior history of diabetes in the DECODE Study. Atherosclerosis 2009;206:298–302.

86. Tominaga M, Eguchi H, Manaka H, et al. Impaired glucose tolerance is a risk factor for cardiovascular disease, but not impaired fasting glucose. The Funagata Diabetes Study. Diabetes Care 1999;22:920–4.

87. Balkau B, Bertrais S, Ducimetière P, et al. Is there a glycemic threshold for mortality risk? Diabetes Care 1999;22:696–9.

88. Resnick HE, Harris MI, Brock DB, et al. American Diabetes Association diabetes diagnostic criteria, advancing age, and cardiovascular disease risk profiles: results from the Third National Health and Nutrition Examination Survey. Diabetes Care 2000;23:176–80.

89. De Marco M, de Simone G, Roman MJ, et al. Cardiac geometry and function in diabetic or prediabetic adolescents and young adults: the strong heart study. Diabetes Care 2011;34:2300–5.

90. Haffner SM, Stern MP, Hazuda HP, et al. Cardiovascular risk factors in confirmed prediabetic individuals. Does the clock for coronary heart disease start ticking before the onset of clinical diabetes? JAMA 1990;263:2893–8.

91. Yan F, Cha E, Lee ET, et al. A self-assessment tool for screening young adults at risk of type 2 diabetes using strong heart family study data. Diabetes Educ 2016;42:607–17.

92. Romeo S, Maglio C, Burza MA, et al. Cardiovascular events after bariatric surgery in obese subjects with type 2 diabetes. Diabetes Care 2012;35:2613–7.

93. Franssen R, Monajemi H, Stroes ES, et al. Obesity and dyslipidemia. Med Clin North Am 2011;95:893–902.

94. Liu T. A comparison of biological and physical risk factors for cardiovascular disease in overweight/obese individuals with and without prediabetes. Clin Nurs Res 2016. [Epub ahead of print].

95. Kim CS, Park HS, Kawada T, et al. Circulating levels of MCP-1 and IL-8 are elevated in human obese subjects and associated with obesity-related parameters. Int J Obes 2006;30:1347–55.

96. Li C, Ford E, Zhao G, et al. Prevalence of pre-diabetes and its association with clustering of cardiometabolic risk factors and hyperinsulinemia among U.S. adolescents: National Health and Nutrition Examination Survey 2005–2006. Diabetes Care 2009;32:342–7.

97. Festa A, Williams K, Hanley AJ, et al. Nuclear magnetic resonance lipoprotein abnormalities in prediabetic subjects in the insulin resistance atherosclerosis study. Circulation 2005;111:3465–72.

98. Zheng S, Zhou H, Han T, et al. Clinical characteristics and beta cell function in Chinese patients with newly diagnosed type 2 diabetes mellitus with different levels of serum triglyceride. BMC Endocr Disord 2015;15:21.

99. Ren X, Chen ZA, Zheng S, et al. Association between triglyceride to HDL-C ratio (TG/HDL-C) and insulin resistance in Chinese patients with newly diagnosed type 2 diabetes mellitus. PLoS One 2016;11:e0154345.

100. Sparks JD, Sparks CE, Adeli K. Selective hepatic insulin resistance, VLDL overproduction, and hypertriglyceridemia. Arterioscler Thromb Vasc Bio 2012;32:2104–12.

101. Bosch J, Yusuf S, Gerstein HC, et al. Effect of ramipril on the incidence of diabetes. N Engl J Med 2006;355:1551–62.

102. Navigator Study Group. Effect of valsartan on the incidence of diabetes and cardiovascular events. N Engl J Med 2010;362:1477–90.

103. The Diabetes Prevention Program Research Group. Impact of intensive lifestyle and metformin therapy on cardiovascular disease risk factors in the diabetes prevention program. Diabetes Care 2005;28:888–94.

104. Moebus S, Hanisch JU, Aidelsburger P, et al. Impact of four different definitions used for assessment of the prevalence of metabolic syndrome in a primary health care setting. The German Metabolic and Cardiovascular Risk Project (GEMCAS). Cardiovasc Diabetol 2007;6:22.

105. Lewington S, Clarke R, Qizilbash N, et al. Age-specific relevance of usual blood pressure to vascular mortality: a meta-analysis of individual data for one million adults in 61 prospective studies. Lancet 2002;360:1903–13.

106. Kahn R, Alperin P, Eddy D. Age at initiation and frequency of screening to detect type 2 diabetes: a cost-effectiveness analysis. Lancet 2010;375:1365–74.

107. Gæde P, Oellgaard J, Carstensen B, et al. Years of life gained by multifactorial intervention in patients with type 2 diabetes mellitus and microalbuminuria: 21

years follow-up on the Steno-2 randomized trial. Diabetologia 2016;59: 2298–307.

108. Knowler WC, Barrett-Connor E, Fowler SE, et al, Diabetes Prevention Program Research Group. Reduction in the incidence of type 2 diabetes with lifestyle intervention or metformin. N Engl J Med 2002;346:393–403.

109. Urbanski P, Wolf A, Herman W. Cost-effectiveness of diabetes education. J Am Diet Assoc 2008;108:S6–11.

110. Stefan N, Staiger H, Wagner R, et al. A high-risk phenotype associates with reduced improvement in glycaemia during a lifestyle intervention in prediabetes. Diabetologia 2015;58:2877–84.

111. The Look AHEAD Research Group. Cardiovascular effects of intensive lifestyle intervention in type 2 diabetes. N Engl J Med 2013;369:145–54.

112. DPP Research Group. Reduction in the incidence of type 2 diabetes with lifestyle intervention or metformin. N Engl J Med 2002;346:393–403.

113. Sprague R, Ellsworth M. Vascular disease in pre-diabetes: new insights derived from systems biology. Mo Med 2010;107:265–9.

114. Hostalek U, Gwilt M, Hildemann S. Therapeutic use of metformin in prediabetes and diabetes prevention. Drugs 2015;75:1071–94.

115. Tuomilehto J, Lindström J, Eriksson JG, et al. Finnish diabetes prevention study group. N Engl J Med 2001;344:1343–50.

116. Anderson J. Achievable cost saving and cost-effective thresholds for diabetes prevention lifestyle interventions in people aged 65 years and older: a single-payer perspective. J Acad Nutr Diet 2012;112:1747–54.

117. Pan XR, Li GW, Hu YH, et al. Effects of diet and exercise in preventing NIDDM in people with impaired glucose tolerance. The Da Qing IGT and diabetes study. Diabetes Care 1997;20:537–44.

118. DeFronzo RA, Tripathy D, Schwenke DC, et al. ACT NOW study. Pioglitazone for diabetes prevention in impaired glucose tolerance. N Engl J Med 2011;364: 1104–15.

119. Chiasson JL, Josse RG, Gomis R, et al. STOP-NIDDM trial research group: acarbose treatment and the risk of cardiovascular disease and hypertension in patients with impaired glucose tolerance: the STOP-NIDDM trial. JAMA 2003;290: 486–94.

120. Torgerson JS, Hauptman J, Boldrin MN, et al. XENical in the prevention of diabetes in obese subjects (XENDOS) study: a randomized study of orlistat as an adjunct to lifestyle changes for the prevention of type 2 diabetes in obese patients. Diabetes Care 2004;27:155–61.

121. DREAM (Diabetes REduction Assessment with ramipril and rosiglitazone Medication) Trial Investigators. Effect of rosiglitazone on the frequency of diabetes in patients with impaired glucose tolerance or impaired fasting glucose: a randomised controlled trial. Lancet 2006;368:1096–105.

122. Zinman B, Harris SB, Neuman J, et al. Low-dose combination therapy with rosiglitazone and metformin to prevent type 2 diabetes mellitus (CANOE trial): a double-blind randomised controlled study. Lancet 2010;376:103–11.

123. NAVIGATOR Study Group. Effect of nateglinide on the incidence of diabetes and cardiovascular events. N Engl J Med 2010;362:1463–76.

124. Ramachandran A, Snehalatha C, Mary S, et al, Indian Diabetes Prevention Programme (IDPP). The Indian diabetes prevention programme shows that lifestyle modification and metformin prevent type 2 diabetes in Asian Indian subjects with impaired glucose tolerance (IDPP-1). Diabetologia 2006;49:289–97.

125. Ramachandran A, Snehalatha C, Mary S, et al. Pioglitazone does not enhance the effectiveness of lifestyle modification in preventing conversion of impaired glucose tolerance to diabetes in Asian Indians: results of the Indian diabetes prevention programme-2 (IDPP-2). Diabetologia 2009;52:1019–26.

126. The Diabetes Prevention Program Research Group. Effects of withdrawal from metformin on the development of diabetes in the diabetes prevention program. Diabetes Care 2003;26:977–80.

127. Tripathy D, Schwenke DC, Banerji M, et al. Diabetes incidence and glucose tolerance after termination of pioglitazone therapy: results from ACT NOW. J Clin Endocrinol Metab 2016;101:2056–62.

128. Li G, Zhang P, Wang J, et al. Cardiovascular mortality, all-cause mortality, and diabetes incidence after lifestyle intervention for people with impaired glucose tolerance in the Da Qing diabetes prevention study: a 23-year follow-up study. Lancet Diabetes Endocrinol 2014;2:474–80.

129. Xiang AH, Hodis HN, Kawakubo M, et al. Effect of pioglitazone on progression of subclinical atherosclerosis in non-diabetic premenopausal Hispanic women with prior gestational diabetes. Atherosclerosis 2008;199:207–14.

130. Salas-Salvadó J, Guasch-Ferré M, Lee CH, et al. Protective effects of the Mediterranean diet on type 2 diabetes and metabolic syndrome. J Nutr 2016;146(4).

131. Mozaffarian D, Marfisi R, Levantesi G, et al. Incidence of new-onset diabetes and impaired fasting glucose in patients with recent myocardial infarction and the effect of clinical and lifestyle risk factors. Lancet 2007;370:667–75.

132. Esposito K, Maiorino MI, Bellastella G, et al. A journey into a Mediterranean diet and type 2 diabetes: a systematic review with meta-analyses. BMJ Open 2015;5(8):e008222.

133. Monlezun DJ, Kasprowicz E, Tosh KW, et al. Medical school-based teaching kitchen improves HbA1c, blood pressure, and cholesterol for patients with type 2 diabetes: results from a novel randomized controlled trial. Diabetes Res Clin Pract 2015;109(2):420–6.

134. Salas-Salvadó J, Bulló M, Estruch R, et al. Prevention of diabetes with Mediterranean diets: a subgroup analysis of a randomized trial. Ann Intern Med 2014;160(1):1–10.

135. Esposito K, Pontillo A, Di Palo C, et al. Effect of weight loss and lifestyle changes on vascular inflammatory markers in obese women: a randomized trial. JAMA 2003;289:1799–804.

136. Perreault L, Temprosa M, Mather KJ, et al, The Diabetes Prevention Program Research Group. Regression from prediabetes to normal glucose regulation is associated with reduction in cardiovascular risk: results from the diabetes prevention program outcomes study. Diabetes Care 2014;37:2622–31.

137. Brannick B, Wynn A, Dagogo-Jack S. Prediabetes as a toxic environment for the initiation of microvascular and macrovascular complications. Exp Biol Med (Maywood) 2016;241:1323–31.

138. Mainous AG 3rd, Tanner RJ, Scuderi CB, et al. Prediabetes screening and treatment in diabetes prevention: the impact of physician attitudes. J Am Board Fam Med 2016;29:663–71.

139. Gopalan A, Lorincz IS, Wirtalla C, et al. Awareness of prediabetes and engagement in diabetes risk-reducing behaviors. Am J Prev Med 2015;49:512–9.

140. Dagogo-Jack S. Preventing diabetes-related morbidity and mortality in the primary care setting. J Natl Med Assoc 2002;94:549–60.

141. Pate RR, Pratt M, Blair SN, et al. Physical activity and public health: recommendation from the centers for disease control and prevention and the American College of Sports Medicine. JAMA 1995;273:402–7.
142. Kimm SY, Glynn NW, Kriska AM, et al. Decline in physical activity in black and white girls during adolescence. N Engl J Med 2002;347:709–15.
143. Dagogo-Jack S. Primary prevention of cardiovascular disease: the glass is half full and half empty. Diabetes Care 2005;28:971–2.

Pathogenesis of Cardiovascular Disease in Diabetes

Andrea V. Haas, MD[a], Marie E. McDonnell, MD[b],*

KEYWORDS

- Cardiac autonomic neuropathy • Diabetic cardiomyopathy • Coronary flow reserve
- Microangiopathy • Diabetic heart disease

KEY POINTS

- Cardiovascular disease is the most common cause of morbidity and mortality in both type 1 and 2 diabetes.
- The "glucose hypothesis" states that hyperglycemia directly contributes to development of cardiovascular disease.
- Insulin resistance and metabolic changes present in diabetes accelerate atherosclerosis development.
- Diabetic cardiomyopathy results in diastolic dysfunction, ventricular hypertrophy, and cardiac remodeling in the absence of coronary artery disease.
- Pathogenesis of cardiac autonomic neuropathy is multifactorial, including metabolic changes, inflammatory cytokines, and autoimmune destruction.

INTRODUCTION

The role of diabetes in the pathogenesis of cardiovascular disease (CVD) was uncovered in the late 1970s when data from the Framingham Heart Study demonstrated a clear link between the 2 conditions. A far greater percentage of patients with diabetes compared with those without the disease have cardiovascular comorbidities (eg, hypertension, dyslipidemia) and complications (eg, heart and vascular disease).[1] The prevalence of CVD among individuals with diabetes overall increased over the last 5 decades but recently appears to be improving presumably because of better adherence to risk factor modification (by both clinicians and patients) in the course of clinical

Disclosure Statement: The authors have nothing to disclose.
[a] Division of Endocrinology, Diabetes, and Hypertension, Brigham and Women's Hospital, Harvard Medical School, 221 Longwood Avenue, Boston, MA 02115, USA; [b] Diabetes Section, Division of Endocrinology, Diabetes, and Hypertension, Brigham and Women's Hospital, Harvard Medical School, 221 Longwood Avenue, Room 381, Boston, MA 02115, USA
* Corresponding author.
E-mail address: mmcdonnell@bwh.harvard.edu

Endocrinol Metab Clin N Am 47 (2018) 51–63
https://doi.org/10.1016/j.ecl.2017.10.010
0889-8529/18/© 2017 Elsevier Inc. All rights reserved.

endo.theclinics.com

care.[2] However, CVD remains the most common cause of death and complications in both type 1 (T1D) and type 2 diabetes (T2D).[2,3] Although it is also known that lifestyle changes, control of blood pressure and lipids, and antiplatelet therapy can reduce the development, progression, and complications associated with diabetes, the timing of these interventions is likely critical to reduce cardiovascular morbidity over a lifetime.[4]

Since these early associations, scientific knowledge of the impact of diabetes on the heart has expanded to address how the diabetes milieu alters the natural history and clinical presentation of heart disease, from the familiar conditions of coronary artery disease (CAD) and congestive heart failure (CHF) to the less familiar conditions of microangiopathy and autonomic dysfunction. In essence, the diabetic state accelerates most cardiac pathologies due to abnormalities in systemic and local vascular inflammation, endothelial and microvascular injury, altered thrombosis, autonomic nerve dysfunction, and likely membrane instability in nerves, smooth muscle, and endothelium. As we continue to learn from genome-wide analyses and functional genomics studies, the influence of genetic and epigenetic susceptibility is also likely important determinants of cardiac health in diabetes. A 2017 *Nature* article found that individuals who had genes known to increase risk of T2D also had an increased risk of heart disease. Furthermore, a new genetic loci, CCDC92, was identified that associated with both T2D and heart disease, implicating a shared pathway in the pathogenesis of these 2 diseases.[5] At this time, however, although multiple single nucleotide polymorphisms have been found to be associated with CVD in genetic association studies, usually their individual influence is small, and genetic contributions to CVD are poorly understood.[6]

In this concise review on pathogenesis of heart disease in diabetes, CVD is considered a class of distinct conditions that involve the heart and blood vessels, with each condition either presenting alone or, commonly, along with others due to overlapping pathophysiologic factors. Although the spectrum of CVD with increased prevalence in diabetes is broad, the authors highlight the pathogenetic factors that are known to contribute to the following conditions that present uniquely in diabetes and often overlap. These conditions include *atherosclerosis*, *microangiopathy*, *diabetic cardiomyopathy*, and *cardiac autonomic neuropathy* (**Fig. 1**). The "glucose hypothesis" linking hyperglycemia to cardiac abnormality is explored in this context, and the unique pathogenic factors are discussed for each condition. Subsequent articles in this issue address some of the conditions (eg, CHF) in more detail as well as the benefit of targeted therapeutic approaches to treat and/or prevent CVD in individuals with diabetes.

THE "GLUCOSE HYPOTHESIS" IN THE HEART

High glucose levels over time play an independent role in the development of CVD, although details on the importance of degree and duration of exposure to the severity of disease are less clear. Perhaps the best evidence of the link between hyperglycemia and cardiac dysfunction due to hyperglycemia is in studies of T1D, a "pure" insulin-deficient state. In one observational study of 20,985 individuals with T1D, each 1% increase in HA1c was associated with a 30% increase in risk of heart failure independent of other factors, including hypertension, smoking, and obesity. The "glucose hypothesis" linking high glucose to cellular damage is based on the concept that for many tissues in the body and/or under certain metabolic conditions, glucose transport across the cell membrane is unregulated by insulin and high glucose concentrations bombard cells with high intracellular glucose and glucose metabolites. These metabolites activate several accessory metabolic

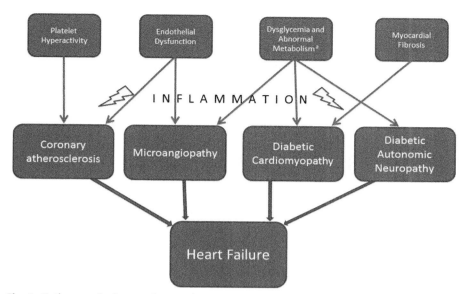

Fig. 1. Pathogenetic factors that are known to contribute to atherosclerosis, microangiopathy, diabetic CM, and cardiac autonomic neuropathy. [a] Combination of defects including impaired insulin signaling, abnormal glucose uptake (increased or decreased), generation of oxidative stress, and formation and deposition of glycation and products.

pathways, for example, the polyol and protein kinase C pathways, that lead to the formation of oxidative free radicals and accumulation of advanced glycation end products (AGEs).[7] AGEs are produced from nonenzymatic glycosylation of lipids, lipoproteins, and amino acids. AGE deposition increases connective tissue cross-linking, fibrosis and cardiac stiffness and contributes to impaired diastolic relaxation.[8] AGE may also directly impact immune cell function, specifically the macrophage, suggesting that part of the acceleration in CAD development in diabetes is due to alteration in macrophage function due in part to AGE.[9] The production of AGEs and reactive oxygen species as the result of hyperglycemia likely has long-term negative effects on the cardiovascular system.

Although these classical mechanisms are important in the microvasculature of the heart, in the myocardium, the hyperglycemic milieu activates different pathologic pathways. Although fatty acid oxidation is an important fuel for the myocardium, normal glucose sensing, uptake, and utilization appear to be critical for normal cardiac cellular function. As in many tissues, in cardiac tissue normal insulin signaling results in glucose uptake via the GLUT4 transporter protein. However, the pure insulin deficiency of T1D and the insulin resistance characteristic of T2D impair normal insulin signaling. The resultant decreased insulin signaling and glucose uptake appear to be important defects along the pathophysiologic pathway to diabetic cardiomyopathy (CM). The result is abnormal intracellular calcium signaling, diminished insulin-stimulated coronary endothelial nitric oxide (NO) synthase activity, and NO production. Added to this is an inappropriate activation of the renin-angiotensin aldosterone system (RAAS) in diabetes and the activation of the maladaptive signaling pathway mTOR-S6K1 due to overnutrition.[10] The end result of these abnormalities is cardiac stiffness and diastolic dysfunction, and over time, clinical heart failure.

Whether controlling glucose using diet, lifestyle, and medications plays a role in modulating the pathogenesis of CVD in diabetes and to what extent has been the subject of much discussion and controversy. In the case of microvascular disease, the "glucose hypothesis" has been tested and proven in rigorous clinical trials of intensive glucose control in both T1D and T2D, namely the Diabetes Control and Complications Trial (DCCT) and UK Prospective Diabetes Study (UKPDS) studies, respectively.[11,12] However, the relationship between glycemic control and CVD outcomes has been more difficult to demonstrate in relatively short trials. The challenge in linking glycemic control and CVD outcomes may be due to unique features in the natural history of glucose-induced cardiovascular damage as well as the difference between the "pure" insulin-deficient state of T1D as noted above versus the additional insulin resistance/metabolic syndrome-related components of T2D. Based on the DCCT and UKPDS trials, the development of clinically significant *microvascular* disease can take less than a decade. Interestingly, however, both the DCCT and the UKPDS trials were only able to show a reduction in cardiovascular events over a decade after the end of the studies. In the DCCT follow-up study in T1D, the CVD event risk was 42% and 30% lower in the intensively treated cohort 18 years and 30 years after the start of the trial, respectively. Similarly, in the UKPDS in new-onset T2D patients, a modest reduction in cardiovascular mortality in the intensive arm did not reach statistical significance until 10 years after the trial ended.[11] Consistent with the hypothesis that early glucose control makes the most impact is the finding from the STOP-NIDDM trial, where a glucose-lowering drug acarbose was used to prevent diabetes; secondary analysis of this trial suggested a reduction in myocardial infarction and total CVD events.[13] Unfortunately, data from studies published 20 years later showed that glucose control may not be an effective strategy to reduce CVD events decades after the diagnosis of diabetes and could potentially cause harm.[14,15]

The totality of the clinical data available suggests that glucose lowering for cardioprotection is effective but probably only when applied early, near the onset of hyperglycemia. As demonstrated by animal studies, the converse may also be true, that poor glucose control early on impedes future attempts to improve outcomes by tighter control. This recognition that the impact of early glucose control, or lack thereof, has a major impact late in the course of both microvascular and macrovascular disease led to the concept of "metabolic memory." The concept was first described from studies performed in the 1980s in diabetic animals and isolated cells exposed to high glucose followed by normal glucose environments.[16] Later, after 2002, findings from large human studies supported the hypothesis. In both the DCCT and the UKPDS trials discussed above, despite both arms arriving at similar glucose control after the study ended, over the subsequent decades the intensive groups continued to have lower risk for both microvascular and macrovascular complications.[17] Subsequent studies designed to investigate potential mechanisms for metabolic memory have indicated that irreversible structural changes might be involved in the progression of late-term hyperglycemic effects.

Another explanation for the observation that early glucose control has the greatest benefit is that hyperglycemia and/or the other elements of the diabetic milieu are often subclinical for years before diagnosis, and the "window" to make a clinical impact through improved control is limited. Because there is a strong genetic predisposition for T2D that becomes clinically manifest in the presence of environmental factors, hyperglycemia typically appears intermittently or gradually over a period of years. Obvious examples of transitory manifestations of diabetes include women who develop gestational diabetes who have remission after delivery and relapse years later as T2D, stress hyperglycemia due to acute illness and other factors, or therapy with glucocorticoids. However, it is also common for asymptomatic, gradually progressive hyperglycemia to occur in the absence of any medical condition other than obesity and thus escape detection for years. An analysis of 2 populations, one in the United States and one in Australia, showed that retinopathy, an easily identified form of asymptomatic microangiopathy, is often present when T2D is diagnosed and then increases in prevalence linearly.[18] Projection of the prevalence slope backward, to a period preceding the diagnosis, showed that hyperglycemia was likely to have been present in these populations for at least 4 to 7 years before diagnosis. Similarly, in the UKPDS, many patients with newly diagnosed T2D were found to have retinopathy visible on retinal examination (21%), an abnormal electrocardiogram (18%), absent pedal pulses (13%), or an abnormal vibration threshold in the feet (7%).[19]

ACCELERATED ATHEROSCLEROSIS IN DIABETES

Atherosclerosis is characterized by focal deposits of cholesterol and lipids in the intimal wall of arteries. It is the most common cause of CAD and hence is a major contributor to CVD in diabetes. Atherosclerosis is a progressive disease that begins before or around the onset of one or more known risk factors and often precedes hyperglycemia, and hence the clinical diagnosis of diabetes, for decades. There are numerous factors that intersect in the pathogenesis of CAD, and many of these are either enhanced by or introduced by diabetes (**Table 1**). Oxidative stress, glyco-oxidation, systemic inflammation, which are all promoted by hyperglycemia, work together to damage endothelial cells lining the arterial wall and promote inflammation in the intimal layer of the coronary artery. This leads to deposition of lipids and oxidized lipoproteins in the wall, which induces a macrophage and T-lymphocyte–driven immune response. The result is a thickened intima and a vicious cycle of local inflammation and apoptosis, leading to progressive endothelial injury and formation of lipid-rich plaques. It is this process, recurring over time with small microinsults, combined with abnormal platelet reactivity and fibrin deposition in diabetes that predisposes to both progressive luminal narrowing (impaired blood flow and chronic ischemia) and plaque rupture with thrombosis that can block blood flow acutely (myocardial infarction).

In diabetes, atherosclerosis is *accelerated* by the unique diabetic milieu and has been a subject of major research and clinical discussion given the high prevalence of the condition in both prediabetes and diabetes.[20] *Insulin resistance* features prominently in this milieu and promotes high levels of circulating lipids as well as plasminogen activator inhibitor-1 (PAI-1) and other factors that reduce the ability to break down accumulated fibrin in the arterial wall. Insulin resistance also contributes to the development and progression of hypertension, which serves to accelerate the process even further. It is unknown whether the abnormally high insulin levels occurring in the setting of insulin resistance plays a direct deleterious role in CAD. Regardless, in the setting of insulin resistance, accelerated atherosclerosis development likely begins more than a decade before dysmetabolic disease is identified through usual preventive care visits that include blood pressure, lipid measurement, and routine diabetes screening. Systemic and dysregulated *inflammation* is also characteristic of diabetes, especially in the setting of obesity. It appears to be a major driver at all phases of atherosclerosis, from the formation of fatty streaks to subsequent rupture of the lesions that cause acute coronary syndromes. Epidemiology and clinical studies have supported this perspective, where systemic inflammatory markers, such as C-reactive protein, interleukin-6, and serum amyloid A, have been shown to be strong predictors of cardiovascular complications in various settings.

The feared complication of coronary atherosclerosis is ischemic CM. Ischemic CM typically develops after myocardial infarction, either clinical or subclinical, which sets

Table 1
Accelerated atherosclerosis in diabetes

Stage of Atherosclerosis Development	Key Pathogenic Factors/Events	Diabetes-Related Pathogenic Accelerator
Foam cells and fatty streak development 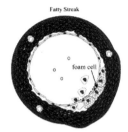	• Endothelial dysfunction • Lipoprotein entry and modification • Leukocyte recruitment • Foam cell formation	• Hyperglycemia • Dyslipidemia (low high-density lipoprotein, high triglycerides, increased small dense low-density lipoprotein) • Microvascular disease, AGEs • Adipocytokines (inter-leukin-1 [IL-1], tumor necrosis factor -α, IL-6) • Insulin resistance with increased fatty acids • Abnormal immune cell function • Secondary kidney dysfunction • *Synergistic accelerator: smoking*
Plaque development 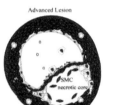	• Intima thickening • Evolution of the fatty streak • Calcification • Fibrous capsule formation • Luminal narrowing of the artery	• Abnormal platelet activation • Autonomic dysfunction, dysregulation of coronary blood flow • Increased sympathetic tone (obesity) • *Synergistic accelerator: smoking*
Plaque progression and disruption 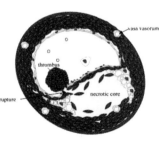	• Plaque size changes, thicker more stable plaques vs thinner less stable plaques, leading to acute coronary syndrome	• Abnormal platelet activation • Hypertension • *Synergistic accelerator: smoking*

The figures show the basic anatomy of a fully formed atherosclerotic plaque (AP). The table indicates the 3 main steps to the formation of the AP and the key pathogenic factors known to promote this process. As indicated in the last column, the diabetic state carries with it specific abnormalities that accelerate the process at each step. Of note, tobacco smoking in the setting of diabetes acts as an additional accelerant throughout AP development.

From Zeadin MG, Petlura CI, Werstuck GH. Molecular mechanisms linking diabetes to the accelerated development of atherosclerosis. Can J Diabetes 2013;37(5):346; with permission.

off interrelated effects that in combination lead to either hypertrophy or dilation and eventually clinical CHF. These 3 effects include neurohormonal overdrive, mechanical overload, and ischemic oxidative injury. Overall, the subject of CHF in diabetes is complex and is reviewed in detail by Anders Jorsal and colleagues' article, "Heart Failure: Epidemiology, Pathophysiology, and Management of Heart Failure in Diabetes Mellitus," in this issue.

MICROANGIOPATHY AND THE MYOCARDIUM

Diabetic microangiopathy is classically described as the contributing factor in major diabetic complications, such as retinopathy, nephropathy, and neuropathy. However, there is good evidence to suggest that diabetes causes impaired coronary microvasculature, similar to other microvascular systems. Diabetic microangiopathy is characterized by abnormal growth and leakage of small blood vessels, resulting in local edema and functional impairment of tissues. Although there are multiple mechanisms leading to the impairment of microcirculation in diabetes, the result is dysregulated vascular regeneration that impacts tissue perfusion independently from coronary arterial flow. In addition, oxidative and hyperosmolar stress, as well as the activation of inflammatory pathways triggered by advanced glycation end-products and toll-like receptors, has been recognized as key pathogenetic factors that impair the microcirculation in the heart.[21,22]

Given the expected overlap in many patients between coronary macrovascular disease and microangiopathy, it has been challenging to tease out the relative importance of each. One of the most common investigative measurements to do this is the coronary flow reserve (CFR). CFR as assessed by PET is a quantitative, reproducible, and sensitive marker of myocardial perfusion and ischemia that integrates the hemodynamic effects of epicardial stenosis, diffuse atherosclerosis, and microvascular dysfunction.[7,8] Interestingly, the addition of CFR has been shown to improve the value of traditional risk assessment for cardiac death in a variety of patient populations, including high-risk cohorts, such as patients with diabetes and patients with mild to moderate chronic kidney disease.[23–27]

When applied to patients without evidence of CAD, the CFR provides a window into the presence or absence of cardiac microangiopathy. One study showed that in the absence of significant epicardial CAD, patients with T2D and impaired myocardial blood flow as defined by a CFR below the median have a 3.2-fold increased rate of cardiac death in comparison with those with CFR above median.[27] Thus, CFR is a good intermediate marker of CVD in diabetes and appears to reflect the unique importance of coronary microangiopathy in understanding the high cardiovascular morbidity and mortality in diabetes.

It is also well established that aldosterone and RAAS play a critical role in the pathophysiology of CVD, and recent studies suggest that this is related to injury to the coronary microvasculature.[28] In the classical RALES study, mineralocorticoid (MR) blockade was established in humans to reduce morbidity and mortality in severe heart failure, although the mechanism was unknown and remains unclear.[29] Interestingly, in a rodent model of angiotensin II–dependent cardiovascular injury, MR blockade reduces coronary microvascular damage, suggesting that excess MR activation promotes injury to the coronary microvasculature.[30] Furthermore, preclinical studies demonstrate that excess MR activation contributes to vascular injury in obesity and diabetes.[31–33] In addition, in a study of 64 men and women with well-controlled diabetes, MR blockade with spironolactone improved CFR.[34] These findings are consistent with current understanding of MR biology in the vasculature. The MR is expressed in endothelium, vascular smooth muscle cell, and cardiomyocytes as well as circulating leukocytes. MR activation has been linked directly to vascular dysfunction and damage, which appears to be due mainly to activation of inflammatory pathways involving increased reactive oxygen species and expression of PAI-1 and intracellular adhesion molecule.[35]

DIABETIC CARDIOMYOPATHY

Diabetic CM is a unique form of heart disease characterized by an early defect in diastolic relaxation that progresses to clinical CHF *in the absence of detectable atherosclerosis or risk factors such as hypertension or dyslipidemia*. Hence, in its pure form, diabetic CM does not develop from ischemia due to the coronary macrovasculature. It was first described as a distinct entity in a 1972 case series, later confirmed by the Framingham Heart Study finding of a 2-fold increased risk of heart failure after adjustment for risk factors, including age, hypertension, obesity, dyslipidemia, and CAD.

As described recently in a comprehensive review, insulin resistance, hyperinsulinemia, and hyperglycemia are each independent risk factors for the development of diabetic CM.[10] The pathophysiologic factors in diabetes that drive the development of CM include systemic metabolic derangement as described in the above section "Alternative glucose hypothesis." Additional factors include inappropriate activation of RAAS, subcellular component abnormalities, oxidative stress, inflammation, and dysfunctional immune modulation. These abnormalities collectively promote cardiac tissue interstitial fibrosis, cardiac stiffness/diastolic dysfunction, and, later, systolic dysfunction, precipitating the syndrome of clinical heart failure. Recent evidence has revealed that dysregulation of coronary endothelial cells and exosomes likely also contribute to the abnormality underlying diabetic CM.[10]

CARDIAC AUTONOMIC NEUROPATHY

Cardiovascular autonomic neuropathy (CAN) is a subtype of diabetic autonomic neuropathy. Diabetic autonomic neuropathy is one of the least recognized yet most common complications of diabetes. Autonomic neuropathy can affect the cardiovascular, gastrointestinal, ocular, and/or genitourinary systems. The parasympathetic and sympathetic nerves are impacted in an ascending, length-dependent fashion.[36] Manifestations can include tachycardia, orthostatic hypotension, exercise intolerance, constipation or diarrhea, urinary retention or incontinence, gastroparesis, and/or erectile dysfunction.[37]

The pathogenesis of autonomic neuropathy is multifactorial and not completely understood. Hyperglycemia, metabolic changes, inflammatory cytokines, autoimmune destruction, and growth factor deficiency all likely contribute.[38] As per the glucose hypothesis described above, hyperglycemia activates alternative metabolic pathways that form toxic AGE and free radicals. All of these effects ultimately result in direct neuronal injury, vascular endothelial damage, and decreased neuronal blood flow.[7] Generation of reactive oxygen species activates genes that promote neurotoxicity.[37] In addition, lymphocyte and macrophage infiltration in autonomic nerves has been identified in a portion of individuals with severe autonomic neuropathy, suggesting an immune cause may be an important factor as well.[39]

CAN, as defined by the CAN Subcommittee of the Toronto Consensus Panel on Diabetic Neuropathy, is the impairment of cardiovascular autonomic control in patients with diabetes after the exclusion of other causes.[40] CAN is present in approximately 25% of individuals with T1D and 33% of individuals with T2D.[41,42] Prevalence increases with age, diabetes duration, and worsening glycemic control.[41]

The vagus nerve is typically affected first because it is the longest autonomic nerve in the human body. It is responsible for 75% of all parasympathetic activity, and loss of parasympathetic tone results in a compensatory increase in sympathetic tone with resultant elevated norepinephrine levels and insulin resistance.[37] These alterations affect glucose utilization by the myocardium because cardiac energy generation favors use of free fatty acids rather than glucose.[43] Free fatty acids, an inefficient energy source, lead to high myocardial oxygen consumption, high oxygen demand, and further generation of reactive oxygen species.[44,45] All of these changes reduce cardiac efficiency and ultimately can contribute to cardiac remodeling.[37] With time, sympathetic denervation ensues, first seen distally at the apex of the heart and with time spreading to the base.[37] More recently, hypoglycemia has also been linked to development of CAN.[46] Evidence suggests that antecedent hypoglycemia impairs generalized autonomic function in healthy subjects.[46]

The natural progression of CAN is not fully known but starts as a subclinical stage with impaired baroreflex sensitivity and reduced heart rate variability mediated by an imbalance between parasympathetic and sympathetic tone.[37] Subclinical autonomic dysfunction has been identified at the time of diabetes diagnosis in 7% of both T1D and T2D.[47] Subclinical autonomic neuropathy progresses to a clinically evident stage over many years.[48] Development is associated with hypertension, smoking, hyperlipidemia, obesity, and poor glucose control.[36] Clinical manifestations include resting tachycardia, postural hypotension, exercise intolerance, intraoperative complications, diabetic CM, silent myocardial infarction, and increased risk of mortality.[36,41]

An increase in resting heart rate is due to vagal nerve damage with resulting unopposed cardiac sympathetic outflow.[49] As autonomic neuropathy progresses, the sympathetic nervous system is also affected. Exercise intolerance results from impairment of heart rate, blood pressure, and cardiac output in response to exercise.[41] Late-stage autonomic neuropathy results in orthostatic hypotension, where damage to the efferent sympathetic nerves causes inability to appropriately increase sympathetic tone and peripheral vascular resistance and thus responds to a decrease in blood pressure.[41,49,50] Diabetic CM is thought to result from relative unopposed sympathetic activity and catecholamine toxicity.[36] This can cause diastolic dysfunction, left ventricular hypertrophy, and cardiac remodeling in the absence of CAD.[36]

CAN increases morbidity and mortality.[44] Individuals have a higher risk of cardiac arrhythmias, silent myocardial ischemia, and sudden death.[44] In the EURODIAB IDDM Complications Study, a cross-sectional study of 3250 patients with T1D, presence of cardiac autonomic neuropathy was the single strongest predictor of mortality.[51] Likewise, among individuals with T2D, the Action to Control Cardiovascular Risk in Diabetes and the Detection of Ischemia in Asymptomatic Diabetics studies showed that cardiac autonomic neuropathy increased rates of silent ischemia and mortality even independent of traditional risk factors (hypertension, dyslipidemia).[52,53]

Cause for increased mortality is attributed to abnormal norepinephrine signaling, resulting in cardiac arrhythmias and sudden death.[54] Autonomic neuropathy is associated with prolonged QT interval, which is also an independent predictor of mortality.[55] Furthermore, the presence of CAN impairs the ability to detect cardiac ischemic pain, leading to silent myocardial ischemia and infarction.[56]

KNOWLEDGE GAPS

There are several areas of investigation that have been proposed to close present knowledge gaps in the understanding of CVD in diabetes. One example is in atherosclerotic plaques in diabetes. Although it is established that there is altered macrophage and T-lymphocyte content in atherosclerosis, it is still not well known if there are significant differences in coronary plaques between subjects with and without diabetes, and with T2D versus T1D. Findings in this regard could help to develop more precise and hence effective therapies for this debilitating disease. Moreover, in this regard, targeted blockade of the appropriate inflammatory pathways known to accelerate most CVD in diabetes continues to elude the clinical armamentarium for diabetes. In another area, the recent findings of reduced cardiovascular mortality in larger cardiovascular outcome trials of modern classes of noninsulin anti-hyperglycemic agents are spawning new areas of investigation. In particular, the sodium-glucose transporter-2 receptor antagonist agents appear to impact CVD morbidity and mortality in less than 6 months, mostly in CHF outcomes even in patients without known CM. This suggests that preclinical CM is a more relevant entity than perhaps once thought. It is also likely that the presence of both diabetic and ischemic CM in an individual alters prognosis and would likely change therapeutic strategy. To address this, more precise approaches to diagnosing cardiac defects in patients with diabetes are on the horizon. Finally, CAN is the most underrecognized form of CVD because it is insidious and, by its nature, painless. Research is needed in this area to assist with identification and treatment of this condition as well as to understand the true nature of the yet unexplained link between CAN and sudden death.

REFERENCES

1. Fox CS, Coady S, Sorlie PD, et al. Increasing cardiovascular disease burden due to diabetes mellitus: the Framingham Heart Study. Circulation 2007;115(12): 1544–50.
2. Gregg EW, Li Y, Wang J, et al. Changes in diabetes-related complications in the United States, 1990-2010. N Engl J Med 2014;370(16):1514–23.
3. Skrivarhaug T, Bangstad HJ, Stene LC, et al. Long-term mortality in a nationwide cohort of childhood-onset type 1 diabetic patients in Norway. Diabetologia 2006; 49(2):298–305.
4. Gaede P, Lund-Andersen H, Parving HH, et al. Effect of a multifactorial intervention on mortality in type 2 diabetes. N Engl J Med 2008;358(6):580–91.
5. Zhao W, Rasheed A, Tikkanen E, et al. Identification of new susceptibility loci for type 2 diabetes and shared etiological pathways with coronary heart disease. Nat Genet 2017;49(10):1450–7.
6. MacRae CA, Vasan RS. The future of genetics and genomics: closing the phenotype gap in precision medicine. Circulation 2016;133(25):2634–9.
7. Kaur N, Kishore L, Singh R. Diabetic autonomic neuropathy: pathogenesis to pharmacological management. J Diabetes Metab 2014;5(7):1–8.
8. Jia G, DeMarco VG, Sowers JR. Insulin resistance and hyperinsulinaemia in diabetic cardiomyopathy. Nat Rev Endocrinol 2016;12(3):144–53.
9. Schmidt AM. 2016 ATVB plenary lecture: receptor for advanced glycation endproducts and implications for the pathogenesis an treatment of cardiometabolic disorders: spotlight on the macrophage. Arterioscler Thromb Vasc Biol 2017; 37(4):613–21.
10. Jia G, Whaley-Connell A, Sowers JR. Diabetic cardiomyopathy: a hyperglycaemia- and insulin-resistance-induced heart disease. Diabetologia 2018;61(1):21–8.
11. UK Prospective Diabetes Study (UKPDS) Group. Intensive blood-glucose control with sulphonylureas or insulin compared with conventional treatment and risk of

complications in patients with type 2 diabetes (UKPDS 33). UK Prospective Diabetes Study (UKPDS) Group. Lancet 1998;352(9131):837–53.

12. The effect of intensive treatment of diabetes on the development and progression of long-term complications in insulin-dependent diabetes mellitus. The Diabetes Control and Complications Trial Research Group. N Engl J Med 1993;329(14): 977–86.

13. Chiasson JL, Josse RG, Gomis R, et al. Acarbose for prevention of type 2 diabetes mellitus: the STOP-NIDDM randomised trial. Lancet 2002;359(9323): 2072–7.

14. Action to Control Cardiovascular Risk in Diabetes Study Group, Gerstein HC, Miller ME, Byington RP, et al. Effects of intensive glucose lowering in type 2 diabetes. N Engl J Med 2008;358(24):2545–59.

15. ADVANCE Collaborative Group, Patel A, MacMahon S, Chalmers J, et al. Intensive blood glucose control and vascular outcomes in patients with type 2 diabetes. N Engl J Med 2008;358(24):2560–72.

16. Ceriello A, Ihnat MA, Thorpe JE. Clinical review 2: the "metabolic memory": is more than just tight glucose control necessary to prevent diabetic complications? J Clin Endocrinol Metab 2009;94(2):410–5.

17. Nathan DM, DCCT/EDIC Research Group. The diabetes control and complications trial/epidemiology of diabetes interventions and complications study at 30 years: overview. Diabetes Care 2014;37(1):9–16.

18. Harris MI, Klein R, Welborn TA, et al. Onset of NIDDM occurs at least 4-7 yr before clinical diagnosis. Diabetes Care 1992;15(7):815–9.

19. UK Prospective Diabetes Study 6. Complications in newly diagnosed type 2 diabetic patients and their association with different clinical and biochemical risk factors. Diabetes Res 1990;13(1):1–11.

20. Beckman JA, Creager MA, Libby P. Diabetes and atherosclerosis: epidemiology, pathophysiology, and management. JAMA 2002;287(19):2570–81.

21. Madonna R, Balistreri CR, Geng YJ, et al. Diabetic microangiopathy: pathogenetic insights and novel therapeutic approaches. Vascul Pharmacol 2017;90:1–7.

22. Di Carli MF, Janisse J, Grunberger G, et al. Role of chronic hyperglycemia in the pathogenesis of coronary microvascular dysfunction in diabetes. J Am Coll Cardiol 2003;41(8):1387–93.

23. Gould KL. Does coronary flow trump coronary anatomy? JACC Cardiovasc Imaging 2009;2(8):1009–23.

24. Gould KL, Johnson NP, Bateman TM, et al. Anatomic versus physiologic assessment of coronary artery disease. Role of coronary flow reserve, fractional flow reserve, and positron emission tomography imaging in revascularization decision-making. J Am Coll Cardiol 2013;62(18):1639–53.

25. Murthy VL, Naya M, Foster CR, et al. Coronary vascular dysfunction and prognosis in patients with chronic kidney disease. JACC Cardiovasc Imaging 2012; 5(10):1025–34.

26. Murthy VL, Naya M, Foster CR, et al. Improved cardiac risk assessment with noninvasive measures of coronary flow reserve. Circulation 2011;124(20): 2215–24.

27. Murthy VL, Naya M, Foster CR, et al. Association between coronary vascular dysfunction and cardiac mortality in patients with and without diabetes mellitus. Circulation 2012;126(15):1858–68.

28. Markowitz M, Messineo F, Coplan NL. Aldosterone receptor antagonists in cardiovascular disease: a review of the recent literature and insight into potential future indications. Clin Cardiol 2012;35(10):605–9.

29. Pitt B, Zannad F, Remme WJ, et al. The effect of spironolactone on morbidity and mortality in patients with severe heart failure. Randomized Aldactone Evaluation Study Investigators. N Engl J Med 1999;341(10):709–17.

30. Oestreicher EM, Martinez-Vasquez D, Stone JR, et al. Aldosterone and not plasminogen activator inhibitor-1 is a critical mediator of early angiotensin II/NG-nitro-L-arginine methyl ester-induced myocardial injury. Circulation 2003;108(20):2517–23.

31. Schafer N, Lohmann C, Winnik S, et al. Endothelial mineralocorticoid receptor activation mediates endothelial dysfunction in diet-induced obesity. Eur Heart J 2013;34(45):3515–24.

32. Pojoga LH, Baudrand R, Adler GK. Mineralocorticoid receptor throughout the vessel: a key to vascular dysfunction in obesity. Eur Heart J 2013;34(45):3475–7.

33. Bender SB, McGraw AP, Jaffe IZ, et al. Mineralocorticoid receptor-mediated vascular insulin resistance: an early contributor to diabetes-related vascular disease? Diabetes 2013;62(2):313–9.

34. Garg R, Rao AD, Baimas-George M, et al. Mineralocorticoid receptor blockade improves coronary microvascular function in individuals with type 2 diabetes. Diabetes 2015;64(1):236–42.

35. Garg R, Adler GK. Aldosterone and the mineralocorticoid receptor: risk factors for cardiometabolic disorders. Curr Hypertens Rep 2015;17(7):52.

36. Dimitropoulos G, Tahrani AA, Stevens MJ. Cardiac autonomic neuropathy in patients with diabetes mellitus. World J Diabetes 2014;5(1):17–39.

37. Kuehl M, Stevens MJ. Cardiovascular autonomic neuropathies as complications of diabetes mellitus. Nat Rev Endocrinol 2012;8(7):405–16.

38. Vinik AI, Freeman R, Erbas T. Diabetic autonomic neuropathy. Semin Neurol 2003;23(4):365–72.

39. Duchen LW, Anjorin A, Watkins PJ, et al. Pathology of autonomic neuropathy in diabetes mellitus. Ann Intern Med 1980;92(2 Pt 2):301–3.

40. Spallone V, Ziegler D, Freeman R, et al. Cardiovascular autonomic neuropathy in diabetes: clinical impact, assessment, diagnosis, and management. Diabetes Metab Res Rev 2011;27(7):639–53.

41. Vinik AI, Ziegler D. Diabetic cardiovascular autonomic neuropathy. Circulation 2007;115(3):387–97.

42. Kempler P, Tesfaye S, Chaturvedi N, et al. Autonomic neuropathy is associated with increased cardiovascular risk factors: the EURODIAB IDDM complications study. Diabet Med 2002;19(11):900–9.

43. An D, Rodrigues B. Role of changes in cardiac metabolism in development of diabetic cardiomyopathy. Am J Physiol Heart Circ Physiol 2006;291(4):H1489–506.

44. Pop-Busui R. What do we know and we do not know about cardiovascular autonomic neuropathy in diabetes. J Cardiovasc Transl Res 2012;5(4):463–78.

45. Hirabara SM, Silveira LR, Alberici LC, et al. Acute effect of fatty acids on metabolism and mitochondrial coupling in skeletal muscle. Biochim Biophys Acta 2006;1757(1):57–66.

46. Adler GK, Bonyhay I, Failing H, et al. Antecedent hypoglycemia impairs autonomic cardiovascular function: implications for rigorous glycemic control. Diabetes 2009;58(2):360–6.

47. Vinik AI, Maser RE, Mitchell BD, et al. Diabetic autonomic neuropathy. Diabetes Care 2003;26(5):1553–79.

48. Pfeifer MA, Weinberg CR, Cook DL, et al. Autonomic neural dysfunction in recently diagnosed diabetic subjects. Diabetes Care 1984;7(5):447–53.

49. Freeman R. Diabetic autonomic neuropathy. Handb Clin Neurol 2014;126:63–79.
50. Low PA, Walsh JC, Huang CY, et al. The sympathetic nervous system in diabetic neuropathy. A clinical and pathological study. Brain 1975;98(3):341–56.
51. Soedamah-Muthu SS, Chaturvedi N, Witte DR, et al. Relationship between risk factors and mortality in type 1 diabetic patients in Europe: the EURODIAB prospective complications study (PCS). Diabetes Care 2008;31(7):1360–6.
52. Pop-Busui R, Evans GW, Gerstein HC, et al. Effects of cardiac autonomic dysfunction on mortality risk in the Action to control cardiovascular risk in diabetes (ACCORD) trial. Diabetes Care 2010;33(7):1578–84.
53. Young LH, Wackers FJ, Chyun DA, et al. Cardiac outcomes after screening for asymptomatic coronary artery disease in patients with type 2 diabetes: the DIAD study: a randomized controlled trial. JAMA 2009;301(15):1547–55.
54. Kleiger RE, Miller JP, Bigger JT Jr, et al. Decreased heart rate variability and its association with increased mortality after acute myocardial infarction. Am J Cardiol 1987;59(4):256–62.
55. Ziegler D, Zentai CP, Perz S, et al. Prediction of mortality using measures of cardiac autonomic dysfunction in the diabetic and nondiabetic population: the MONICA/KORA Augsburg cohort study. Diabetes Care 2008;31(3):556–61.
56. Ambepityia G, Kopelman PG, Ingram D, et al. Exertional myocardial ischemia in diabetes: a quantitative analysis of anginal perceptual threshold and the influence of autonomic function. J Am Coll Cardiol 1990;15(1):72–7.

Intensive Diabetes Treatment and Cardiovascular Outcomes in Type 1 Diabetes Mellitus

Implications of the Diabetes Control and Complications Trial/Epidemiology of Diabetes Interventions and Complications Study 30-Year Follow-up

Savitha Subramanian, MD*, Irl B. Hirsch, MD

KEYWORDS

- Diabetes • Cardiovascular • Mortality • Risk • DCCT • EDIC

KEY POINTS

- The Diabetes Control and Complications Trial (DCCT)/Epidemiology of Diabetes Interventions and Complications (EDIC) study has effectively demonstrated that early intensive insulin therapy in type 1 diabetes mellitus (T1D) decreases cardiovascular mortality and several cardiovascular risk factors.
- Despite this, limited evidence exists for management of cardiovascular risk in T1D.
- Management of increased cardiovascular risk involves excellent glycemic, blood pressure, lipid control, and management of kidney disease.

INTRODUCTION

As the 100th anniversary of the discovery of insulin fast approaches, globally the prevalence of type 1 diabetes mellitus (T1D) is increasing.[1] T1D is a heterogeneous disorder characterized by autoimmune destruction of insulin-secreting pancreatic beta cells, and exogenous insulin replacement is crucial for metabolic optimization,

Disclosure Statement: Dr S. Subramanian is an ad hoc consultant Intarcia, Akcea. Dr I.B. Hirsch is a consultant with Abbott Diabetes Care, Roche, Intarcia, Big Foot, and Adocia.
Division of Metabolism, Endocrinology and Nutrition, University of Washington, 4245 Roosevelt Way Northeast, Box 354691, Seattle, WA 98105, USA
* Corresponding author.
E-mail address: ssubrama@uw.edu

Endocrinol Metab Clin N Am 47 (2018) 65–79
https://doi.org/10.1016/j.ecl.2017.10.012
0889-8529/18/© 2017 Elsevier Inc. All rights reserved.

typically achieved using insulin analogs and mechanical technologies. The actual prevalence of T1D is unknown, although one estimate by the Juvenile Diabetes Research Foundation (JDRF) suggests that there are up to 3 million individuals in the United States with T1D (http://www.jdrf.org/about/what-is-t1d/facts/).

Complications in T1D can be microvascular, neuropathic, or macrovascular. Atherosclerotic cardiovascular disease (CVD) is a long-term macrovascular complication that is a major concern when caring for individuals with T1D. It is now well established that T1D is associated with an accelerated risk of CVD compared with individuals without diabetes, leading to increased morbidity and mortality in both men and women.[2] In the past 2 decades, rates of complications in T1D have declined, with the largest relative declines in acute myocardial infarction (MI) and stroke.[3] Data from Canada and the United Kingdom document a 3% to 5% yearly decline in the rates of acute MI, stroke, cardiovascular mortality, and all-cause mortality in patients with diabetes since the early 1990s.[4,5] Despite a decline in mortality rates and consequent increase in life expectancy,[6] however, individuals with T1D still experience a 10-times higher cardiovascular risk than those without. Women are disproportionately affected,[7–9] and one estimate suggests that cardiovascular risk for young adults with childhood-onset T1D is increased more than 30-fold.[10] Thus the mortality burden remains high, and cardiovascular complications are the major contributor later in life.

The Diabetes Control and Complications Trial (DCCT) was a prospective randomized control trial comparing intensive versus standard glycemic control in individuals with recently diagnosed T1D.[11] This landmark study demonstrated that intensive blood glucose control with hemoglobin A_{1c} (HbA$_{1c}$) close to 7% reduced the incidence of microvascular complications of T1D. The long-term follow up trial Epidemiology of Diabetes Interventions and Complications (EDIC), which followed participants from the DCCT over 11 years for complications of T1D, demonstrated that early intensive therapy aimed at near-normal glycemia compared with conventional therapy decreased the risk of cardiovascular complications by 42%.[12] This article reviews the current evidence on CVD in T1D, primarily focusing on 30-year results from the DCCT/EDIC, and discusses implications for clinical care. CVD, for purposes of this review, is defined as coronary heart disease (CHD), cerebrovascular disease, and peripheral arterial disease.

EPIDEMIOLOGY OF CARDIOVASCULAR DISEASE IN TYPE 1 DIABETES MELLITUS

The prevalence of CVD in T1D in the EURODIAB IDDM Complications Study, which included 3250 patients from 16 European countries, was approximately 9% in men and 10% in women, increasing with age and duration of diabetes.[13] A large Finnish database report, which included 86 individuals with T1D, revealed that CVD mortality in T1D increases by 52% for every 1% increase in HbA$_{1C}$.[14]

When considered separately, CHD is the most common manifestation of CVD. CHD mortality rates are reported as between 6% and 8% and are higher in those over 40 years of age than in those under 40 years of age.[15] The reported average cumulative incidence of CHD ranges is approximately 15% over 15 years of follow-up.[16] Cerebrovascular disease occurs less commonly than CHD in T1D and, although incidence rates are low,[16] associated mortality is high.[17] The EURODIAB study reported an incidence of 0.74% per year, which is higher than the incidence in the general population.[13] A United Kingdom cohort study revealed increased hazard ratios for stroke in men and women with T1D.[18] PAD has been shown to be a predictor of CHD and cardiovascular mortality. Most available data in diabetes focus on lower extremity amputations. In a meta-analysis that included 5 studies of T1D patients, the risk of lower extremity amputation increased by 26% for every 1% increase in HbA$_{1C}$.[19]

Thus, CVD prevalence rates in T1D vary based on duration of diabetes, age, gender, and race or ethnic background. In general, CVD events are more common and occur earlier in patients with T1D than in people without diabetes.[16] Women with T1D experience greater relative risks of CVD than men compared with those without diabetes.[18] African Americans with T1D experience significantly higher mortality rates due to diabetes or related complications.[20,21]

PATHOPHYSIOLOGY OF CARDIOVASCULAR DISEASE IN TYPE 1 DIABETES MELLITUS

The increased risk of CVD in T1D seems primarily due to accelerated atherosclerosis, but how this occurs in humans is unclear — for example, it is unknown if diabetes is associated with increased lipoprotein retention in the artery wall or if hyperglycemia results in endothelial cell activation.[22] Contributors to accelerated atherosclerosis in T1D include glucose, lipoproteins, glyco-oxidation, inflammatory mediators, prothrombotic factors, and excess visceral adiposity (**Fig. 1**). Data on atherosclerotic lesion morphology in humans are sparse. Individuals with T1D show evidence of multivessel disease, increased plaque burden, and severe stenotic and distal lesions compared with patients without diabetes.[23] Small postmortem studies have revealed soft, fibrous, and concentric lesions with increased T-cell and macrophage infiltration in individuals with T1D compared with those without.[24] Presence of larger necrotic cores due to dying macrophages in lesions suggests a larger contribution of immune cells to the pathogenesis of diabetic atherosclerotic lesions compared with individuals without T1D.[25] There

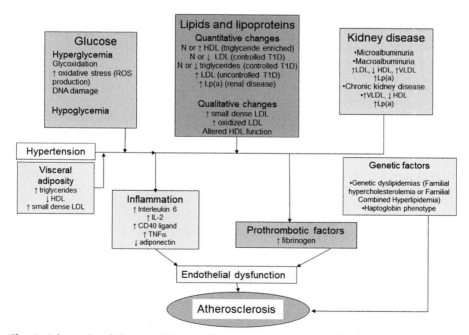

Fig. 1. Schematic of the possible contributors to pathogenesis of atherosclerosis in T1D. Several players contribute to the atherosclerotic process in T1D, eventually leading to endothelial dysfunction and propagation of the atherosclerotic process. HDL, high density lipoprotein; IL2, interleukin 2; LDL, low density lipoprotein; Lp(a), lipoprotein (a); N, normal; ROS, reactive oxygen species; TNF, tumor necrosis factor alpha; VLDL, very low density lipoprotein.

are few human data linking inflammation as a factor in atherosclerotic CVD in T1D that demonstrate increased systemic inflammation based on markers, such as C-reactive protein, interleukin 6, and fibrinogen.[16] Diabetic kidney disease (DKD) manifested as albuminuria and/or impaired glomerular filtration and can contribute to progression of atherosclerosis (see **Fig. 1**). T1D cohort studies suggest that increased mortality and CVD risks are directly related to the presence of DKD.[26] Mechanisms by which DKD worsens CVD risk may be related to accompanying lipid abnormalities and worsening of traditional risk factors as well as novel pathways.[16] The progression of CVD in T1D also seems influenced by certain genetic polymorphisms, the most well studied of these being the haptoglobin (Hp) genotype (see **Fig. 1**). Hp, an acute-phase plasma protein, irreversibly binds free hemoglobin, preventing heme release and ensuing oxidative tissue damage, and facilitates its macrophage-mediated removal from circulation.[27] Of the 3 major human genotypes, Hp 1-1 genotype is the most efficient in preventing heme release and macrophage uptake, and Hp 2-2 the least. In the Pittsburgh Epidemiology of Diabetes Complications study, the proportions of individuals with T1D with the Hp 1-1, 2-1, and 2-2 genotypes were 12%, 40.7%, and 47.3%, respectively, with the Hp 2-2 genotype associated with increased CAD incidence.[28,29]

EVIDENCE FROM THE DIABETES CONTROL AND COMPLICATIONS TRIAL/ EPIDEMIOLOGY OF DIABETES INTERVENTIONS AND COMPLICATIONS

The DCCT examined whether intensive treatment could decrease the frequency and severity of long-term complications of diabetes.[11] A total of 1441 individuals with T1D were recruited from 29 medical centers between 1983 and 1989 and followed for long-term microvascular, neuropathic, and macrovascular complications. The average age for the group at DCCT closeout visit was 35 ± 5.7 years; 45% were female and 97% were white. Subjects were randomly assigned to 1 of 2 groups. The conventional diabetes therapy group (n = 730) received 1 or 2 daily injections of insulin. The intensive therapy group (n = 711) frequently monitored blood glucose levels and received at least 3 daily insulin injections; a few used continuous insulin infusion through an external pump. Dose adjustments based on at least 4 self-monitored glucose measurements per day. Daily glucose goals were 70 mg/dL to 120 mg/dL before meals and 180 mg/dL peak levels after meals. After a mean follow-up of 6.5 years in the United States and Canada, the intensive therapy group achieved an HbA_{1C} of 7.2% compared with 9% in the group who received conventional therapy. At the end of the DCCT, participants in the intensive therapy group were encouraged to continue intensive therapy practices, and the conventional group participants were taught intensive therapy. The patients were then followed in the EDIC observational study, which offered the opportunity to evaluate the impact of earlier intensive therapy on more advanced outcomes; 1394 participants (representing 97% of the entire cohort) joined EDIC (1994–present) and received subsequent diabetes care from their personal physicians and were followed longitudinally for complications.[12] During EDIC, HbA_{1C} differences between the treatment groups dissipated. At year 11 of EDIC follow-up and most recently at 19 years to 20 years of EDIC follow-up, there was only a trivial difference between the original intensive and conventional treatment groups in the mean level of HbA_{1C}.[30]

Evidence pertaining to macrovascular complications from the DCCT/EDIC is summarized.

Mortality

The DCCT/EDIC examined the differences in all-cause and cause-specific mortality between the original treatment groups that received 6.5 years of intensive versus conventional therapy during the clinical trial.[31] After an overall follow-up of approximately 27 years, overall all-cause mortality was low at 0.29% per year, and overall mortality risk in the intensive treatment group was lower than in the conventional group. Mortality between treatment groups did not differ until after the first 15 years of follow-up. The most common cause of death was cardiovascular (24 events or 22.4%) and the intensive treatment group had fewer cardiovascular deaths (9 vs 15).

Major Adverse Cardiac Events

The 17-year follow-up of the effects of intensive therapy on long-term incidence of CVD was reported in 2005.[12] The primary outcome was the time to the first of any cardiovascular event defined as nonfatal MI or stroke, death secondary to CVD, silent MI detected on an annual electrocardiogram (ECG), angina-confirmed exercise tolerance testing or by clinically significant obstruction on coronary angiography, congestive heart failure, or need for revascularization with angioplasty and/or coronary artery bypass. Intensive diabetes therapy reduced the risk of a cardiovascular event by 42% and reduced the risk of severe clinical events, including nonfatal MI, stroke, or death from CVD, by 57%. Older age, longer duration of diabetes, presence of retinopathy, smoking, higher low-density lipoprotein cholesterol (LDL-C) levels, higher body mass index (BMI), higher HbA_{1C}, albuminuria, and assignment to conventional therapy were all associated with development of CVD.

The 30-year risk of CVD, which included follow-up until December 2013, was recently published.[30] At the end of this analysis, 366 adjudicated cardiovascular events had occurred in 184 subjects, 149 among 82 former intensive treatment group subjects, and 217 among 102 former conventional treatment group subjects. The incidence of any cardiovascular event within the original DCCT intensive therapy cohort was 30% lower than that of the conventional therapy group. The incidence of the first occurrence of a nonfatal MI, stroke, or cardiovascular death (major adverse cardiac event [MACE]) was reduced 32% in the intensive compared with conventional therapy. Early intensive treatment protected against fatal rather than nonfatal CHD.

Risk Factors for Cardiovascular Disease in Type 1 Diabetes Mellitus

The analyses of established and putative risk factors for CVD, including glycemic control, after a mean of 27 years of follow-up of the DCCT/EDIC cohort has also been reported.[32] In this analysis, the association of traditional and novel risk factors with MACE and any-CVD (MACE plus confirmed angina, silent MI, revascularization, or congestive heart failure) was evaluated. The risk factors studied included age, gender, BMI, systolic blood pressure, smoking, lipids, HbA_{1C}, and current use of angiotensin-converting enzyme (ACE) inhibitor as well as diabetes-related risk factors, including duration of diabetes, hypoglycemia, and albuminuria. Age and mean HbA_{1C} were strongly associated with any-CVD and with MACE. For each percentage point increase in mean HbA_{1C}, the risk for any-CVD and for MACE increased by 31% and 42%, respectively. After adjustment for age and HbA_{1C}, CVD and MACE were also associated with other conventional factors, such as higher systolic blood pressure, triglycerides, mean LDL-C, and diabetes duration. Current use of an ACE inhibitor was protective. There were no significant differences between men and women. At year 11, 14% in the intensive therapy group and 11% in conventional treatment group were current smokers. Obesity or BMI, an established CVD risk factor in type 2 diabetes mellitus (T2D), did not emerge in this study. Although recent studies have supported an important role, albuminuria also did not emerge as a risk factor in this study. The investigators extrapolated that the strong relationship between glycemia and CVD in this study could be explained by better assessment of glycemia, lack of inclusion of individuals with CVD risk, younger age, and infrequent smoking history. These factors may have allowed the role of glycemia to be manifest compared with older studies, which did not show such a relationship. Additionally, the absence of albuminuria as a risk factor could be related to lack of power or due to common use of ACE inhibitors in the cohort.

Blood Pressure

Long-term changes in CVD risk factors observed over a 30-year period of follow-up in the DCCT/EDIC study were recently reported.[30] Systolic blood pressure increased steadily over the 30-year period, whereas the diastolic blood pressure rose during the first 17 years and began to fall thereafter. There was an increasing prevalence of antihypertensive medication use during EDIC study (6% at year 10%–60% by year 30).

Hypertension, an established and modifiable risk factor for CVD and mortality, is particularly common among people with T2D. The effect of intensive therapy on development of hypertension has been examined in the DCCT/EDIC cohort.[33] During a median of 15.8 years of follow-up, 630 participants met the definition of incident hypertension (systolic blood pressure >140 mm Hg, diastolic blood pressure >90 mm Hg). At hypertension diagnosis, 395 participants (62.7% of incident cases) had elevated blood pressure and 277 (44.0%) reported use of antihypertensive medications to treat high blood pressure. During the DCCT itself, intensive therapy did not lead to a statistically significant reduction in the risk of incident hypertension.[11] The intensive therapy group, however, had a 24% reduction in the risk of incident hypertension during the EDIC follow-up. During the entire combined period of DCCT/EDIC, intensive therapy reduced the overall long-term incidence of hypertension by 20%. This incidence rate of hypertension is higher than that for an age-matched cohort in the general population.[34] Higher HbA_{1C} level at baseline or throughout follow-up was a risk factor for development of hypertension, and the antihypertensive effect of intensive insulin therapy was explained by improved glycemic control. Other risk factors in this group included older age, family history of hypertension, and higher BMI, similar to those described in other studies.[35,36]

Overall, these data suggest that hyperglycemia contributes to the pathogenesis of hypertension in T1D and emphasizes the importance of long-term prevention of hypertension as an additional benefit of intensive insulin therapy.

Lipids

Lipid changes over 30 years have been reported.[30] During the DCCT, participants in the intensive treatment group had lower LDL-C and triglyceride levels compared with the conventional therapy group. The pattern reversed during the EDIC follow-up, with both groups experiencing decreasing LDL-C levels from year 12 onward as the use of lipid-lowering medication increased (2% at year 10%–62% by year 30). Overall, serum triglyceride levels were remarkably stable throughout the DCCT/EDIC study. There were no treatment group differences in HDL cholesterol levels: the levels were stable throughout the DCCT and actually increased by 24% by year 30 in the EDIC study.

Weight or Body Mass Index

Intensive therapy in T1D results in excess weight gain[37] and is amplified in women compared with men. This group difference in weight among women persisted during the EDIC study, whereas there was a negligible group difference among men in the EDIC follow-up.

Individuals with T1D who had a family history of T2D gain more weight with intensive therapy than those with no family history. This increased weight gain is centrally distributed, accompanied by a greater insulin requirement, and associated with dyslipidemia commonly observed in T2D.[38] The relationships between this excess weight gain, components of metabolic syndrome, and other nontraditional CVD risk factors in T1D have been examined.[39] Individuals were classified as excess gainers if the BMI increased by at least 4.39 kg/m^2 in both the intensive and conventional treated groups. In the intensive treatment group, excess gainers showed a greater increase in HbA$_{1C}$ in the EDIC follow-up. This group also had higher LDL-C levels, systolic blood pressure, and diastolic blood pressure and greater use of lipid-lowering medications. More individuals in this group also met the metabolic syndrome criteria and developed incremental increase in carotid intima–media thickness (CIMT) but association with coronary artery calcium (CAC) showed a trend toward increase did not reach statistical significance.

Thus, excessive weight gain with intensive therapy was sustained during 6 years of EDIC follow-up and continued to be associated with central adiposity, higher insulin requirements, a progressive rise in blood pressure, and dyslipidemia.

EVIDENCE FOR SURROGATE MARKERS OF CARDIOVASCULAR DISEASE FROM THE DIABETES CONTROL AND COMPLICATIONS TRIAL/EPIDEMIOLOGY OF DIABETES INTERVENTIONS AND COMPLICATIONS STUDY
Carotid Intima–Media Thickness

CIMT is considered a surrogate marker for subclinical atherosclerosis and a predictor of cardiovascular events in the general population.[40] As part of the EDIC observational study, 1229 patients underwent ultrasonography of the internal and common carotid arteries in 1994 to 1996 and again in 1998 to 2000.[41] At year 1 of the EDIC study, the CIMT was similar to that in an age-matched and gender-matched nondiabetic population. After 6 years, the CIMT was significantly greater in the T1D cohort than in the controls, for each gender, even after adjustment for smoking status. The CIMT progression was significantly less in the intensive therapy group during the DCCT than in the group that had received conventional therapy after adjustment for other risk factors. CIMT progression was associated with age, baseline systolic blood pressure, smoking, the LDL/HDL ratio, urinary albumin excretion rate, and mean HbA$_{1C}$ value during the mean duration of the DCCT.

Thus, intensive therapy during the DCCT resulted in decreased progression of CIMT 6 years after the end of the trial, which suggests that structural and vascular changes occur early on in T1D[42] and that these changes can have long-lasting effects.[43]

Coronary Artery Calcium Scores

CAC is measured by CT and is also considered a quantitative marker of atherosclerotic burden. In general, the absence of CAC (a score of zero) in asymptomatic individuals identifies individuals at low risk for CVD and events in individuals without diabetes.[44,45] In T1D, the risk of having any CAC is increased by 50% compared with individuals without diabetes.[43] Prevalence of CAC and CAC scores increase with age and are higher in men than in women as well as in individuals with higher BMI in T1D. In the DCCT/EDIC cohort, CAC was measured 1 time in 1205 subjects at approximately 7 years to 9 years after the end of the DCCT.[46] Overall, 31% had CAC scores greater than zero at baseline. The prevalence of CAC and CAC scores were significantly lower in the former intensive treatment compared with the former conventional treatment group. The prevalence of a clinically significant CAC score of greater than 200 Agatston units was 7.0% in the former intensive treatment group and 9.9% in the former conventional treatment group. No baseline CAC assessment was performed, however, and in general the majority of patients had no detectable levels of calcification, a likely reflection of the younger age of the study cohort. Additionally, macroalbuminuria was associated with a greater degree of CAC.[47] Intensive glycemic control in also reduced the incidence of peripheral arterial calcification but did not decrease rates of peripheral arterial occlusion.[48]

ECG Changes

In a study of 1306 individuals from the DCCT/EDIC study, the presence of major ECG abnormalities at the time of enrollment and progression of these abnormalities over 16 years was assessed.[49] At baseline, more men with T1D had an abnormality on ECG. Individuals with any ECG abnormality also had lower lipids and BMI at baseline. During 16 years of follow-up, 77.3% participants developed new ECG abnormalities. Patients age 40 years and older or with higher baseline HbA_{1C} were more likely to develop new major ECG abnormalities. The most common new ECG abnormalities that developed during follow-up were incomplete bundle branch block, major ST/T abnormalities, and ECG evidence of definite or possible MI. The study suggests that the occurrence of new ECG abnormalities is common in the course of T1D, some of the associated risk factors being older age, increased systolic blood pressure, smoking, and higher HbA_{1C}.

Using the same cohort, the participants were also followed for development of CVD events.[50] During a median follow-up of 19 years, 155 participants (11.9%) developed CVD events. Presence of a major ECG abnormality (major ST/T wave abnormalities or ECG evidence of a definite or possible MI) was associated with a 2-fold increase in risk of CVD event. The investigators suggest a potential role for ECG screening in patients with T1D to identify individuals at risk for CVD.

CLINICAL IMPLICATIONS FROM THE DIABETES CONTROL AND COMPLICATIONS TRIAL/EPIDEMIOLOGY OF DIABETES INTERVENTIONS AND COMPLICATION: STRATEGIES TO REDUCE CARDIOVASCULAR RISK IN TYPE 1 DIABETES MELLITUS

The fact that T1D is associated with increased atherosclerotic CVD risk, one that is evident at an early age, is now well established. The DCCT/EDIC evidence suggests that early intensive glycemic control results in decreased mortality, fewer cardiovascular events, lesser incidence of hypertension, and decreased CIMT and CAC scores. Limitations of the DCCT/EDIC include the younger age group of patients, and 95% of EDIC participants are white, which limits generalizability of results to other races/ethnicities. Nevertheless, the ethnic makeup of the DCCT/EDIC cohort is not dissimilar from the general white T1D population.

Despite the evidence, in general, management of cardiovascular risk in T1D is based on limited clinical trial evidence, often extrapolated from studies in T2D or the general population. This approach is suboptimal because it is clear that the pathogenesis of atherosclerosis in T1D is different from T2D and the general population.[51,52] The age at which CVD becomes evident differs between T1D and T2D, where it occurs typically in older patients. Importantly, differences in the duration and natural history of CVD in patients with T1D and T2D raise the need to initiate preventative cardiovascular therapies earlier in the former.

Several major associations, including the American Diabetes Association and the American College of Cardiology/American Heart Association, have made recommendations on managing CVD risk in individuals with T1D.[53,54] These guidelines do not recommend routine screening for CVD in asymptomatic patients with diabetes due to lack of evidence for benefit. Several risk calculators are available for calculating CVD risk but diabetes itself confers increased risk; none of the available risk engines is specific for T1D and they are largely based on data from studies of the general population. Recently, a prediction model for CVD events in T1D to help decision making for primary prevention that has been developed shows promise but needs further validation.[55] Similarly, there are few controlled studies of the effect of aspirin, and lipid and blood pressure–lowering therapy in T1D patients.

In the absence of clear-cut data for cardiovascular risk management, what does a clinician do? Some expert opinion, extrapolated from existing evidence and clinical experience (**Box 1, Table 1**), is offered.

Achieve Excellent Glycemic Control

The overarching implication of the DCCT/EDIC study is that achieving excellent glycemic control, especially in the first decade after diabetes diagnosis, results in early changes that are protective from a cardiovascular standpoint. Thus, achieving an HbA_{1c} of 7% or lower should be attempted whenever possible with room for individualization based on comorbidities.

Achieve Target Blood Pressure and Management of Kidney Disease

In T1D, hypertension is often the result of underlying DKD. Patients with T1D should be treated to a systolic blood pressure less than 140 mm Hg and diastolic blood pressure less than 90 mm Hg, with lower blood pressure targets appropriate in individuals with cardiovascular risk.[54] Treatment should be promptly initiated and titrated to achieve the appropriate goal blood pressure. Lifestyle intervention strategies should be encouraged. With any degree of albuminuria in patients with T1D with or without hypertension, ACE inhibitors or angiotensin receptor blockers decrease loss of glomerular filtration rate and delay progression of nephropathy and hence are the

---

Box 1
Risk factor assessment

Diabetes related
  Glycemic control
  Longer duration of T1D

Hypertension

Lipids
  Family history of premature atherosclerotic CVD
  Genetic dyslipidemia
    Familial hypercholesterolemia
    Familial combined hyperlipidemia
    Elevated lipoprotein(a)

Kidney disease
  Macroalbuminuria
  Chronic kidney disease

Weight
  Central adiposity

Solid organ transplantation

Smoking

Table 1 Recommended cardiovascular risk factor targets in adults with type 1 diabetes mellitus	
Target	**Goal**
Glucose	HbA_{1c} <7% for many nonpregnant adults; goals can be adjusted based on age (less stringent HbA_{1c} with greater age), duration of diabetes (less stringent HbA_{1c} with greater duration), comorbidities (less stringent HbA_{1c})
Blood pressure	<140/90 mm Hg; 130/80 mm Hg in individuals with high ASCVD risk or known renal disease
Lipids	Age <40 y, add high-intensity statin if known ASCVD Age 40–75 y and no additional ASCVD risk factors, consider moderate-intensity statin Age 40–75 y, with additional ASCVD risk factors, add high-intensity statin Age >75 y and no additional ASCVD risk factors, consider moderate-intensity statin Age >75 y, with additional ASCVD risk factors, add moderate-intensity statin
Aspirin	75–162 mg, if known ASCVD; if aspirin allergy, use clopidogrel, 75 mg daily Age >50 y, 75–162 mg in the presence of 1 additional risk factor Age <50 y without ASCVD risk — do not use

Abbreviation: ASCVD, atherosclerotic cardiovascular disease.

recommended first-line agents. Multiple-drug therapy may be necessary. Individuals with DKD should be closely evaluated for CVD.

General Lifestyle Measures

Nutrition therapy is a key aspect in the management of T1D and is typically individualized based on schedules and food preferences and involves carbohydrate estimation. From a CVD risk aspect, however, reduction of excess body weight by calorie restriction; decreasing saturated fat, trans fat, and cholesterol intake; and increase of dietary ω-3 fatty acids and viscous fiber should be encouraged. Exercise (aerobic) should be a standard recommendation as it is for individuals without diabetes. Smoking cessation has broad benefits in general and should be strongly advised. Decreased sodium intake should be recommended in the setting of hypertension.

Lipid Management

Little clinical trial evidence for lipid targets in T1D exists. Significant dyslipidemia, when it occurs in T1D, usually occurs in the setting of poor glycemic control, nephropathy, central adiposity, or genetic factors.

In the Heart Protection Study (lower age limit 40 years), which included 615 patients with T1D, statin therapy resulted in a proportionately similar, although not statistically significant, reduction in cardiovascular risk as in patients with T2D.[56] The American Diabetes Association recommends that "even though the data are not definitive, similar statin treatment approaches should be considered for patients with T1D or T2D, particularly in the presence of other cardiovascular risk factors."[54] Based on the 2013 American College of Cardiology/American Heart Association guidelines, high-intensity statin therapy is recommended for all patients with diabetes and atherosclerotic CVD.[53] Treatment with a moderate dose of statin should be considered in patients without clinical atherosclerotic CVD but has additional cardiovascular risk factors (see **Table 1**). Like statins, there is no evidence on use of nonstatin therapies, such as ezetimibe or PCSK9 inhibitors, in T1D, but these agents can be considered in certain situations, such as intolerance to statins, renal disease with proteinuria, or familial hypercholesterolemia.

Management considerations

Age under 40 years There is no clinical trial evidence for cardiovascular risk reduction in the under–40 years age group. In the absence of risk factors, such as hypertension, smoking, dyslipidemia, or a strong family history of premature or early atherosclerotic CVD, it may be reasonable to defer therapy or offer low-dose statin therapy as appropriate, especially in young women of childbearing age. In certain clinical settings, however, such as genetic dyslipidemias (see **Table 1**), strong family history of premature atherosclerotic CVD, presence of heavy proteinuria, and solid organ transplantation, statin therapy is indicated for cardiovascular risk reduction.

Age over 40 years Besides the Heart Protection Study discussed previously, there is limited evidence for atherosclerotic CVD risk reduction in T1D. Statin therapy is recommended at moderate or high intensity based on other risk factors (see **Box 1**, **Table 1**). Aspirin, ACE inhibitors, angiotensin receptor blockers, and β-blockers are generally not recommended for primary prevention without other risk factors.

Advanced Cardiovascular Risk Assessment

There are no CVD risk-prediction algorithms for patients with T1D in widespread use. Cardiovascular stress testing is not routinely recommended, unless there is an indication for testing, such as symptoms suggestive of CHD or an abnormal resting ECG. Advanced testing may be useful in individuals with T1D, specifically CAC, although there are no data available that have assessed its clinical utility of for risk prediction in this setting. Applying the current guidelines for the use of CAC assessment in T1DM, as recommended for the general population, is an acceptable approach.[16,57] In T1D, the authors use CAC scores in certain settings, for example in men over age 40 with no evidence of dyslipidemia or other cardiovascular risk factors to assess need for statin therapy.

Other CVD testing modalities are less useful in assessing CVD in individual patients. As discussed previously, increased duration of T1D is associated with increased CIMT; however, the association between increased CIMT and subsequent CHD risk in this patient population is unknown, and its routine clinical use is not recommended.

SUMMARY

Despite an increase in life expectancy in individuals with T1D, CVD risk burden continues to be high and associated with increased mortality. Contributors to this enhanced risk include traditional modifiable risk factors, such as blood pressure, lipids, cigarette smoking, and adiposity as well as disease-specific elements, such as renal disease and genetic factors. Evidence from the DCCT/EDIC shows an undoubted benefit for early intensive glycemic control in reducing CV risk whereas relative contributions of other factors, such as inflammation, oxidative stress, and lipids, is less clear. Further evidence is required for use of surrogate markers, such as CIMT and CAC scores, in individuals with T1D. Based on current evidence, management strategies at this time primarily should involve ensuring rigorous glycemic, blood pressure, and lipid control.

REFERENCES

1. Atkinson MA, Eisenbarth GS, Michels AW. Type 1 diabetes. Lancet 2014; 383(9911):69–82.
2. Harjutsalo V, Forsblom C, Groop PH. Time trends in mortality in patients with type 1 diabetes: nationwide population based cohort study. BMJ 2011;343:d5364.
3. Gregg EW, Li Y, Wang J, et al. Changes in diabetes-related complications in the United States, 1990-2010. N Engl J Med 2014;370(16):1514–23.
4. Booth GL, Kapral MK, Fung K, et al. Recent trends in cardiovascular complications among men and women with and without diabetes. Diabetes Care 2006; 29(1):32–7.
5. Lind M, Garcia-Rodriguez LA, Booth GL, et al. Mortality trends in patients with and without diabetes in Ontario, Canada and the UK from 1996 to 2009: a population-based study. Diabetologia 2013;56(12):2601–8.
6. Miller RG, Secrest AM, Sharma RK, et al. Improvements in the life expectancy of type 1 diabetes: the Pittsburgh epidemiology of diabetes complications study cohort. Diabetes 2012;61(11):2987–92.
7. Lee SI, Patel M, Jones CM, et al. Cardiovascular disease and type 1 diabetes: prevalence, prediction and management in an ageing population. Ther Adv Chronic Dis 2015;6(6):347–74.
8. Schnell O, Cappuccio F, Genovese S, et al. Type 1 diabetes and cardiovascular disease. Cardiovasc Diabetol 2013;12:156.
9. Huxley RR, Peters SA, Mishra GD, et al. Risk of all-cause mortality and vascular events in women versus men with type 1 diabetes: a systematic review and meta-analysis. Lancet Diabetes Endocrinol 2015;3(3):198–206.
10. Miller RG, Mahajan HD, Costacou T, et al. A contemporary estimate of total mortality and cardiovascular disease risk in young adults with type 1 diabetes: the Pittsburgh epidemiology of diabetes complications study. Diabetes Care 2016; 39(12):2296–303.
11. Diabetes Control and Complications Trial Research Group, Nathan DM, Genuth S, Lachin J, et al. The effect of intensive treatment of diabetes on the development and progression of long-term complications in insulin-dependent diabetes mellitus. N Engl J Med 1993;329(14):977–86.
12. Nathan DM, Cleary PA, Backlund JY, et al. Intensive diabetes treatment and cardiovascular disease in patients with type 1 diabetes. N Engl J Med 2005;353(25): 2643–53.
13. Koivisto VA, Stevens LK, Mattock M, et al. Cardiovascular disease and its risk factors in IDDM in Europe. EURODIAB IDDM Complications Study Group. Diabetes Care 1996;19(7):689–97.
14. Juutilainen A, Lehto S, Ronnemaa T, et al. Similarity of the impact of type 1 and type 2 diabetes on cardiovascular mortality in middle-aged subjects. Diabetes Care 2008;31(4):714–9.
15. Laing SP, Swerdlow AJ, Slater SD, et al. Mortality from heart disease in a cohort of 23,000 patients with insulin-treated diabetes. Diabetologia 2003;46(6): 760–5.
16. de Ferranti SD, de Boer IH, Fonseca V, et al. Type 1 diabetes mellitus and cardiovascular disease: a scientific statement from the American Heart Association and American Diabetes Association. Diabetes Care 2014;37(10):2843–63.
17. Laing SP, Swerdlow AJ, Carpenter LM, et al. Mortality from cerebrovascular disease in a cohort of 23 000 patients with insulin-treated diabetes. Stroke 2003; 34(2):418–21.

18. Soedamah-Muthu SS, Fuller JH, Mulnier HE, et al. High risk of cardiovascular disease in patients with type 1 diabetes in the U.K.: a cohort study using the general practice research database. Diabetes Care 2006;29(4):798–804.
19. Adler AI, Erqou S, Lima TA, et al. Association between glycated haemoglobin and the risk of lower extremity amputation in patients with diabetes mellitus-review and meta-analysis. Diabetologia 2010;53(5):840–9.
20. Roy M, Rendas-Baum R, Skurnick J. Mortality in African-Americans with type 1 diabetes: the New Jersey 725. Diabet Med 2006;23(6):698–706.
21. Secrest AM, Becker DJ, Kelsey SF, et al. All-cause mortality trends in a large population-based cohort with long-standing childhood-onset type 1 diabetes: the Allegheny County type 1 diabetes registry. Diabetes Care 2010;33(12): 2573–9.
22. Bornfeldt KE. Uncomplicating the macrovascular complications of diabetes: the 2014 Edwin Bierman award lecture. Diabetes 2015;64(8):2689–97.
23. Valsania P, Zarich SW, Kowalchuk GJ, et al. Severity of coronary artery disease in young patients with insulin-dependent diabetes mellitus. Am Heart J 1991;122(3 Pt 1):695–700.
24. Burke AP, Kolodgie FD, Zieske A, et al. Morphologic findings of coronary atherosclerotic plaques in diabetics: a postmortem study. Arterioscler Thromb Vasc Biol 2004;24(7):1266–71.
25. Virmani R, Burke AP, Kolodgie F. Morphological characteristics of coronary atherosclerosis in diabetes mellitus. Can J Cardiol 2006;22(Suppl B):81B–4B.
26. Chronic Kidney Disease Prognosis Consortium, Matsushita K, van der Velde M, Astor BC, et al. Association of estimated glomerular filtration rate and albuminuria with all-cause and cardiovascular mortality in general population cohorts: a collaborative meta-analysis. Lancet 2010;375(9731):2073–81.
27. Bowman BH, Kurosky A. Haptoglobin: the evolutionary product of duplication, unequal crossing over, and point mutation. Adv Hum Genet 1982;12:189–261, 453–4.
28. Costacou T, Ferrell RE, Orchard TJ. Haptoglobin genotype: a determinant of cardiovascular complication risk in type 1 diabetes. Diabetes 2008;57(6):1702–6.
29. Costacou T, Orchard TJ. The Haptoglobin genotype predicts cardio-renal mortality in type 1 diabetes. J Diabetes Complications 2016;30(2):221–6.
30. Writing Group for the DCCT/EDIC Research Group. Coprogression of cardiovascular risk factors in type 1 diabetes during 30 years of follow-up in the DCCT/EDIC study. Diabetes Care 2016;39(9):1621–30.
31. Writing Group for the DCCT/EDIC Research Group, Orchard TJ, Nathan DM, Zinman B, et al. Association between 7 years of intensive treatment of type 1 diabetes and long-term mortality. JAMA 2015;313(1):45–53.
32. Diabetes Control and Complications Trial/Epidemiology of Diabetes Interventions and Complications (DCCT/EDIC) Research Group. Risk factors for cardiovascular disease in type 1 diabetes. Diabetes 2016;65(5):1370–9.
33. de Boer IH, Kestenbaum B, Rue TC, et al. Insulin therapy, hyperglycemia, and hypertension in type 1 diabetes mellitus. Arch Intern Med 2008;168(17):1867–73.
34. Dyer AR, Liu K, Walsh M, et al. Ten-year incidence of elevated blood pressure and its predictors: the CARDIA study. Coronary Artery Risk Development in (Young) Adults. J Hum Hypertens 1999;13(1):13–21.
35. Sonne-Holm S, Sorensen TI, Jensen G, et al. Independent effects of weight change and attained body weight on prevalence of arterial hypertension in obese and non-obese men. BMJ 1989;299(6702):767–70.

36. Lauer RM, Burns TL, Clarke WR, et al. Childhood predictors of future blood pressure. Hypertension 1991;18(3 Suppl):I74–81.
37. Purnell JQ, Hokanson JE, Marcovina SM, et al. Effect of excessive weight gain with intensive therapy of type 1 diabetes on lipid levels and blood pressure: results from the DCCT. Diabetes control and complications trial. JAMA 1998; 280(2):140–6.
38. Purnell JQ, Dev RK, Steffes MW, et al. Relationship of family history of type 2 diabetes, hypoglycemia, and autoantibodies to weight gain and lipids with intensive and conventional therapy in the diabetes control and complications trial. Diabetes 2003;52(10):2623–9.
39. Purnell JQ, Zinman B, Brunzell JD, DCCT/EDIC Research Group. The effect of excess weight gain with intensive diabetes mellitus treatment on cardiovascular disease risk factors and atherosclerosis in type 1 diabetes mellitus: results from the Diabetes Control and Complications Trial/Epidemiology of Diabetes Interventions and Complications Study (DCCT/EDIC) study. Circulation 2013; 127(2):180–7.
40. Lorenz MW, Markus HS, Bots ML, et al. Prediction of clinical cardiovascular events with carotid intima-media thickness: a systematic review and meta-analysis. Circulation 2007;115(4):459–67.
41. Nathan DM, Lachin J, Cleary P, et al. Intensive diabetes therapy and carotid intima-media thickness in type 1 diabetes mellitus. N Engl J Med 2003;348(23): 2294–303.
42. Chahal H, Backlund JY, Cleary PA, et al. Relation between carotid intima-media thickness and left ventricular mass in type 1 diabetes mellitus (from the Epidemiology of Diabetes Interventions and Complications [EDIC] Study). Am J Cardiol 2012;110(10):1534–40.
43. Orchard TJ, Costacou T, Kretowski A, et al. Type 1 diabetes and coronary artery disease. Diabetes Care 2006;29(11):2528–38.
44. Burge MR, Eaton RP, Schade DS. The role of a coronary artery calcium scan in type 1 diabetes. Diabetes Technol Ther 2016;18(9):594–603.
45. Sarwar A, Shaw LJ, Shapiro MD, et al. Diagnostic and prognostic value of absence of coronary artery calcification. JACC Cardiovasc Imaging 2009;2(6): 675–88.
46. Cleary PA, Orchard TJ, Genuth S, et al. The effect of intensive glycemic treatment on coronary artery calcification in type 1 diabetic participants of the Diabetes Control and Complications Trial/Epidemiology of Diabetes Interventions and Complications (DCCT/EDIC) study. Diabetes 2006;55(12):3556–65.
47. de Boer IH, Gao X, Cleary PA, et al. Albuminuria changes and cardiovascular and renal outcomes in type 1 diabetes: the DCCT/EDIC study. Clin J Am Soc Nephrol 2016;11(11):1969–77.
48. Carter RE, Lackland DT, Cleary PA, et al. Intensive treatment of diabetes is associated with a reduced rate of peripheral arterial calcification in the diabetes control and complications trial. Diabetes Care 2007;30(10):2646–8.
49. Soliman EZ, Backlund JY, Bebu I, et al. Progression of electrocardiographic abnormalities in type 1 diabetes during 16 years of follow-up: the epidemiology of diabetes interventions and complications (EDIC) study. J Am Heart Assoc 2016;5(3):e002882.
50. Soliman EZ, Backlund JC, Bebu I, et al. Electrocardiographic abnormalities and cardiovascular disease risk in type 1 diabetes: the epidemiology of diabetes interventions and complications (EDIC) study. Diabetes Care 2017; 40(6):793–9.

51. Moreno PR, Murcia AM, Palacios IF, et al. Coronary composition and macrophage infiltration in atherectomy specimens from patients with diabetes mellitus. Circulation 2000;102(18):2180–4.
52. Pajunen P, Taskinen MR, Nieminen MS, et al. Angiographic severity and extent of coronary artery disease in patients with type 1 diabetes mellitus. Am J Cardiol 2000;86(10):1080–5.
53. Stone NJ, Robinson JG, Lichtenstein AH, et al. 2013 ACC/AHA guideline on the treatment of blood cholesterol to reduce atherosclerotic cardiovascular risk in adults: a report of the American College of Cardiology/American Heart Association Task Force on Practice Guidelines. J Am Coll Cardiol 2014;63(25 Pt B): 2889–934.
54. American Diabetes Association. 8. Cardiovascular disease and risk management. Diabetes Care 2016;39(Suppl 1):S60–71.
55. Vistisen D, Andersen GS, Hansen CS, et al. Prediction of first cardiovascular disease event in type 1 diabetes mellitus: the steno type 1 risk engine. Circulation 2016;133(11):1058–66.
56. Collins R, Armitage J, Parish S, et al, Heart Protection Study Collaborative Group. MRC/BHF Heart Protection Study of cholesterol-lowering with simvastatin in 5963 people with diabetes: a randomised placebo-controlled trial. Lancet 2003; 361(9374):2005–16.
57. Greenland P, Alpert JS, Beller GA, et al. 2010 ACCF/AHA guideline for assessment of cardiovascular risk in asymptomatic adults: a report of the American College of Cardiology Foundation/American Heart Association Task Force on Practice Guidelines. Circulation 2010;122(25):e584–636.

Intensive Blood Glucose Control and Vascular Outcomes in Patients with Type 2 Diabetes Mellitus

 CrossMark

Marian Sue Kirkman, MD[a], Hussain Mahmud, MD[b],
Mary T. Korytkowski, MD[c],*

KEYWORDS

- Type 2 diabetes mellitus • Cardiovascular disease • Glycemic control
- Hypoglycemia

KEY POINTS

- Cardiovascular disease (CVD) is the primary cause of excess morbidity and mortality observed in people with type 2 diabetes mellitus.
- Prior studies have demonstrated a direct association between hyperglycemia and risk for CVD events.
- Intensive glucose-lowering strategies that target hemoglobin A_{1c} (HbA_{1c}) levels less than 7% (53 mmol/mol) may reduce CVD risk in younger patients with recent-onset type 2 diabetes mellitus but not in high-risk older individuals with advanced disease.
- Hypoglycemia that occurs more frequently with intensive glycemic control strategies may be associated with a higher frequency of adverse outcomes in those with higher HbA_{1c}.
- Medications used to lower HbA_{1c} influence CVD risk.

INTRODUCTION

People with type 2 diabetes mellitus have excess morbidity and mortality from cardiovascular disease (CVD) compared with age-matched and gender-matched populations without diabetes.[1–4] CVD accounts for much of the observed increase in morbidity, mortality, and economic costs associated with this disorder.[5] A U-shaped

Disclosure Information: Dr M.S. Kirkman receives research support from Novo Nordisk, Theracos, and Bayer. Dr M.T. Korytkowski has served as a consultant to Novo Nordisk. Dr H. Mahmud has nothing to disclose.
[a] Division of Endocrinology, University of North Carolina at Chapel Hill, 8025 Burnett Womack Building, Campus Box #7172 UNC-CH, Chapel Hill, NC 27599-7170, USA; [b] Division of Endocrinology, University of Pittsburgh Medical Center, 3601 Fifth Avenue, Suite 562, Pittsburgh, PA 15213, USA; [c] Division of Endocrinology, Department of Medicine, University of Pittsburgh, Falk Medical Building, Room 560, 3601 Fifth Avenue, Pittsburgh, PA 15213, USA
* Corresponding author.
E-mail address: mtk7@pitt.edu

Endocrinol Metab Clin N Am 47 (2018) 81–96
https://doi.org/10.1016/j.ecl.2017.10.002
endo.theclinics.com

curve has been described between measures of fasting and postprandial glucose levels and hemoglobin A_{1c} (HbA_{1c}) with mortality in individuals with diabetes, demonstrating increased CVD risk at the lower and higher ends of these glycemic measures.[6-8] These associations persist after controlling for other known CVD risk factors, including blood pressure (BP), body weight, and lipid measures.[8] These observed relationships between measures of glycemia and CVD led to several large interventional studies seeking to investigate the hypothesis that CVD risk could be reduced by using strategies to reduce mean glucose levels in patient populations with type 2 diabetes mellitus.

The first studies that explored this glycemic control hypothesis in people with type 2 diabetes mellitus were the University Group Diabetes Program (UGDP) and the United Kingdom Prospective Diabetes Study (UKPDS).[9-11] Controversial findings in regard to CVD outcomes from each of these studies prompted several small-scale and large-scale follow-up studies targeting near-euglycemia as part of an intensive diabetes management program in populations with type 2 diabetes mellitus at high risk for CVD.[12-17] The Action to Control Diabetes Risk in Diabetes (ACCORD), Action in Diabetes and Vascular Disease: Preterax and Diamicron Modified Release Controlled Evaluation (ADVANCE), and the Veterans Affairs Diabetes Trial (VADT) in turn generated further controversy and questions regarding the cardiovascular (CV) benefit of strategies targeting tight, or near-normal, levels of glycemic control in high-risk individuals with type 2 diabetes mellitus.[14,18] These studies together challenged the glycemic control hypothesis as a CVD risk reduction strategy and prompted modification of treatment guidelines for hyperglycemia management that place an increased emphasis on individualized glycemic goals.[18-20]

In this article, the findings from ACCORD, ADVANCE, and VADT, together with contributing data from subgroup analyses and other published studies, are reviewed. Factors that may have contributed to absence of significant CVD benefit with tight glycemic control, such as hypoglycemia and CV safety of specific agents used to achieve glycemic control, are discussed. Finally, a suggested approach for glycemic targets according to a patient's overall health status and expected benefit are addressed.

THE GLYCEMIC CONTROL HYPOTHESIS AND VASCULAR OUTCOMES

The UGDP was the first study to investigate the effect of the long-term use of available diabetes treatments on preventing or delaying vascular outcomes in type 2 diabetes mellitus. Participants were randomly assigned to receive fixed doses of the short-acting sulfonylurea (SU) tolbutamide, insulin, or placebo.[11,12] An increase in CVD events observed in participants receiving tolbutamide created significant controversy, in part due to the fact that SUs were the only noninsulin therapies available for therapeutic use in the United States until metformin was first approved for clinical use in 1994.[21] Questions were raised regarding flaws in the design and conduct of the UGDP, but this study nevertheless resulted in a black box warning from the Food and Drug Administration (FDA) that persists today stating that use of SU could increase risk for CVD events.[22,23] This prompted recommendations from the American Diabetes Association and other groups for a well-controlled multicenter study, resulting in the design and implementation of the UKPDS.[24]

The UKPDS randomized 4209 participants below age 65 years with newly diagnosed type 2 diabetes mellitus to intensive therapy with one of 2 SU agents (glibenclamide or chlorpropamide), insulin, or metformin (n = 342 obese patients).[24] All UKPDS participants received a 3-month dietary intervention primary to randomization. The glycemic goal in the intensively treated group was to achieve and maintain a fasting glucose 108 mg/dL (less than 6 mmol/L), whereas the conventional therapy group received education regarding diet approaches to avoid hyperglycemic symptoms and maintain fasting glucose less than 270 mg/dL (15 mmol/L). One of the several pre-specified goals of the UKPDS was to determine whether targeting near-normal BG levels reduced morbidity and improved life expectancy.[24] These outcome measures encompassed several diabetes-related microvascular and macrovascular endpoints, diabetes-related death, and total mortality.[24,25] Over a period of 10 years, a program of intensive glucose control significantly reduced microvascular events by 25% (largely due to a reduction in the need for laser photocoagulation) but not diabetes-related or total mortality.[9,10] There was a borderline reduction in myocardial infarction (MI) with intensive therapy with SU or insulin that did not reach statistical significance ($P = .052$).[9] What was noteworthy when examined in context of the UGDP was that mortality among participants receiving an SU was not increased as was suggested by the UGDP.

Obese participants randomly assigned to receive metformin in the UKPDS did experience significant reductions in risk for MI and coronary death as well as for diabetes-related and total mortality.[10] Although the number of subjects receiving met-formin was small, these findings were the first demonstration of a CV benefit with glucose-lowering therapy and served as part of the rationale for updated guidelines recommending metformin therapy as first-line therapy for type 2 diabetes mellitus.[10,20] In the 10-year follow-up of UKPDS participants, despite loss of between-group differences in HbA_{1c} levels, intensively treated subjects continued to experience reductions in microvascular and macrovascular complications that were again more pronounced with those receiving metformin.[26] These favorable findings suggest that a strategy targeting near-normal glycemic control early in type 2 diabetes mellitus may be associated with a favorable legacy effect.[26,27]

An epidemiologic analysis of all participants in the UKPDS demonstrated a direct association between glycemic control and risk for CV events, where each 1% (10.9 mmol/mol) increase in glycated hemoglobin was associated with an 18% increase in risk for a CV event and a 12% increase in for death.[28] These results fostered plans to definitively test the glycemic control hypothesis for reducing CVD outcomes in patients with longstanding type 2 diabetes mellitus at high risk for CVD.[13,17,29] The ACCORD, ADVANCE, and VADT studies were conducted between 2001 and 2009 (**Table 1**). In contrast to the UGDP and the UKPDS, each of these 3 studies investigated the effects of intensive glycemic control on CVD outcomes during a period of increased recognition of the importance of other interventions, such as BP management, lipid-lowering, and aspirin therapy for primary and secondary CV protection.[30]

Subjects enrolled in ACCORD, ADVANCE, and VADT (mean age 60–66 years) were older and had longer duration of diabetes than those enrolled in the UKPDS (mean age 53 years) (see **Table 1**).[14] In addition, participants in these more recent trials either had a history of CVD events or were at high CV risk due to the presence of multiple risk factors. All 3 trials randomized participants to an intensive (HbA_{1c} targets <6% or < 6.5% [42 mmol/mol or 48 mmol/mol]) or a conventional glycemic control arm with less stringent targets (see **Table 1**). Study investigator groups achieved and maintained a significant separation of HbA_{1c} between the glycemic control arms over the duration of each of these studies. ACCORD and ADVANCE embedded trials investigating targeted treatment of other risk factors (hypertension in both; dyslipidemia in ACCORD), whereas the VADT protocol called for use of statins and aspirin, with a BP goal less than 130/80 mm Hg, for all participants.[17,29,31,32] The primary outcome of ACCORD was time to first major adverse cardiac event (MACE) that included nonfatal MI, nonfatal stroke, or CV death.[13] ADVANCE had an aggregate of both

Table 1
Findings from 3 large randomized controlled trials of the effects of intensive glycemic control versus standard glycemic control on cardiovascular outcomes

	ACCORD (Unless Otherwise Cited in Table, All Data from Ref.[13])	ADVANCE (Unless Otherwise Cited in Table, All Data from Ref.[16])	VADT (Unless Otherwise Cited in Table, All Data from Ref.[17])
Participant characteristics at trial baseline	N = 10,251 Mean age 62 y Mean duration 10 y 39% male 35% history of CVD Median HbA$_{1c}$ 8.1%	N = 11,140 Mean age 66 y Mean duration 8 y 42% male 32% history of CVD Median HbA$_{1c}$ 7.2%	N = 1791 Mean age 60 y Mean duration 11.5 y 97% male 40% history of CVD Median HbA$_{1c}$ 9.4%
Protocol characteristics	HbA$_{1c}$ goals (intensive glycemic control vs standard glycemic control): <6.0% vs 7.0%–7.9% Medications: multiple in both arms	HbA$_{1c}$ goals (intensive glycemic control vs standard glycemic control): ≤6.5 vs "based on local guidelines" Medications: gliclazide plus other medications vs no gliclazide plus other medications	HbA$_{1c}$ goals (intensive glycemic control vs standard glycemic control): <6.0% (action if ≥6.5%) vs planned separation between arms of 1.5% Medications: multiple in both arms
On-study characteristics	Mean duration of follow-up 3.5 y (terminated early) Median achieved HbA$_{1c}$ 6.4% vs 7.5%	Median duration of follow-up 5.0 y Mean achieved HbA$_{1c}$ 6.5% vs 7.3%	Median duration of follow-up 5.6 y Median achieved HbA$_{1c}$ 6.9% vs 8.4%
Outcomes	Definition of primary CVD outcome: nonfatal MI, nonfatal stroke, CV death (MACE) Blinded adjudication of all outcomes HR (95% CI) for primary outcome: 0.9 (0.78–1.04); P = .16 HR (95% CI) for death: 1.22 (1.01–1.46); P = .004	Definition of primary CVD outcome: nonfatal MI, nonfatal stroke, CV death (MACE) Blinded adjudication of all outcomes HR (95% CI) for primary outcome: 0.94 (0.84–1.06); P = .32 HR (95% CI) for death: 0.93 (0.83–1.06); P = .28	Definition of primary CVD outcome: MACE plus CHF, surgery for vascular disease, amputation for ischemia Blinded adjudication of all outcomes HR (95% CI) for primary outcome: 0.88 (0.74–1.05); P = .14 HR (95% CI) for death: 1.07 (0.81–1.42); P = .62

Prespecified subgroup analyses	Significant interaction (intensive glycemic control with CV benefit) if no known CVD and if baseline HbA$_{1c}$ ≤8.0%	No interactions	No prespecified subgroups
Ancillary studies or post hoc analyses	Severe hypoglycemia associated with mortality in both arms; association stronger in control arm[36]	Severe hypoglycemia associated with CV events, CV and total mortality, and many nonvascular events. No association of repeated episodes with CV outcomes or mortality[75]	Subset of participants had CAC scores at baseline. Significant reduction of CVD outcome in those with low CAC scores[45]
	Baseline characteristics associated with increased mortality with INT: self-reported neuropathy, HbA$_{1c}$ >8.5%, use of aspirin; all others nonsignificant[38]		U-shaped relationship between benefits of intensive glycemic control and duration of diabetes, suggesting benefit if duration <15 y and harm if >21 y[46]
	Older participants had more severe hypoglycemia in both arms; association of intensive glycemic control with increased mortality only seen in participants under age 65 y at baseline[37]		
Follow-up of study cohorts	Follow-up from study onset: 5 y[33]; 8.8 y[40] No significant reduction in primary outcome; continued significant increase in death in original intensive glycemic control arm	Follow-up from study onset: 10.9 y[41] No significant reduction in primary outcome	Follow-up from study onset: 9.8 y[42] Small but significant reduction in primary outcome (HR 0.83; 95% CI, 0.70–0.99; $P = .04$); no significant difference in mortality

Adapted from Skyler JS, Bergenstal R, Bonow RO, et al. Intensive glycemic control and the prevention of cardiovascular events: implications of the ACCORD, ADVANCE, and VA diabetes trials: a position statement of the American Diabetes Association and a scientific statement of the American College of Cardiology Foundation and the American Heart Association. Diabetes Care 2009;32(1):187–92. © 2016 by the American Diabetes Association. *Reprinted with permission from American Diabetes Association.*

microvascular and macrovascular events as a primary outcome, although MACE was assessed separately as a primary macrovascular outcome.[16] The VADT used an expanded primary CVD outcome that included MACE plus non-MACE events.[17]

There were no observed reductions in the primary aggregate CV outcomes with intensive compared with conventional glycemic control strategies in any of these studies.[13,16,17] In ACCORD, the glycemic control intervention was terminated early due to a significant (22%) increase in mortality in participants randomized to intensive therapy. Intensively treated participants were subsequently transitioned to the conventional glycemic control protocol, with a goal HbA_{1c} of 7.0% to 7.9% (53–63 mmol/mol) and followed until the planned original end date of the study. The hypertension and dyslipidemia randomized interventions were continued.[31–33]

The increase in total and CV mortality with intensive glycemic control in ACCORD has been the subject of additional investigations but has not been fully explained.[34,35] Among potential contributors to mortality in ACCORD, hypoglycemia has been most closely examined. Both moderate and severe hypoglycemia occurred more frequently in the intensively treated subjects in ACCORD.[34,36] The occurrence of severe hypoglycemia in ACCORD, defined as an episode requiring third-party assistance, was associated with excess mortality in both intensively and conventionally treated subjects with a larger hazard ratio (HR) for death observed in conventionally treated participants.[34,36] It is, therefore, unlikely that hypoglycemia alone explains the mortality findings observed in ACCORD. The excess mortality with intensive glycemic control was limited to participants who were less than age 65 years at baseline and was not greater in those with known CVD.[37,38] A post hoc epidemiologic analysis of factors related to mortality in ACCORD showed that mortality increased linearly with higher average on-study HbA_{1c} in the intensive glycemic control arm and that mortality was greater in the intensive versus standard arm only when average on-study HbA_{1c} was greater than 7.0% (53 mmol/mol). Neither the degree of reduction nor the rapidity of reduction of HbA_{1c} in the intensive arm was a predictor of mortality.[39] Hypoglycemia was identified as causative for mortality in less than 1% of all deaths, which clouds any connection between hypoglycemia and CV mortality with intensive therapy. Other factors, including excess weight gain, which was also observed in ACCORD; drug effects; or intensity of the intervention, are potential alternative explanations. The role of hypoglycemia and CV outcomes, which also occurred more frequently with intensive therapy in ADVANCE and the VADT, has also been examined and is discussed in more detail later.

The study cohorts of ACCORD, ADVANCE, and VADT continued to be followed after the cessation of the randomized interventions. Follow-up analyses of the ACCORD[33,40] and ADVANCE[41] cohorts found no emergence of significant CV benefit approximately 10 years after initiation of the randomized trials. The VADT follow-up study showed a small but statistically significant reduction in the primary outcome (HR 0.83; 95% CI, 0.70–0.99) with no reduction in total or CV mortality.[42] This suggests that in patients with more advanced type 2 diabetes mellitus at high CV risk, benefits of tighter glycemic control may primarily be in reducing nonfatal events.

Although ACCORD, ADVANCE, and the VADT suggest that intensive glycemic control may not result in significant benefits at a population level in terms of CVD prevention in type 2 diabetes mellitus, subgroup analyses, ancillary, and post hoc analyses raise interesting hypotheses about the types of patients who might realize a benefit. In ACCORD, prespecified subgroup analyses showed significant heterogeneity of the primary outcome based on baseline HbA_{1c} and history of CV events (in which benefit was seen in those with baseline HbA_{1c} $\leq$8.0% [64 mmol/mol] but not in those with higher HbA_{1c} as well as in those with no history of CVD but not those with prior history of CVD).[37,43] This suggests that intensive glycemic control may be beneficial in a primary prevention cohort for those with baseline HbA$_{1c}$ less than or equal to 8.0% (64 mmol/mol).[13,37,43] Another report examined outcomes according to group assignment based on a hemoglobin glycation index (HGI), calculated by subtracting a predicted (based on a linear regression model using fasting glucose measures) from the observed HbA$_{1c}$.[44] In this study, significant reductions in the primary outcomes were observed in intensively compared with conventionally treated subjects with low or moderate, but not high, HGI, where the risk for hypoglycemia was higher.

In an ancillary study from the VADT, intensive glycemic control reduced the primary CV outcome in the subset of patients with low compared with high coronary artery calcium (CAC) scores at baseline.[45] Another analysis of VADT outcomes based on duration of diabetes at baseline showed a U-shaped relationship for CVD events, suggesting a benefit of intensive glycemic control in those with diabetes less than 15 years and possible harm for those with diabetes greater than 22 years.[46]

The main and ancillary results of ACCORD, ADVANCE, and VADT, combined with the results of the UKPDS follow-up study, suggest several principles. The first is that intensive glycemic control in those with an established diagnosis of type 2 diabetes mellitus is not likely to offer major benefit for preventing CVD events. Those with a shorter duration of diabetes who do not have a history of CVD events prior to glycemic intensification may benefit from intensification of diabetes therapy, provided that attention is paid to minimizing risk for weight gain and hypoglycemia (**Box 1**).[47] As was observed in the UKPDS and VADT, any reduction in CV events may take years to manifest and may be limited to nonfatal events.[9,10,26,42] As further evidence emerges about types of patients who are more likely to have experience a CV benefit from stringent glycemic control, such therapy should be undertaken with the knowledge that the primary benefit may be to prevent microvascular complications, as has been demonstrated in the majority of intensive therapy trials in type 2 diabetes mellitus.[27] Evidence-based interventions for nonglycemic risk factors, such as BP management, statin therapy and cessation of smoking, should be the focus of efforts to reduce CVD burden in most patients with type 2 diabetes mellitus.[27,30,48] This includes following

---

Box 1
Candidates with type 2 diabetes mellitus for whom intensive glycemic control can be considered

Patients with recent-onset type 2 diabetes mellitus[18,26]

Patients with type 2 diabetes mellitus for less than 15 years[46]

Patients with baseline HbA$_{1c}$ $\leq$8.0%[37,43]

Patients at low risk for hypoglycemia[18]

Patients with no prior history of a CVD event[37]

Patients with low CAC scores[45]

Patients with low or moderate HGI[44]

These are clinical characteristics that have been derived from the described studies investigating the glycemic control hypothesis as a contributor to CVD risk reduction and emphasize recommendations by the American Diabetes Association for an individualized approach for establishing glycemic targets.

Data from Ismail-Beigi F, Moghissi E, Tiktin M, et al. Individualizing glycemic targets in type 2 diabetes mellitus: implications of recent clinical trials. Ann Intern Med 2011;154(8):554–9.

current recommendations for glycemic control that take into account an individual's overall health status, presence of other comorbidities, and patient preference[48,49]

GLUCOSE-LOWERING MEDICATIONS AND THE GLYCEMIC CONTROL HYPOTHESIS

Differentiating between studies that seek to achieve desired levels of glycemic control studies with specific diabetes medications and those that use a strategy of combining available therapies to achieve tight glycemic targets can be difficult. ACCORD, ADVANCE, and the VADT are more representative of studies that used a strategy of using multiple medications to achieve intensive glycemic goals. ADVANCE stands out as a study of a specific medication as part of the glycemic-lowering strategy, given that subjects randomized to intensive therapy received gliclazide in addition to other glucose-lowering medications used in both the intensive and control groups.[16] Several other trials have bridged the glycemic control hypothesis with specific diabetes medications.

The Bypass Angioplasty Revascularization Investigation 2 Diabetes study used the glycemic control hypothesis as part of intensive medical therapy for reducing CVD events and mortality in 2368 participants with type 2 diabetes mellitus.[50] In this study, subjects with angiographic documentation of coronary artery disease were randomized to intensive medical therapy alone or in combination with prompt revascularization with either percutaneous coronary intervention or coronary artery bypass graft. A glycemic target for an HbA_{1c} less than 7% (53 mmol/mol) was pursued for all participants by randomization to an insulin-providing (SU and/or insulin) or insulin-sensitizing (IS) (metformin and/or thiazolidinedione [predominantly rosiglitazone]) therapy. All participants received intensive medical management with lipid-lowering and BP-lowering medications in addition to antiplatelet therapy. There were no differences in the primary CV outcome with either glucose management strategy; however, subgroup analyses revealed some potential advantages with IS therapy on HbA_{1c}, weight gain, markers of inflammation, selected vascular outcomes, and risk for hypoglycemia.[50–52] Despite identical glycemic goals, the IS group achieved better glycemic control than the insulin-providing group (7.0% ± 1.2% vs 7.5% ± 1.4% [53 mmol/mol ± 13 mmol/mol vs 58 mmol/mol ± 15 mmol/mol]; P<.001), which may have contributed to any potential advantage.

The PROspective pioglitAzone Clinical Trial In macroVascular Events (PROactive) study investigated CV outcomes in more than 5000 participants with type 2 diabetes mellitus and known macrovascular disease randomly assigned to receive the IS medication, pioglitazone, or placebo in addition to other diabetes medications.[53] PROactive investigators were encouraged to target an HbA_{1c} of less than 6.5% (48 mmol/mol) in both treatment groups, achieving mean levels of 7.0% versus 7.6% (53 mmol/mol vs 60 mmol/mol) in the pioglitazone and control groups, respectively. There were no significant differences in the composite primary endpoint that included all-cause mortality, nonfatal MI, stroke, acute coronary syndrome, vascular interventions, and amputations. A statistically significant reduction in the composite secondary endpoint, however, that included all-cause mortality, nonfatal MI, and stroke (HR 0.84; 95% CI, 0.72–0.98; P = .027) was observed. Subgroup analysis of participants with a prior history of stroke demonstrated significant reductions in recurrence of both fatal and nonfatal stroke in PROactive.[54]

Interest in use of thiazolidinediones for type 2 diabetes mellitus waned after controversial publication of a meta-analysis demonstrating an increase in MI and CV death with rosiglitazone.[55] This resulted in the FDA-directed imposition of restrictions on use of this medication.[56,57] Subsequent publication of results from the Rosiglitazone Evaluated for Cardiovascular Outcomes in Oral Agent Combination Therapy for

Type 2 Diabetes (RECORD) study, a prospective randomized controlled trial evaluating the CV safety of rosiglitazone, did not confirm the results of the meta-analysis.[58] In RECORD, there were no differences in MI, stroke, or CV death over 5.5 years of follow-up. There was an increase in the number of hospitalizations for congestive heart failure (CHF), however, as well as an increase in fractures among those randomly assigned to receive rosiglitazone. Based in part on the results of this trial, an FDA mandated reanalysis of the CV safety of rosiglitazone resulted in a reversal of the restrictions on use of this agent in 2013. Despite this reversal, there has not been a rebound in the frequency of its use.[57]

The controversy surrounding rosiglitazone did not affect the use of pioglitazone to the same extent.[57,59] There has in fact been a renewed interest in use of pioglitazone for CV risk reduction after recent publication of the Insulin Resistance Intervention after Stroke (IRIS) study.[60] In IRIS, insulin-resistant subjects without diabetes randomly assigned to receive pioglitazone after a stroke experienced significant improvements in insulin sensitivity with a reduction in the combined primary outcome of stroke and MI compared with placebo. Studies of rosiglitazone, as well as favorable findings with studies using pioglitazone, have been accompanied by weight gain, edema, reductions in bone mineral density and increased fracture risk, and a higher frequency of CHF-related hospitalizations.[58,60,61]

The controversy surrounding rosiglitazone prompted a mandate from the FDA that CV outcome trials be performed on all new hypoglycemic agents submitted for review.[62] These recent trials have focused on studies where patients with type 2 diabetes mellitus were randomized to receive a specific medication versus placebo, in combination with other glycemic-lowering medications, to maintain equivalent HbA$_{1c}$ among participants. These trials are briefly addressed in this article and discussed in more detail in Hertzel C. Gerstein and Reema Shah's article, "Cardiovascular Outcomes Trials of Glucose-Lowering Drugs or Strategies in Type 2 Diabetes," in this issue.

The dipeptidyl peptidase 4 inhibitors (sitagliptin, saxagliptin, and alogliptin) have been studied with primarily neutral results with regard to CV outcomes.[63–65] The only exception was an unexplained increase in the number of CHF hospitalizations using saxagliptin in 1 but not all reports.[64,66] Among the CV outcome trials using the glucagon-like peptide 1 receptor, the Liraglutide Effect and Action in Diabetes: Evaluation of Cardiovascular Outcomes Results (LEADER) trial demonstrated significant reductions in the composite primary outcome of CV death, nonfatal MI, or stroke with liraglutide in a patient population at high risk for CVD.[67] When the components of the primary outcome were examined individually, the primary benefit was for all-cause and CV mortality, without significant reductions in nonfatal MI or stroke. Semaglutide, which is not currently approved for clinical use in the United States, was also associated with reductions in a similar composite primary outcome as used in LEADER.[68] When examined by individual components of the primary outcome, there was a significant reduction in nonfatal stroke but not for nonfatal MI or mortality. Of concern was an increase in retinopathy complications with more vitreous hemorrhage and blindness in those receiving semaglutide. The use of lixisenatide in subjects with type 2 diabetes mellitus after a recent acute coronary event offered no CV benefit or detriment compared with placebo in this very-high-risk group of patients.[69]

Favorable findings relating to CV outcomes have been observed with the new class of glucose-lowering agents, the sodium glucose cotransporter 2 inhibitors. In the EMPA-REG Outcome study, subjects randomly assigned to 1 of 2 doses of a significant reduction in hospitalization for heart failure, CV, and all-cause mortality despite a modest reduction in HbA$_{1c}$ of approximately 0.6% (approximately 6.6 mmol/mol).[70]

The use of canagliflozin also showed reductions in a composite of CV outcomes (CV death, nonfatal MI, and stroke), which were not significant when investigated individually.[71] Of concern was an observed increase in fractures and risk for amputations at the toe or metatarsals among participants treated with canagliflozin.[71,72] In the studies using both empagliflozin and canagliflozin, significant reductions in BP were observed, which may have contributed to the favorable CV results.[73]

These studies investigating the efficacy of specific glucose-lowering agents used may influence risk for CV events in the population of patients with type 2 diabetes mellitus with prior CVD or at very high CV risk. It will be important, however, to monitor risk for other potential diabetes-related complications, including fracture risk, retinopathy, amputations, and diabetic ketoacidosis, as the use of these newer agents increases. Individuals with advanced diabetes often have other diabetes-related complications or comorbidities that have the potential to increase the risks associated with these newer agents.

HYPOGLYCEMIA AND THE GLYCEMIC CONTROL HYPOTHESIS FOR CARDIOVASCULAR RISK REDUCTION

The greater incidence of both moderate and severe hypoglycemia in intensively treated subjects in ACCORD, ADVANCE, and VADT has been closely examined as a potential explanation for the inability to achieve clear evidence of CV benefit in these trials.[34,36,74,75] In the UKPDS, hypoglycemia occurred more frequently in the intensively treated groups treated with SU or insulin, but no association was observed for mortality.[9] This discrepancy between the UKPDS and the more recent trials can be explained in part by the fact that the UKPDS population was at least 10 years younger with a lower prevalence of CVD or CVD risk factors at study entry.[24] Participants in ACCORD, ADVANCE, and VADT were older, with longer duration of diabetes, and had either had a history of a CVD event or had multiple CV risk factors[14] (see **Table 1**). The medications used in these later trials also differed from those used in the UKPDS, in that a high percentage of patients (particularly in ACCORD and VADT) were treated with insulin in combination with a thiazolidinedione (primarily rosiglitazone). No adverse effect was observed, however, between use of any particular medication and CV events.[76,77]

As discussed previously, severe hypoglycemia was more common in ACCORD, but detailed analyses have not shown it to explain the mortality or CV outcomes in that trial. In ADVANCE, severe hypoglycemia was associated with an increased incidence of microvascular and macrovascular events, including mortality, as well as several nonvascular events (including respiratory and skin diseases).[75] In a post hoc analysis, no clear relationship was identified between severe hypoglycemia and CV mortality, leading the investigators to conclude that severe hypoglycemia may serve as a marker of frailty and increased vulnerability to adverse events. In VADT, a recent hypoglycemic event was identified as cause of mortality at 90 days, but severe hypoglycemia was associated with progression of coronary artery calcifications only in those receiving standard but not intensive glycemic management.[42,78]

This discussion is not intended to vindicate hypoglycemia as a contributor to morbidity and mortality in type 2 diabetes mellitus. Hypoglycemia remains an undesirable consequence of intensified glycemic control in all patients, but questions remain as to role of hypoglycemia in provoking adverse CV outcomes.[79] It is possible that recurrent episodes of mild or moderate hypoglycemia, which are more difficult to capture and quantify, may have contributed to the adverse outcomes observed in ACCORD, ADVANCE, and VADT. Based on the requirement for outside intervention, episodes of severe hypoglycemia are easier to capture than mild events.[34,80] Recent studies using continuous glucose monitoring in conjunction with cardiac monitoring devices demonstrated an increase in cardiac arrhythmias and prolonged QT intervals during periods of hypoglycemia that did not require outside assistance.[79,81,82] Other potential mechanisms that have been proposed for hypoglycemia as a contributor to CV morbidity and mortality include enhanced sympathetic nervous system activation, catecholamine excess, induction of cardiac ischemia, increased thrombogenesis and inflammation, and cardiac autonomic neuropathy.[35] In ACCORD, subjects with baseline evidence of cardiac autonomic neuropathy were more likely to die than those without in both randomization groups.[82]

SUMMARY

The UPKDS and the UKPDS legacy studies demonstrated that early implementation of a strategy of intensive glycemic control in younger individuals with recent-onset type 2 diabetes mellitus can effectively reduce the risk for CV complications over the long term.[26] ACCORD, ADVANCE, and VADT each demonstrated that there is no clear benefit with aggressive strategies directed at intensification of glycemic control in older individuals with established type 2 diabetes mellitus identified as at high risk for CVD and mortality.[14] Although not definitively related to CV morbidity or mortality, the increased frequency of severe hypoglycemia with intensified therapy in each of these studies has potential to not only have an impact on CV outcomes but also provoke other undesirable adverse events, including an increase in fall risk or cognitive impairment.[49,80] These studies have alerted the diabetes community to the importance of paying attention to risks associated with hypoglycemia with glucose lowering regimens in vulnerable individuals at any level of glycemic control.

U-shaped curves for HbA_{1c} with all-cause mortality and cardiac events demonstrate a favorable window for glycemic goals of 7.5% to 8.0% (58–64 mmol/mol) using regimens with and without insulin therapy.[6] These results are consistent with targets achieved in the conventionally treated groups in ACCORD and ADVANCE as well as with current recommendations for individualizing glycemic goals based on a combination of factors, including age, other comorbidities, life expectancy, and patient preference.[13,16,48,49]

Control of glycemia has been demonstrated to effectively reduce risk for microvascular and neuropathic complications in people with type 2 diabetes mellitus.[16] For reduction in CVD events and mortality, it is important to focus on control of BP, use of statins, and smoking cessation for primary and secondary prevention as well as aspirin for secondary prevention.[48] Lessons can be learned from the Steno study, which randomly assigned 160 patients with type 2 diabetes mellitus to a multifactorial or control intervention that addressed a composite of CVD factors, including glycemic control on all-cause and CV mortality over a period of approximately 13 years.[15] The glycemic goal in this study was to achieve an HbA_{1c} less than 6.6% (42 mmol/mol), which is considered intensive by current standards. This goal was achieved by a small percentage of subjects in each treatment group. The mean HbA_{1c} levels achieved at the end of the 7-year intervention and 5-year follow-up periods were 7.9% versus 9.0% and 7.7% versus 8.0% (63 mmol/mol vs 75 mmol/mol and 61 mmol/mol vs 64 mmol/mol), respectively. A majority of patients were receiving insulin in combination with oral diabetes medications by the end of the study period. Although this is a small study, the significant reductions in primary outcomes as well as secondary outcomes that included CV events and microvascular endpoints lend support to recommendations for a comprehensive strategy that embraces attention to glycemic control together with attention to all other CV risk factors.[15]

REFERENCES

1. Juutilainen A, Kortelainen S, Lehto S, et al. Gender difference in the impact of type 2 diabetes on coronary heart disease risk. Diabetes Care 2004;27(12): 2898–904.
2. Available at: http://www.cdc.gov/diabetes/statistics/dmany/fig1.htm. Accessed July 21, 2017.
3. The Emerging Risk Factors Collaboration. Diabetes mellitus, fasting glucose, and risk of cause-specific death. N Engl J Med 2011;364(9):829–41.
4. Rawshani A, Rawshani A, Franzen S, et al. Mortality and cardiovascular disease in type 1 and type 2 diabetes. N Engl J Med 2017;376(15):1407–18.
5. American Diabetes Association. Economic costs of diabetes in the U.S. in 2012. Diabetes Care 2013;36(4):1033–46.
6. Currie CJ, Peters JR, Tynan A, et al. Survival as a function of HbA(1c) in people with type 2 diabetes: a retrospective cohort study. Lancet 2010;375(9713):481–9.
7. Takao T, Suka M, Yanagisawa H, et al. Impact of postprandial hyperglycemia at clinic visits on the incidence of cardiovascular events and all-cause mortality in patients with type 2 diabetes. J Diabetes Investig 2017;8(4):600–8.
8. Selvin E, Steffes MW, Zhu H, et al. Glycated hemoglobin, diabetes, and cardio-vascular risk in nondiabetic adults. N Engl J Med 2010;362(9):800–11.
9. The UK Prospective Diabetes Study (UKPDS) Group. Intensive blood-glucose control with sulphonylureas or insulin compared with conventional treatment and risk of complications in patients with type 2 diabetes (UKPDS 33). Lancet 1998;352(9131):837–53.
10. The UK Prospective Diabetes Study (UKPDS) Group. Effect of intensive blood-glucose control with metformin on complications in overweight patients with type 2 diabetes (UKPDS 34). UK Prospective Diabetes Study (UKPDS) Group. Lancet 1998;352(9131):854–65.
11. Meinert CL, Knatterud GL, Prout TE, et al. A study of the effects of hypoglycemic agents on vascular complications in patients with adult-onset diabetes. II. Mortal-ity results. Diabetes 1970;19(Suppl):789–830.
12. Whitehouse FW, Arky RA, Bell DI, et al. American diabetes association policy statement: the UGDP controversy. Diabetes Care 1979;2(1):1–3.
13. The ACCORD Study Group. Effects of intensive glucose lowering in type 2 dia-betes. N Engl J Med 2008;358(24):2545–59.
14. Skyler JS, Bergenstal R, Bonow RO, et al. Intensive glycemic control and the pre-vention of cardiovascular events: implications of the ACCORD, ADVANCE, and VA diabetes trials: a position statement of the American Diabetes Association and a scientific statement of the American College of Cardiology Foundation and the American Heart Association. Diabetes Care 2009;32(1):187–92.
15. Gaede P, Lund-Andersen H, Parving HH, et al. Effect of a multifactorial interven-tion on mortality in type 2 diabetes. N Engl J Med 2008;358(6):580–91.
16. Patel A, MacMahon S, Chalmers J, et al. Intensive blood glucose control and vascular outcomes in patients with type 2 diabetes. N Engl J Med 2008; 358(24):2560–72.
17. Duckworth W, Abraira C, Moritz T, et al. Glucose control and vascular complica-tions in veterans with type 2 diabetes. N Engl J Med 2009;360(2):129–39.

18. Ismail-Beigi F, Moghissi E, Tiktin M, et al. Individualizing glycemic targets in type 2 diabetes mellitus: implications of recent clinical trials. Ann Intern Med 2011; 154(8):554–9.

19. Inzucchi SE, Bergenstal RM, Buse JB, et al. Management of hyperglycemia in type 2 diabetes, 2015: a patient-centered approach: update to a position statement of the American Diabetes Association and the European Association for the Study of Diabetes. Diabetes Care 2015;38(1):140–9.

20. Inzucchi SE, Bergenstal RM, Buse JB, et al. Management of hyperglycemia in type 2 diabetes: a patient-centered approach: position statement of the American Diabetes Association (ADA) and the European Association for the Study of Diabetes (EASD). Diabetes Care 2012;35(6):1364–79.

21. Metformin approved for U.S. market. Am J Health Syst Pharm 1995;52(7):676.

22. Seltzer HS. A summary of criticisms of the findings and conclusions of the University Group Diabetes Program (UGDP). Diabetes 1972;21(9):976–9.

23. Riddle MC. Modern sulfonylureas: dangerous or wrongly accused? Diabetes Care 2017;40(5):629–31.

24. UK Prospective Diabetes Study Group. UK Prospective Diabetes Study (UKPDS). VIII. Study design, progress and performance. Diabetologia 1991;34(12):877–90.

25. King P, Peacock I, Donnelly R. The UK prospective diabetes study (UKPDS): clinical and therapeutic implications for type 2 diabetes. Br J Clin Pharmacol 1999;48(5):643–8.

26. Holman RR, Paul SK, Bethel MA, et al. 10-year follow-up of intensive glucose control in type 2 diabetes. N Engl J Med 2008;359(15):1577–89.

27. Cefalu WT, Rosenstock J, LeRoith D, et al. Getting to the "Heart" of the matter on diabetic cardiovascular disease: "Thanks for the Memory". Diabetes Care 2016; 39(5):664–7.

28. Stratton IM, Adler AI, Neil HA, et al. Association of glycaemia with macrovascular and microvascular complications of type 2 diabetes (UKPDS 35): prospective observational study. Br Med J 2000;321(7258):405–12.

29. Patel A, MacMahon S, Chalmers J, et al. Effects of a fixed combination of perindopril and indapamide on macrovascular and microvascular outcomes in patients with type 2 diabetes mellitus (the ADVANCE trial): a randomised controlled trial. Lancet 2007;370(9590):829–40.

30. American Diabetes Association. Cardiovascular disease and risk management. Diabetes Care 2017;40(Suppl 1):S75–87.

31. Accord Study Group, Cushman WC, Evans GW, Byington RP, et al. Effects of intensive blood-pressure control in type 2 diabetes mellitus. N Engl J Med 2010;362(17):1575–85.

32. Accord Study Group, Ginsberg HN, Elam MB, Lovato LC, et al. Effects of combination lipid therapy in type 2 diabetes mellitus. N Engl J Med 2010;362(17): 1563–74.

33. Accord Study Group, Gerstein HC, Miller ME, Genuth S, et al. Long-term effects of intensive glucose lowering on cardiovascular outcomes. N Engl J Med 2011; 364(9):818–28.

34. Seaquist ER, Miller ME, Bonds DE, et al. The impact of frequent and unrecognized hypoglycemia on mortality in the ACCORD study. Diabetes Care 2012; 35(2):409–14.

35. Paty BW. The role of hypoglycemia in cardiovascular outcomes in diabetes. Can J Diabetes 2015;39(Suppl 5):S155–9.

36. Bonds DE, Miller ME, Bergenstal RM, et al. The association between symptomatic, severe hypoglycaemia and mortality in type 2 diabetes: retrospective epidemiological analysis of the ACCORD study. Br Med J 2010;340:b4909.

37. Miller ME, Williamson JD, Gerstein HC, et al. Effects of randomization to intensive glucose control on adverse events, cardiovascular disease, and mortality in older versus younger adults in the ACCORD Trial. Diabetes Care 2014;37(3):634–43.

38. Calles-Escandon J, Lovato LC, Simons-Morton DG, et al. Effect of intensive compared with standard glycemia treatment strategies on mortality by baseline subgroup characteristics: the Action to Control Cardiovascular Risk in Diabetes (ACCORD) trial. Diabetes Care 2010;33(4):721–7.

39. Riddle MC, Ambrosius WT, Brillon DJ, et al. Epidemiologic relationships between A1C and all-cause mortality during a median 3.4-year follow-up of glycemic treatment in the ACCORD trial. Diabetes Care 2010;33(5):983–90.

40. The ACCORD Study Group. Nine-year effects of 3.7 years of intensive glycemic control on cardiovascular outcomes. Diabetes Care 2016;39(5):701–8.

41. Zoungas S, Chalmers J, Neal B, et al. Follow-up of blood-pressure lowering and glucose control in type 2 diabetes. N Engl J Med 2014;371(15):1392–406.

42. Hayward RA, Reaven PD, Wiitala WL, et al. Follow-up of glycemic control and cardiovascular outcomes in type 2 diabetes. N Engl J Med 2015;372(23):2197–206.

43. Miller ME, Bonds DE, Gerstein HC, et al. The effects of baseline characteristics, glycaemia treatment approach, and glycated haemoglobin concentration on the risk of severe hypoglycaemia: post hoc epidemiological analysis of the ACCORD study. Br Med J 2010;340:b5444.

44. Hempe JM, Liu S, Myers L, et al. The hemoglobin glycation index identifies subpopulations with harms or benefits from intensive treatment in the ACCORD trial. Diabetes Care 2015;38(6):1067–74.

45. Reaven PD, Moritz TE, Schwenke DC, et al. Intensive glucose-lowering therapy reduces cardiovascular disease events in veterans affairs diabetes trial participants with lower calcified coronary atherosclerosis. Diabetes 2009;58(11):2642–8.

46. Duckworth WC, Abraira C, Moritz TE, et al. The duration of diabetes affects the response to intensive glucose control in type 2 subjects: the VA diabetes trial. J Diabetes Complications 2011;25(6):355–61.

47. American Diabetes Association. Approaches to glycemic treatment. Diabetes Care 2016;39(Suppl 1):S52–9.

48. Korytkowski MT, Forman DE. Management of atherosclerotic cardiovascular disease risk factors in the older adult patient with diabetes. Diabetes Care 2017;40(4):476–84.

49. Kirkman MS, Briscoe VJ, Clark N, et al. Diabetes in older adults. Diabetes Care 2012;35(12):1–15.

50. BARI 2D Study Group. A randomized trial of therapies for type 2 diabetes and coronary artery disease. N Engl J Med 2009;360(24):2503–15.

51. Wolk R, Bertolet M, Brooks MM, et al. Differential effects of insulin sensitization and insulin provision treatment strategies on concentrations of circulating adipokines in patients with diabetes and coronary artery disease in the BARI 2D trial. Eur J Prev Cardiol 2016;23(1):50–8.

52. Althouse AD, Abbott JD, Sutton-Tyrrell K, et al. Favorable effects of insulin sensitizers pertinent to peripheral arterial disease in type 2 diabetes: results from the Bypass Angioplasty Revascularization Investigation 2 Diabetes (BARI 2D) trial. Diabetes Care 2013;36(10):3269–75.

53. Dormandy JA, Charbonnel B, Eckland DJ, et al. Secondary prevention of macrovascular events in patients with type 2 diabetes in the PROactive Study (PROspective pioglitAzone Clinical Trial In macroVascular Events): a randomised controlled trial. Lancet 2005;366(9493):1279–89.

54. Wilcox R, Bousser MG, Betteridge DJ, et al. Effects of pioglitazone in patients with type 2 diabetes with or without previous stroke: results from PROactive (PROspective pioglitAzone Clinical Trial In macroVascular Events 04). Stroke 2007;38(3):865–73.

55. Nissen SE, Wolski K. Effect of rosiglitazone on the risk of myocardial infarction and death from cardiovascular causes. N Engl J Med 2007;356(24):2457–71.

56. Jain R, Mullins CD, Lee H, et al. Use of rosiglitazone and pioglitazone immediately after the cardiovascular risk warnings. Res Social Adm Pharm 2012;8(1):47–59.

57. Hsu JC, Ross-Degnan D, Wagner AK, et al. How did multiple FDA actions affect the utilization and reimbursed costs of thiazolidinediones in US medicaid? Clin Ther 2015;37(7):1420–32.e1.

58. Home PD, Pocock SJ, Beck-Nielsen H, et al. Rosiglitazone evaluated for cardiovascular outcomes in oral agent combination therapy for type 2 diabetes (RECORD): a multicentre, randomised, open-label trial. Lancet 2009;373(9681):2125–35.

59. Ryder RE. Pioglitazone: reports of its death are greatly exaggerated - it is alive and ready to resume saving lives. Diabet Med 2015;32(4):e9–15.

60. Kernan WN, Viscoli CM, Furie KL, et al. Pioglitazone after ischemic stroke or transient ischemic attack. N Engl J Med 2016;374(14):1321–31.

61. Erdmann E, Charbonnel B, Wilcox RG, et al. Pioglitazone use and heart failure in patients with type 2 diabetes and preexisting cardiovascular disease: data from the PROactive study (PROactive 08). Diabetes Care 2007;30(11):2773–8.

62. Hirshberg B, Katz A. Cardiovascular outcome studies with novel antidiabetes agents: scientific and operational considerations. Diabetes Care 2013;36(Suppl 2):S253–8.

63. Green JB, Bethel MA, Armstrong PW, et al. Effect of sitagliptin on cardiovascular outcomes in type 2 diabetes. N Engl J Med 2015;373(3):232–42.

64. Scirica BM, Bhatt DL, Braunwald E, et al. Saxagliptin and cardiovascular outcomes in patients with type 2 diabetes mellitus. N Engl J Med 2013;369(14):1317–26.

65. White WB, Cannon CP, Heller SR, et al. Alogliptin after acute coronary syndrome in patients with type 2 diabetes. N Engl J Med 2013;369(14):1327–35.

66. Toh S, Hampp C, Reichman ME, et al. Risk for hospitalized heart failure among new users of saxagliptin, sitagliptin, and other antihyperglycemic drugs: a retrospective cohort study. Ann Intern Med 2016;164(11):705–14.

67. Marso SP, Daniels GH, Brown-Frandsen K, et al. Liraglutide and cardiovascular outcomes in type 2 diabetes. N Engl J Med 2016;375(4):311–22.

68. Marso SP, Bain SC, Consoli A, et al. Semaglutide and cardiovascular outcomes in patients with type 2 diabetes. N Engl J Med 2016;375(19):1834–44.

69. Pfeffer MA, Claggett B, Diaz R, et al. Lixisenatide in patients with type 2 diabetes and acute coronary syndrome. N Engl J Med 2015;373(23):2247–57.

70. Zinman B, Wanner C, Lachin JM, et al. Empagliflozin, cardiovascular outcomes, and mortality in type 2 diabetes. N Engl J Med 2015;373(22):2117–28.

71. Neal B, Perkovic V, Mahaffey KW, et al. Canagliflozin and cardiovascular and renal events in type 2 diabetes. N Engl J Med 2017;377(7):644–57.

72. Stenlof K, Cefalu WT, Kim KA, et al. Efficacy and safety of canagliflozin monotherapy in subjects with type 2 diabetes mellitus inadequately controlled with diet and exercise. Diabetes Obes Metab 2013;15(4):372–82.

73. Ingelfinger JR, Rosen CJ. Cardiovascular risk and sodium–glucose cotransporter 2 inhibition in type 2 diabetes. N Engl J Med 2015;373(22):2178–9.

74. Boussageon R, Bejan-Angoulvant T, Saadatian-Elahi M, et al. Effect of intensive glucose lowering treatment on all cause mortality, cardiovascular death, and microvascular events in type 2 diabetes: meta-analysis of randomised controlled trials. BMJ 2011;343:d4169.

75. Zoungas S, Patel A, Chalmers J, et al. Severe hypoglycemia and risks of vascular events and death. N Engl J Med 2010;363(15):1410–8.

76. Siraj ES, Rubin DJ, Riddle MC, et al. Insulin dose and cardiovascular mortality in the ACCORD trial. Diabetes Care 2015;38(11):2000–8.

77. Florez H, Reaven PD, Bahn G, et al. Rosiglitazone treatment and cardiovascular disease in the Veterans Affairs Diabetes Trial. Diabetes Obes Metab 2015;17(10): 949–55.

78. Saremi A, Bahn GD, Reaven PD. A link between hypoglycemia and progression of atherosclerosis in the Veterans Affairs Diabetes Trial (VADT). Diabetes Care 2016;39(3):448–54.

79. Desouza CV, Bolli GB, Fonseca V. Hypoglycemia, diabetes, and cardiovascular events. Diabetes Care 2010;33(6):1389–94.

80. Seaquist ER, Anderson J, Childs B, et al. Hypoglycemia and diabetes: a report of a workgroup of the American Diabetes Association and the Endocrine Society. Diabetes Care 2013;36(5):1384–95.

81. Chow E, Bernjak A, Williams S, et al. Risk of cardiac arrhythmias during hypoglycemia in patients with type 2 diabetes and cardiovascular risk. Diabetes 2014; 63(5):1738–47.

82. Clark AL, Best CJ, Fisher SJ. Even silent hypoglycemia induces cardiac arrhythmias. Diabetes 2014;63(5):1457–9.

Cardiovascular Outcomes Trials of Glucose-Lowering Drugs or Strategies in Type 2 Diabetes

Hertzel C. Gerstein, MD, MSc*, Reema Shah, MD

KEYWORDS

- Type 2 diabetes • Cardiovascular complications • Glucose-lowering drugs
- Cardioprotective agents

KEY POINTS

- Diabetes affects approximately 1 in 10 adults worldwide, most with type 2 diabetes, which is characterized by an inability to make sufficient insulin to prevent glucose levels from increasing.
- Type 2 diabetes arises from various factors including genetic predisposition, aging, obesity, diet, family history, ethnicity, culture, economics, and lifestyle.
- As recently as 20 years ago there were essentially no randomized controlled trials of potentially cardiovascular protective therapies in people with type 2 diabetes.
- More than 120,000 people to date have been recruited into the trials studying diabetes and cardiovascular disease.
- The discovery of at least 4 agents with cardioprotective properties, represents a remarkable addition to the evidence for cardiovascular protection in people with type 2 diabetes.

Diabetes is a metabolic disease characterized by persistently elevated fasting and/or postprandial glucose levels that are at or above carefully defined diagnostic thresholds. In addition to suffering from the symptoms of hyperglycemia, including fatigue, changes in weight, nocturia, polyuria, polyphagia, and polydipsia, people with diabetes are at high risk of developing a wide variety of serious health outcomes. These

Disclosure: Dr H.C. Gerstein is supported by the McMaster-Sanofi Population Health Institute Chair in Diabetes Research and Care. Dr Gerstein has received research grant support from Sanofi, Lilly, AstraZeneca, and Merck, honoraria for speaking from Sanofi, Novo Nordisk, and AstraZeneca, and consulting fees from Sanofi, Lilly, AstraZeneca, Merck, Novo Nordisk, Abbot, Amgen, Janssen, and Boehringer Ingelheim. Dr R. Shah has nothing to disclose.
Department of Medicine, Population Health Research Institute, McMaster University, Hamilton Health Sciences, HSC 3V38, 1280 Main Street West, Hamilton, Ontario L8S 4K1, Canada
* Corresponding author.
E-mail address: gerstein@mcmaster.ca

Endocrinol Metab Clin N Am 47 (2018) 97–116
https://doi.org/10.1016/j.ecl.2017.10.003
0889-8529/18/© 2017 Elsevier Inc. All rights reserved.

include retinal disease and vision loss, renal failure, nerve damage and neuropathic pain, cardiovascular diseases (ischemic heart disease, heart failure, and cardiovascular death), cerebrovascular disease, peripheral vascular disease, cancers, cirrhosis, cognitive decline, erectile dysfunction, and premature mortality. Some of these health problems, such as retinopathy, are highly specific to diabetes, whereas others occur earlier in people with diabetes than in people without diabetes. The fact that the retinal changes associated with diabetic retinopathy only occur with hyperglycemia was used as the basis for establishing the diagnostic thresholds for diabetes (ie, fasting and 2 hour post oral glucose load plasma glucose levels of 7 and 11.1 mmol/L respectively or a hemoglobin A1c [HbA1c] of $\geq$6.5%).[1] These diagnostic thresholds, therefore, represent glucose levels above which the risk of retinopathy increases exponentially, and below which the relationship is fairly flat. Notably, they are much higher than the fasting, 2 hour postglucose load, and HbA1c levels of 5.59 mmol/L, 7.79 mmol/L and 5.6%, respectively, that characterize normal glucose physiology.[1]

Diabetes affects approximately 1 in 10 adults worldwide. The vast majority (>90%) of affected individuals have type 2 diabetes, which is characterized by an inability to make sufficient insulin to prevent glucose levels from rising. Type 2 diabetes arises from various combinations of factors including aging, obesity, diet, family history, ethnicity, culture, economics, and lifestyle, factors that have contributed to its rapid increase in prevalence over the last 20 years.

CARDIOVASCULAR DISEASES PROMOTED BY DIABETES

Diabetes is an independent risk factor for cardiovascular diseases. Compared with people without diabetes, the incidence of myocardial infarctions, strokes, coronary death, peripheral vascular disease, and heart failure are all increased by approximately 100%.[2,3] Not surprisingly, diabetes also doubles the risk of cardiovascular death[4] and reduces life expectancy. In a recent metaanalysis of data from 689,300 participants from 91 cohorts followed for a median of 12.8 years, during which 128,843 deaths occurred, the incidence of death in people with diabetes was similar to that of people without prior diabetes who had a prior myocardial infarction or a prior stroke (about double the incidence of death in people with none of these risk factors). In the same study, people with both prior diabetes and either a prior myocardial infarction or stroke had about a 4-fold greater incidence of death than people with none of these risk factors.[5] Moreover, in an international registry of people aged 45 years or older with prior cardiovascular disease or related risk factors, the risk for heart failure hospitalization was 33% greater in people with diabetes versus those without diabetes, and 470% higher in people with both prior heart failure and diabetes versus prior heart failure alone.[6] These relationships reduce life expectancy by 5.7 years for a 60-year-old man and 6.7 years for a 60-year-old woman with diabetes alone, and 12 and 13 years for a 60-year-old man or woman, respectively, in the setting of diabetes plus either a prior myocardial infarction or stroke, with 59% of the excess deaths owing to cardiovascular diseases.[5] Finally, despite evidence of decreasing incidence rates of myocardial infarction and stroke over the last 20 years in the United States, a large gap between people with diabetes and the general population persists for these outcomes.[7]

LINK BETWEEN DYSGLYCEMIA AND CARDIOVASCULAR DISEASE

Compared with retinal disease, the link between dysglycemia and incident cardiovascular (CV) disease (ischemic heart disease, cerebrovascular disease, cardiovascular death, and heart failure) starts well below the diabetes threshold (ie, at the upper limit of the normal fasting glucose, postload glucose, and HbA1c levels[8–14]), and increases progressively after it surpasses the diagnostic thresholds for diabetes.[15,16] The progressive relationship between glucose levels and/or the HbA1c above the diabetes thresholds and cardiovascular death is best illustrated by a large, population-based analysis using Swedish national health data,[17] in which 435,369 adults with diabetes were each matched with 5 controls without diabetes (n = 2,117,483) and followed within the database for a mean period of 4.6 years. After stratification for diabetes duration and adjustment for time-updated age, sex, birth country, education, and comorbidity, the hazard of cardiovascular death (**Fig. 1**) and the hazard of death increased progressively with each time-updated category of HbA1c varying from 6.9% or less to 9.7% or more across all age ranges. The observation that the relationship persisted across all age ranges reflects a robust link between dysglycemia and cardiovascular disease. The observation that it nevertheless becomes attenuated with age is likely attributable to the impact of other, "competing" causes of cardiovascular death that increase in incidence with age.

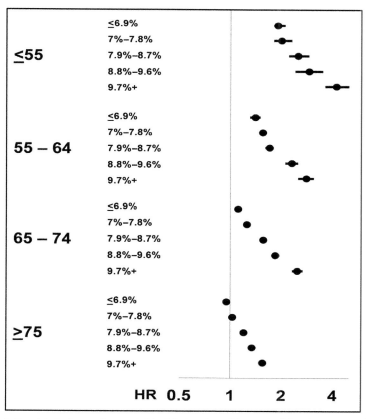

Fig. 1. Relationship between hemoglobin A1c levels and hazard of death. Data are based on an analysis of the Swedish registry, comprising 435,369 cases of diabetes and 2,117,483 controls without diabetes, followed for a mean of 4.6 years. Hazard ratios (HR) are adjusted for sex, time-updated age, birth country, education, and diabetes duration.

THE CRUCIAL NEED FOR RANDOMIZED CONTROLLED CARDIOVASCULAR OUTCOMES TRIALS

These observational studies clearly demonstrate that diabetes and indeed, any degree of dysglycemia are important independent risk factors for cardiovascular outcomes, and support the search for strategies to reduce or eliminate the excess risk. Whereas such studies excel at identifying and quantifying risk factors for outcomes, they cannot be used to determine whether intervening on the risk factor by either changing its level or by adding a drug can reduce the cardiovascular outcome. This is because the relationship between the risk factor or any drug therapy and cardiovascular outcomes in observational studies may be as likely to reflect the effect of the risk factor or drug as it is to reflect some other measured or unmeasured factor or drug indication or contraindication that accounted for the relationship between the risk factor and outcome or the drug and outcome. This "confounding" factor may be totally invisible to researchers and clinicians alike. Therefore, the most reliable way to determine the effect of the therapy is to identify 2 large groups of individuals that are, on average, identical, to give the therapy to only 1 of the 2 groups, and to follow all participants until sufficient outcomes have accrued to detect a difference (if one indeed exists). The only proven reliable way of creating 2 such groups is to use the randomization process to distribute every measured and unmeasured or unimagined confounder equally between 2 groups. It is important that the groups are large enough to ensure that the randomization truly achieves this balance, and to ensure that enough outcomes will accrue over time to ensure that any difference between groups is unlikely to be spurious. The actual size and follow-up duration depends on the anticipated annual event rate in the control group, and the minimum difference between groups that is judged important to detect.

Cardiovascular outcomes trials have generally shown that therapies that reduce cardiovascular outcomes in the general population also do so in the subgroup with diabetes. These include reducing low-density lipoprotein cholesterol, reducing blood pressure, and adding statins, renin–angiotensin system modulators, and other therapies in specific subpopulations. However, a comprehensive review of the literature in support of these therapies is beyond the scope of this paper, which is limited to the large cardiovascular outcomes trials that have assessed the effect of glucose lowering, glucose-lowering strategies, and/or specific glucose-lowering drugs on cardiovascular outcomes. Such trials are crucial to both identify novel preventive therapies and to ensure that the glucose-lowering therapies that have been shown to reduce other consequences of diabetes such as eye and kidney disease do not promote cardiovascular diseases.

GLUCOSE LOWERING AND CARDIOVASCULAR OUTCOMES

A more extensive discussion of this question can be found in the article in this issue. Briefly, only 4 large trials randomly allocated people to a strategy of more versus less intensive glucose lowering.[18] Completed between 1997 and 2008, these 4 trials studied participants with either newly diagnosed[19] or well-established type 2 diabetes plus additional cardiovascular risk factors,[20–22] allocated them to more intense versus less intense glucose control using a menu of drugs, and prospectively followed them for the occurrence of cardiovascular outcomes. In a metaanalysis of these 4 trials comprising 27,049 people that was published in 2009,[18] participants allocated to intensive glucose control experienced a modest, statistically significant 9% reduced hazard of the composite outcome of the first occurrence of nonfatal myocardial infarction, nonfatal stroke, or death from cardiovascular causes (referred to as major adverse cardiovascular events), and a 2- to 3-fold increased hazard of severe hypoglycemia. Data from the longest trial[19] was truncated at 5 years in keeping with the other 3 shorter trials. As such, this effect occurred during a mean follow-up period of 4.4 years and in response to an achieved overall between-group difference in HbA1c of 0.88%.[18]

The evidence, however, is not nearly as clear as the metaanalysis suggests because one of the trials, the ACCORD trial (Action to Control Cardiovascular Risk in Diabetes), was stopped early by the Independent Data Safety and Monitoring Board because of increased mortality (owing to cardiovascular mortality) in the intervention group. No clear explanation for this signal have emerged, and possibilities such as the degree of glucose lowering, hypoglycemia, weight gain, and the drugs used have not been supported by exploratory analyses. Remaining possibilities include chance alone[23] or persistent hyperglycemia despite attempts to normalize glucose levels.[24] Regardless of the reason, this finding has tempered clinical practice guideline recommendations such that intensive glucose lowering in type 2 diabetes is now recommended in patients who are otherwise reasonably healthy.[25] Further trials assessing this question are clearly indicated but not yet underway.

EFFECT OF GLUCOSE-LOWERING STRATEGIES ON CARDIOVASCULAR OUTCOMES

Many epidemiologic studies have suggested that a reduced physiologic response to insulin (insulin resistance) is a risk factor for cardiovascular outcomes. Whether this relationship is modifiable such that strategies that increase responsiveness to insulin (insulin sensitization strategies) can reduce cardiovascular outcomes was explicitly tested in one well-conducted large study. The BARI-2D (Bypass Angioplasty Reduction Investigation in type 2 Diabetes)[26] trial studied 2368 people (mean age 63 years; 30% women) with type 2 diabetes and a median HbA1c 7.7% who had proven coronary artery disease requiring revascularization. Providers and participants all targeted a HbA1c of less than 7% and were randomly allocated to achieve this using either insulin sensitizing drugs (including metformin and/or thiazolidinediones) or insulin providing drugs (including sulfonylureas and/or insulin). Compared with the insulin sensitizing group, participants in the insulin providing group had a higher mean HbA1c (7.5% vs 7.0%) and median insulin level (10 vs 6.3 uU/L) at the 3 year follow-up visit. During a mean trial follow-up period of 5.3 years, the glucometabolic strategy used had a neutral effect on both survival and the composite outcome of cardiovascular death, myocardial infarction, or stroke. These findings suggest that insulin resistance or hyperinsulinemia is not a modifiable risk factor for cardiovascular disease in high-risk individuals.

EFFECT OF GLUCOSE-LOWERING DRUGS ON CARDIOVASCULAR OUTCOMES

The possibility that glucose-lowering drugs may have cardiovascular or other effects that are distinct or independent of their glucose-lowering effects has been assessed in several large trials. A common design element for all of these trials was the targeting of guideline-recommended glucose control in all participants, regardless of their allocated group, along with the freedom to use glucose-lowering agents other than the ones being tested to achieve this level of glucose control. Such an approach seeks to achieve similar HbA1c levels in all participants (ie, regardless of allocated group) to support the inference that any observed cardiovascular effect of the drug (ie, benefit or harm) is attributable to its nonglycemic actions. Clearly, the more that the postrandomization glycemic profile of the intervention and control groups overlap, the more confidence there will be in this inference. For these trials, a summary of the characteristics of the included participants is provided in **Table 1**, the key cardiovascular results are shown in **Fig. 2** and **Table 2**, and the effect of the interventions in key subgroups is summarized in **Table 3**.

Insulin

Because people with type 2 diabetes are unable to make sufficient insulin, exogenous insulin could potentially restore normal glucose levels. Such an approach has been limited by the fact that exogenous insulin is given systemically and not into the hepatic portal circulation, is not regulated by initial delivery to the liver, is dosed according to intermittently measured versus continuously detected glucose levels, and has varying absorption owing to injection techniques, intraindividual and interindividual factors, and the formulation of the insulin being administered. These considerations, and concerns about injections and the risk of hypoglycemia and modest weight gain, meant that exogenous insulin tended to be given late in the course of diabetes when patients had developed cardiovascular and other consequences, which in turn raised concerns regarding whether insulin was promoting some of these consequences. These concerns were explicitly addressed in the ORIGIN (Outcomes Reduction with an Initial Glargine INtervention) trial of basal insulin glargine.[27]

The ORIGIN trial recruited 12,537 people (mean age 64 years; 35% women, 59% with previous cardiovascular disease) with either impaired fasting glucose or impaired glucose tolerance (11%) or diabetes (89%) who were unlikely to need insulin to control glucose levels over the subsequent 7 years, and whose baseline median HbA1c was 6.4%. Participants were allocated to the addition of a once daily injection of insulin glargine titrated to a fasting plasma glucose of 5.3 mmol/L or less (95 mg/dL) or standard care without insulin. During a median follow-up of 6.2 years, the incidence of the composite primary outcome of cardiovascular death, myocardial infarction, or stroke in the control group was 2.9% per year and the hazard for this outcome in people allocated to insulin versus standard care was 1.02 (95% confidence interval [CI], 0.94–1.11). Insulin also had a neutral effect on all other serious outcomes, and the only adverse effects were hypoglycemia and modest weight gain.

Once ORIGIN was completed, it provided a benchmark against which the cardiovascular and other effects of basal insulins could be assessed. Thus, in the DEVOTE trial (Trial comparing cardiovascular safety of insulin degludec vs insulin glargine in patients with type 2 diabetes at high risk of cardiovascular events),[28,29] 7637 people (mean age 65 years; 33% women) with established diabetes (mean HbA1c of 8.4%) at high risk for a cardiovascular event were randomly allocated to receive either masked insulin degludec U100 or insulin glargine U100, and were instructed to target fasting glucose levels of 4.0 to 5.0 mmol/L. During a median follow-up of 2 years, the incidence of the composite primary outcome of cardiovascular death, myocardial infarction, or stroke in the insulin glargine group was 4.7% per year and the hazard for this outcome in people allocated to insulin degludec was 0.91 (95% CI, 0.78–1.06).

One much smaller study assessed the cardiovascular effects of prandial versus basal insulin. The HEART-2D Trial (Hyperglycemia and Its Effect After Acute Myocardial Infarction on Cardiovascular Outcomes in Patients With Type 2 Diabetes Mellitus) studied 1115 people (mean age 61 years; 37% women) with type 2 diabetes.[30] Participants who had a myocardial infarction within the prior 21 days stopped their oral glucose-lowering drugs and were randomly allocated to either insulin Lispro given 3 xtimes daily targeting a postprandial glucose of less than 7.5 mmol/L or basal insulin with either NPH or glargine given twice or once daily targeting a fasting glucose level of less than 6.7 mmol/L. During a mean follow-up period of 2.7 years, the incidence of the composite primary outcome of cardiovascular death, myocardial infarction, or stroke

Table 1
Key features of randomized controlled cardiovascular outcomes trials of glucose-lowering drugs

Trial Acronym[a]	n	Characteristics			Factors Relevant to Participant's Response				
		Age	Women	Follow-up (y)	Prior CVD	Baseline HbA1c (%)	Glycemia Contrast (%)[g]	Cardiovascular Outcome	Cardiovascular Outcome Incidence in Controls (%/y)
NAVIGATOR[a]	9306	64	51	6.3[d]	24	5.8	FG 0.03 mmol/L	MACE or HF	1.4
HEART 2D	1115	61	37	2.7[d]	100[e]	8.3	0.1	MACE	12[k]
ORIGIN[b]	12,537	64	35	6.2[d]	59	6.4	0.3 at 2 y[d]	MACE	2.9
DEVOTE	7637	65	37	2.0[d]	85	8.4	FG 0.40 mmol/L at 2 y	MACE	4.7
PROACTIVE	5238	62	34	2.9	98	8.1	0.6 at end	MACE Plus[j]	7.5[k]
IRIS[c]	3876	64	35	4.8[d]	100[f]	5.8	FG 0.26 mmol/L at 1 y	MACE	2.5[k]
EXAMINE	5380	61	32	1.5[d]	100[e]	8.0	0.4 at end	MACE	7.9[k]
TECOS	14,671	66	29	3.0[d]	74	7.2	0.3	MACE	4.2
SAVOR	16,492	65	33	2.1[d]	78	8.0	0.2 at end	MACE	3.7
ELIXA	6068	60	31	2.1[d]	100[e]	7.7	0.3	MACE or UA	6.3
LEADER	9340	64	36	3.8[d]	81	8.7	0.4 at 3 y	MACE	3.9
SUSTAIN 6	3297	65	39	2.1	59	8.7	0.7 and 1.1[h] at end	MACE	4.4
EMPA-REG	7020	63	29	3.1[d]	99	8.1	0.2 and 0.4[i] at end	MACE	4.4
CANVAS	10,142	63	36	2.4[d]	66	8.2	0.58	MACE	3.2

Data in cells are percentages for categorical variables and (unless otherwise stated) mean values for continuous variables.

Abbreviations: CVD, cardiovascular disease; FG, fasting plasma glucose; HbA1c, hemoglobin A1c; HF, heart failure hospitalization; MACE, nonfatal myocardial infarction (MI), or nonfatal stroke or cardiovascular (CV) death; UA, unstable angina.

[a] All participants had impaired glucose tolerance at randomization.
[b] Eighty-eight percent of participants had diabetes at randomization.
[c] No patients had diabetes, but 86% had a FG ≥5.6 mmol/L and a HbA1c ≥5.7% at baseline.
[d] Median value (others are means).
[e] Recent acute coronary syndrome.
[f] Recent stroke or transient ischemic attack.
[g] Unless otherwise indicated, the between-group difference in achieved glycemic levels after randomization (the timing varies across trials) is expressed as the mean hemoglobin A1c difference (%).
[h] For 0.5 mg and 1.0 mg semaglutide versus placebo, respectively.
[i] For 10 mg and 25 mg empagliflozin versus placebo, respectively.
[j] Includes all-cause mortality, acute coronary syndrome, endovascular or surgical intervention on the coronary or leg arteries, or amputation above the ankle.
[k] Annual rate was estimated from the overall rate divided by the years of follow-up.

Drug "Class"	Trial Acronym	Drug	n	Follow-up (y)		Primary Outcome	HR (95% CI)
Meglitinide	NAVIGATOR	Nateglinide	9306	6.3		MACE/HF	0.94 (0.82–1.09)
Insulin	HEART 2D	Prandial vs basal	1115	2.7		MACE	0.98 (0.80–1.21)
	ORIGIN	Glargine vs no insulin	12537	6.2		MACE	1.02 (0.94–1.11)
	DEVOTE	Degludec vs glargine	7637	2.0		MACE	0.91 (0.78–1.06)
Thiazolidine-dione	PROACTIVE	Pioglitazone	5238	2.9*		MACE/other	0.90 (0.80–1.02)
	IRIS	Pioglitazone	3876	4.8		MACE	0.76 (0.62–0.93)
DPP4 inhibitor	EXAMINE	Alogliptin	5380	1.5		MACE	0.96 (<1.16)
	TECOS	Sitagliptin	14671	3.0		MACE	0.98 (0.89–1.08)
	SAVOR	Saxagliptin	16492	2.1		MACE	1.00 (0.89–1.12)
GLP1 receptor agonist	ELIXA	Lixisenatide	6068	2.1		MACE/UA	1.02 (0.89–1.17)
	LEADER	Liraglutide	9340	3.8		MACE	0.87 (0.78–0.97)
	SUSTAIN 6	Semaglutide	3297	2.1*		MACE	0.74 (0.58–0.95)
SGLT2 inhibitor	EMPA-REG OUTCOME	Empagliflozin	7020	3.1		MACE	0.86 (0.74–0.99)
	CANVAS	Canagliflozin	10142	2.4		MACE	0.86 (0.75–0.97)

0.5   1   HR   2

Fig. 2. Summary of outcomes trials. The data shown in **Tables 1** and **2** are summarized graphically. DPP4, dipeptidyl peptidase 4; GLP-1, glucagon-like peptide 1; HF, heart failure; MACE, nonfatal myocardial infarction, or nonfatal stroke or cardiovascular death; UA, unstable angina. Median follow-up data are shown, except as indicated by * (which denotes the mean).

in the basal insulin group was approximately 12% per year, and the hazard for this outcome in people allocated to prandial versus basal insulin was 0.98 (95% CI, 0.80–1.21).

The ORIGIN and DEVOTE trials provide compelling data regarding the cardiovascular safety of basal insulin. Moreover, the fact that the upper limit of the 95% CI for the composite cardiovascular outcome from the HEART 2D trial is 1.21, suggests that prandial insulin is noninferior to basal insulin. Taken together, these 3 trials very strongly support the conclusion that insulin has a neutral effect on cardiovascular and other serious health outcomes.

Metformin and Sulfonylureas

Metformin and a variety of sulfonylureas have been available for treating diabetes for more than 50 years. It is noteworthy, therefore, that no dedicated large outcomes trials have been conducted to ascertain whether either metformin or the various sulfonylurea agents have cardiovascular effects that are independent of their glucose-lowering effects in ambulatory settings. Indeed, the best information currently comes from the trials of more versus less intense glucose lowering, in which people allocated to the more intense glucose-lowering group used more of these agents than those allocated to the less intense glucose-lowering group.

The major source of information regarding metformin comes from the United Kingdom Prospective Diabetes Study[31] in which 753 overweight people (mean age 53 years; 53% women, and mean body mass index of 32 kg/m^2) with newly diagnosed diabetes who were overweight were randomized to an intensive metformin-based glucose-lowering policy (n = 342) versus a conventional, diet-based glucose-lowering policy (n = 411) with diet standard approaches to glucose lowering. During a median

Table 2
Hazard ratios (95% confidence intervals) for the effect of the interventions on cardiovascular outcomes

| Outcomes Trial | Primary | Other Key Cardiovascular Outcomes | | | | |
Acronym	Composite	CV Death	Nonfatal MI	Nonfatal Stroke	Heart Failure	Death
NAVIGATOR	0.94 (0.82–1.09)	1.07 (0.83–1.38)	0.95 (0.75–1.20)[a]	0.89 (0.69–1.15)[a]	0.85 (0.64–1.14)	1.00 (0.85–1.17)
HEART 2D	0.98 (0.80–1.21)	1.05 (0.69–1.60)	1.01 (0.45–1.60)[b]	1.21 (0.62–2.35)	0.90 (0.56–1.44)	1.00 (0.68–1.48)
ORIGIN	1.02 (0.94–1.11)	1.00 (0.89–1.13)	1.02 (0.88–1.19)[a]	1.03 (0.89–1.21)[a]	0.90 (0.77–1.05)	0.98 (0.90–1.08)
DEVOTE	0.91 (0.78–1.06)	0.96 (0.69–1.20)	0.85 (0.68–1.06)[c]	0.90 (0.65–1.23)	N/A	0.91 (0.76–1.11)
PROACTIVE	0.90 (0.80–1.02)	N/A (NS)	0.83 (0.65–1.06)[c]	0.81 (0.61–1.07)[a]	N/A (NS)	0.96 (0.78–1.18)
IRIS	0.76 (0.62–0.93)	N/A	0.75 (0.52–1.07)[a]	0.82 (0.61–1.10)[a]	N/A (NS)	0.93 (0.73–1.17)
EXAMINE	0.96 (≤1.16)	0.85 (0.66–1.10)	1.08 (0.88–1.33)	0.91 (0.55–1.50)	N/A (NS)	0.88 (0.71–1.09)
TECOS	0.98 (0.89–1.08)	1.03 (0.89–1.19)	0.95 (0.81–1.11)[a]	0.97 (0.79–1.19)[a]	1.00 (0.83–1.20)	1.01 (0.90–1.14)
SAVOR	1.00 (0.89–1.12)	1.03 (0.87–1.22)	0.95 (0.80–1.12)[a]	1.11 (0.88–1.39)[a]	1.27 (1.07–1.51)	1.11 (0.96–1.27)
ELIXA	1.02 (0.89–1.17)	0.98 (0.78–1.22)	1.03 (0.87–1.22)[a]	1.12 (0.79–1.58)[a]	0.96 (0.75–1.23)	0.94 (0.78–1.13)
LEADER	0.87 (0.78–0.97)	0.78 (0.66–0.93)	0.88 (0.75–1.03)	0.89 (0.72–1.11)	0.87 (0.73–1.05)	0.85 (0.74–0.97)
SUSTAIN 6	0.74 (0.58–0.95)	0.98 (0.65–1.48)	0.74 (0.51–1.08)	0.61 (0.38–0.99)	1.11 (0.77–1.61)	1.05 (0.74–1.05)
EMPA-REG	0.86 (0.74–0.99)	0.62 (0.49–0.77)	0.87 (0.70–1.09)[b]	1.24 (0.92–1.67)	0.65 (0.50–0.85)	0.68 (0.57–0.82)
CANVAS	0.86 (0.75–0.97)	0.87 (0.72–1.06)	0.85 (0.69–1.05)[b]	0.90 (0.71–1.15)	0.67 (0.52–0.87)	0.87 (0.74–0.77)

Abbreviations: CV, cardiovascular; MI, myocardial infarction; N/A, not available; NS, no significant effect.
[a] Includes fatal MI or stroke.
[b] Excludes silent MI.
[c] Includes silent MI.

Table 3
HRs for the effect of the interventions on cardiovascular outcomes in specific subgroups

Outcomes Trial	Age		Sex		Prior CVD		Glycemia	
Acronym	Group	HR (95% CI)	Group	HR (95% CI)	Group	HR (95% CI)	Group	HR (95% CI)
NAVIGATOR	<60	1.01 (0.74–1.37)	M	0.90 (0.75–1.07)	Yes	0.89 (0.72–1.09)	FG ≤ med	0.96 (0.79–1.17)
	60–67	1.05 (0.81–1.36)	F	1.05 (0.82–1.33)	No	1.00 (0.82–1.22)	FG > med	0.92 (0.75–1.14)
	>67	0.87 (0.71–1.07)	N/A	N/A	N/A	N/A	N/A	N/A
HEART 2D	≤67.4	1.24 (0.95–1.63)[a]	N/A	N/A	N/A	N/A	N/A	N/A
	>67.4	0.69 (0.49–0.96)[a]	N/A	N/A	N/A	N/A	N/A	N/A
ORIGIN	<65	1.06 (0.93–1.21)	M	0.98 (0.89–1.09)	Yes	0.97 (0.87–1.07)	<6.4	1.11 (0.97–1.27)
	≥65	0.99 (0.88–1.11)	F	1.11 (0.94–1.31)[b]	No	1.17 (1.00–1.37)	≥6.4	0.95 (0.85–1.07)
DEVOTE	<65	0.84 (0.67–1.05)	M	0.99 (0.83–1.20)	Yes	0.89 (0.76–1.04)	<8.0	0.89 (0.70–1.13)
	≥65	0.97 (0.79–1.19)	F	0.76 (0.59–0.99)	No	1.03 (0.62–1.72)	≥8.0	0.91 (0.75–1.11)
IRIS	<65	0.73 (0.55–0.97)	M	0.81 (0.64–1.03)	Yes	0.70 (0.45–1.08)	<5.7	0.67 (0.47–0.95)
	≥65	0.79 (0.60–1.03)	F	0.65 (0.46–0.93)	No	0.77 (0.62–0.93)	≥5.7	0.81 (0.64–1.02)
EXAMINE	<65	0.91 (0.73–1.13)	M	1.02 (0.84–1.24)	Yes	1.01 (0.79–1.29)	<8.0	0.98 (0.78–1.22)
	≥65	0.98 (0.78–1.24)	F	0.87 (0.67–1.12)	No	0.91 (0.74–1.12)	≥8.0	0.93 (0.74–1.16)
TECOS	<65	0.95 (0.81–1.12)	M	0.99 (0.88–1.10)	N/A	N/A	≤med	0.95 (0.83–1.09)
	≥65	1.01 (0.90–1.15)	F	0.95 (0.78–1.15)	N/A	N/A	>med	1.00 (0.88–1.14)
SAVOR	<75	1.01 (0.89–1.15)	M	1.01 (0.89–1.16)	Yes	0.96 (0.86–1.09)	<7	1.01 (0.78–1.31)
	≥75	0.96 (0.75–1.22)	F	0.97 (0.78–1.20)	No	1.34 (0.95–1.90)	7–<8	0.98 (0.80–1.20)
	N/A	N/A	N/A	N/A	N/A	N/A	8–<9	1.09 (0.85–1.39)
	N/A	N/A	N/A	N/A	N/A	N/A	≥9	0.95 (0.77–1.18)

Trial	Age	HR (95% CI)	Sex	HR (95% CI)	Clinical	HR (95% CI)	A1c	HR (95% CI)
ELIXA	<65	1.10 (0.90–1.32)	M	0.95 (0.75–1.20)	NSTEMI	1.05 (0.77–1.25)	<7.5	1.05 (0.87–1.38)
	≥65	0.98 (0.80–1.25)	F	1.10 (0.90–1.30)	STEMI	0.90 (0.70–1.15)	≥7.5	0.98 (0.80–1.20)
	N/A	N/A	N/A	N/A	UA	1.20 (0.84–1.70)	N/A	N/A
LEADER	<60	0.78 (0.62–0.97)	M	0.86 (0.75–0.98)	Yes	0.83 (0.74–0.93)[d]	≤8.3	0.89 (0.76–1.05)
	≥60	0.90 (0.79–1.02)	F	0.88 (0.72–1.08)	No	1.20 (0.86–1.67)	>8.3	0.84 (0.72–0.98)
SUSTAIN 6	<65	0.74 (0.52–1.05)	M	0.68 (0.50–0.92)	Yes	0.72 (0.55–0.93)	≤8.5	0.72 (0.50–1.03)
	≥65	0.72 (0.51–1.02)	F	0.84 (0.54–1.31)	No	1.00 (0.41–2.46)	>8.5	0.74 (0.52–1.04)
EMPA-REG	<65	1.04 (0.89–1.29)[c]	M	0.87 (0.73–1.02)	CeVD	1.15 (0.74–1.78)	<8.5	0.76 (0.64–0.90)[c]
	≥65	0.71 (0.59–0.87)	F	0.83 (0.62–1.11)	CAD	0.83 (0.68–1.02)	≥8.5	1.14 (0.86–1.50)
	N/A	N/A	N/A	N/A	PAD	0.94 (0.47–1.88)	N/A	N/A
CANVAS	<65	0.91 (0.76–1.10)	M	0.86 (0.74–1.00)	Yes	0.82 (0.72–0.95)	<8.0	0.94 (0.77–1.15)
	≥65	0.80 (0.67–0.95)	F	0.84 (0.66–1.06)	No	0.98 (0.74–1.30)	≥8.0	0.80 (0.68–0.94)

For the ELIXA trial's subgroups, the numbers are estimated from a figure in the paper's appendix. Subgroup analyses were not provided by the PROACTIVE trial, although the paper reports no interaction in any of 25 subgroups assessed. Unless otherwise specified, there were no interactions between the intervention and subgroup (ie, the nominal *P* value for the interaction term was >.05), and glycemia is presented as hemoglobin A1c levels.

Abbreviations: CAD, coronary artery disease; CeVD, cerebrovascular disease; CI, confidence interval; CVD, cardiovascular disease; F, female; FG, fasting plasma glucose; HR, hazard ratio; M, male; med, median; N/A, not available; NS, not significant; NSTEMI, non–ST elevation myocardial infarction; PAD, peripheral artery disease; STEMI, ST elevation myocardial infarction; UA, unstable angina.

[a] Interaction tests were not reported.
[b] *P* (interaction) = .05.
[c] *P* (interaction) = .01.
[d] *P* (interaction) = .04.

follow-up period of 10.7 years, the incidence of a diabetes-related endpoint and all-cause mortality in the control group was 4.3% and 2.1% per year, respectively, and the hazard for these outcomes in people allocated to metformin-based glucose lowering was 0.68 (95% CI–0.53, 0.87) and 0.64 (95% CI–0.45, 0.91), respectively.

Similarly, in the major portion of the UKPDS trial (UK Prospective Diabetes Study)[19] and in the ADVANCE trial (Action in Diabetes and Vascular Disease: Preterax and Diamicron Controlled Evaluation)[21] of people with established type 2 diabetes and other cardiovascular risk factors, individuals allocated to the more intense glucose-lowering group were prescribed sulfonylureas in addition to other glucose-lowering drugs. As noted, however, the results of these trials cannot be used to draw any conclusions about the nonglycemic cardiovascular effects of these drugs.

Notably, 2 ongoing trials will together provide important information regarding the cardiovascular effects of the sulfonylurea glimepiride. One trial is testing the effect of linagliptin versus glimepiride in 6041 people with type 2 diabetes and other cardiovascular risk factors,[32] and the other is testing the cardiovascular effect of linagliptin versus placebo in a similar population of more than 8000 individuals (NCT01897532). If linagliptin is shown to be equivalent to placebo and either superior or inferior to glimepiride, it may be possible to draw clear conclusions regarding the cardiovascular effects of the sulfonylurea glimepiride.

Thiazolidinediones

Rosiglitazone and pioglitazone are TZDs that bind to the peroxisome proliferator–activated gamma receptors located and expressed on adipocytes as well as a variety of other tissues. These drugs have multiple effects, including a reduction in glucose, insulin resistance, insulin levels, free fatty acid levels, blood pressure, urinary albumin excretion, visceral fat, hemoglobin, and inflammation, and an increase in adiponectin, weight, fluid retention, pulmonary edema, and fractures.[33–35] They also both dramatically reduce the incidence of diabetes.[36,37] Whereas many of these effects suggested that they may be cardioprotective, other effects highlighted possible hazards and the importance of conducting large randomized trials to explicitly test their overall risks versus benefits.[38]

Rosiglitazone was assessed in 4447 people (mean age 58 years; 48% women) on either a sulfonylurea or metformin in the RECORD trial (Rosiglitazone Evaluated for Cardiovascular Outcomes and Regulation of Glycemia in Diabetes).[39] Participants were allocated to either open-label rosiglitazone (up to 8 mg/d) or a combination of metformin (up to 2550 mg/d) and a sulfonylurea. During a mean follow-up of 5.5 years, the incidence of the composite primary outcome of cardiovascular death or cardiovascular hospitalization in the control group was an estimated 2.6% per year with no difference between groups (hazard ratio [HR] 0.99; 95% CI, 0.85–1.16), but with a 2-fold higher hazard of heart failure (from a control rate of approximately 0.24% per year) and an increase in fractures (particularly in women). Widely publicized concerns that rosiglitazone actually increased myocardial infarctions and cardiovascular death (that were based on epidemiologic analyses and metaanalyses of trials with few events[40]) led to intense scrutiny of all of this trial's events and its reanalysis, which subsequently validated the findings.[41] Unfortunately, these same concerns also led to the premature cessation of an ongoing blinded, 16,000-person cardiovascular outcomes trial of people with diabetes who were being allocated randomly to rosiglitazone, pioglitazone, or placebo.[42,43]

Pioglitazone was assessed in 2 placebo-controlled outcomes trials. The PROACTIVE (Prospective Pioglitazone Clinical Trial in Macrovascular Events) trial was conducted in people with diabetes and either a recent myocardial infarction, acute coronary syndrome, stroke, revascularization, or anatomic evidence of cardiovascular disease. A total of 5238 people (mean age 62 years; 34% women) were allocated to either pioglitazone (up to 45 mg/d) or placebo and followed for a mean of 2.9 years, during which the incidence of the composite primary outcome of all-cause mortality, nonfatal myocardial infarction (including silent myocardial infarction), stroke, acute coronary syndrome, endovascular or surgical intervention on the coronary or leg arteries, or amputation above the ankle was an estimated 7.5% per year. Pioglitazone had a neutral effect on this endpoint (HR, 0.90; 95% CI, 0.80–1.02), but modestly reduced the secondary endpoint of all-cause death, nonfatal myocardial infarction, or stroke (HR, 0.84; 95% CI, 0.72–0.98). It also increased the risk of heart failure requiring hospitalization by approximately 50% from an estimated placebo rate of 1.4% per year.

The IRIS trial (Insulin Resistance Intervention after Stroke) was conducted in people with biochemical evidence of insulin resistance without diabetes (of whom 76% had a fasting glucose of ≥5.6 mmol/L or an HbA1c of ≥5.7%) who had an ischemic stroke or a transient ischemic attack within 6 months of randomization. A total of 3876 people (mean age 64 years; 35% women) were allocated to either pioglitazone (up to 45 mg/d) or placebo. During a median follow-up of 4.8 years, the incidence of the composite primary outcome of fatal or nonfatal myocardial infarction or stroke in controls was an estimated 2.5% per year. Pioglitazone reduced the hazard of this endpoint (HR, 0.76; 95% CI, 0.62–0.93).

Meglitinides

Nateglinide and replaglinide are short-acting insulin secretagogues. Whereas the cardiovascular effect of neither one has been assessed in people with diabetes, nateglinide was assessed in 9306 people (mean age 64 years; 51% women) in the NAVIGATOR trial (Nateglinide and Valsartan in Impaired Glucose Tolerance Outcomes Research).[44] Participants with impaired glucose tolerance and additional cardiovascular risk factors were allocated randomly to receive either nateglinide (60 mg 3 times per day) or matching placebo. During a median follow-up period of 5.0 years, the incidence of the composite primary outcome of cardiovascular death, myocardial infarction, stroke, or heart failure requiring hospitalization in the control group was 1.4% per year, and the hazard for this outcome in people allocated to nateglinide versus placebo was 0.94 (95% CI, 0.82–1.09).

Glucagon-Like Peptide 1 Receptor Agonists

Glucagon-like peptide 1 (GLP1) is a hormone secreted by the L-cells of the distal ileum that increases pancreatic insulin secretion in response to glucose elevation, slows gastric emptying, increases satiety, reduces weight, and suppresses pancreatic glucagon levels.[45,46] As endogenous GLP1 has a short half-life, analogues of this hormone have been created that resist degradation by the dipeptidyl peptidase 4 (DPP4) enzyme.[47] The GLP1 properties as noted plus evidence that these drugs have antiarrhythmic, blood pressure–lowering, antiinflammatory, diuretic and, other cardiovascular properties are consistent with cardioprotective effects,[46] and 3 of these drugs have been tested in large cardiovascular outcomes trials.

Lixisenatide was assessed in 6068 people (mean age 60 years; 30% women) at very high risk for a cardiovascular event in the ELIXA (Evaluation of Lixisenatide in Acute Coronary Syndrome) Trial.[48] Participants with type 2 diabetes and acute coronary syndrome within the prior 180 days were allocated randomly to receive a once daily injection of either lixisenatide (up to 20 μg/d) or placebo. During a median follow-up period of 2.1 years, the incidence of the composite primary outcome of cardiovascular death, myocardial infarction, stroke, or hospitalization for unstable angina in the control group was 6.3% per year, and the hazard for this outcome in people allocated to lixisenatide versus placebo was 1.02 (95% CI, 0.89–1.17).

Liraglutide was assessed in 9340 people (mean age 64 years; 36% women) at high risk for a cardiovascular event in the LEADER trial (Liraglutide Effect and Action in Diabetes: Evaluation of cardiovascular outcome Results).[49] Participants with type 2 diabetes (81% with prior cardiovascular disease) were allocated randomly to receive a once-daily injection of either liraglutide (up to 1.8 mg/d) or placebo. During a median follow-up period of 3.8 years, the incidence of the composite primary outcome of cardiovascular death, myocardial infarction, or stroke in the control group was 3.9% per year, and the hazard for this outcome in people allocated to liraglutide versus placebo was 0.87 (95% CI, 0.78–0.97). Moreover, liraglutide significantly reduced the expanded composite outcome that included the primary outcome plus either coronary revascularization or hospitalization for heart failure or unstable angina (HR, 0.88; 95% CI, 0.81–0.96). The observed effect on other secondary outcomes is noted in **Table 2**.

Semaglutide is a biochemically similar GLP1 receptor that can be given once weekly. Its cardiovascular effects were assessed in the SUSTAIN-6 trial (Trial to Evaluate Cardiovascular and Other Long-term Outcomes with Semaglutide in Subjects with Type 2 Diabetes) of 3297 people with type 2 diabetes (mean age 65 years; 39% women; 83% with prior cardiovascular disease). Participants were randomly allocated to receive 5 or 10 mg of semaglutide (5 or 10 mg/wk) or placebo. During a mean follow-up of 2.1 years, the incidence of the composite primary outcome of cardiovascular death, myocardial infarction, or stroke in the control group was 4.4% per year, and the hazard for this outcome in people allocated to semaglutide (doses combined) versus placebo was 0.74 (95% CI, 0.58–0.95). The observed effect on secondary outcomes is noted in **Table 2**.

The absence of a clear cardiovascular benefit of lixisenatide in light of the benefits of liraglutide and semaglutide remains unknown and highlights the importance of requiring evidence for each drug being tested, rather than assigning a "class effect" to all similar drugs. The difference may be owing to the different populations studied (acute coronary syndrome vs high risk for events), differences in the cardiovascular effect of exendin-based analogues like lixisenatide versus human-based analogues, or other unmeasured factors.

Dipeptidyl Peptidase Inhibitors

Endogenous GLP1 has a very short half-life and is inactivated through the actions of the DPP4 enzyme. DPP4 inhibitor drugs share the ability to inhibit the activity of this enzyme, and thereby prolong the half-life and clinical effect of endogenous GLP1. The effect of DPP4 inhibitors on cardiovascular outcomes has been studied in individuals at high risk for cardiovascular events who have had recent acute coronary syndrome, in individuals with evidence of cardiovascular disease, and in individuals with either a prior cardiovascular event or cardiovascular risk factors. The results are summarized in **Table 2**.

Alogliptin was assessed in 5380 people (mean age 61 years; 32% women) at very high risk for a cardiovascular event in the EXAMINE trial (Examination of Cardiovascular Outcomes with Alogliptin versus Standard of Care).[50] Participants with type 2 diabetes and acute coronary syndrome within the prior 15 to 90 days were allocated randomly to receive either alogliptin (25 mg/d) or matching placebo. During a median follow-up period of 1.5 years, the incidence of the composite primary outcome of cardiovascular death, myocardial infarction, or stroke in the control group was approximately 7.9% per year, and the hazard for this outcome in people allocated to alogliptin versus placebo was 0.96 with an upper bound of a 97.5% CI of 1.16 (ie, establishing noninferiority).

Sitagliptin was assessed in 14,671 people (mean age 66 years; 29% women) at high risk for a cardiovascular event in TECOS (Trial Evaluating Cardiovascular Outcomes with Sitagliptin).[51] Participants with type 2 diabetes and established coronary artery, cerebrovascular, and/or peripheral vascular disease were randomly allocated to receive either sitagliptin (100 mg/d) or matching placebo. During a median follow-up period of 3.0 years, the incidence of the composite primary outcome of cardiovascular death, myocardial infarction, stroke, or unstable angina requiring hospitalization in the control group was 3.8% per year, and the hazard for this outcome in people allocated to sitagliptin versus placebo was 0.98 (95% CI, 0.88–1.09).

Saxagliptin was assessed in 16,492 people (mean age 65 years; 33% women) with a lower prevalence of established cardiovascular disease in the SAVOR trial (Saxagliptin Assessment of Vascular Outcomes Recorded in Patients with Diabetes Mellitus).[52] Participants with type 2 diabetes and either established cardiovascular disease (79%) or who were at least age 55 years of age (men) or 60 years of age (women) with either dyslipidemia, hypertension, or active smoking were randomly allocated to receive either saxagliptin (5 mg/d) or matching placebo. During a median follow-up period of 2.1 years, the incidence of the composite primary outcome of cardiovascular death, myocardial infarction, or ischemic stroke was 3.7% per year, and the hazard for this outcome in people allocated to saxagliptin versus placebo was 1.00 (95% CI, 0.89–1.12).

Saxagliptin's effect on the SAVOR trial's secondary outcomes has been the focus of particular scrutiny. As noted in the protocol, if saxagliptin was shown to reduce the primary outcome, its effect on the secondary outcome that was to be tested first was a composite of the primary outcome, hospitalization for heart failure, coronary revascularization, or hospitalization for unstable angina. The effect on the all-cause mortality was to be tested next.[52] No testing order was prespecified for the other efficacy outcomes that comprised the 6 individual components of the primary and secondary outcomes plus 7 other outcomes (for a total of 13). In light of this testing strategy, saxagliptin's neutral effect on the primary outcome precluded formal testing of its effect on any of the subsequent outcomes, but permits estimates of its effect for these outcomes. Not surprisingly, the HRs for its effect on the composite secondary outcome and mortality were 1.02 (95% CI, 0.94–1.11) and 1.11 (95% CI, 0.96–1.27), respectively. What was unexpected was the estimated HR of 1.27 (95% CI, 1.07–1.51) for the heart failure component of the secondary outcome. Whereas the statistical significance of this observation could not strictly be assessed (owing to the possibility of a type 1 error, as noted), whether it reflects a true effect of the drug on heart failure or a spurious finding is controversial. There is no question that it advanced a hypothesis regarding the effects of the drug on heart failure. Arguments suggesting that it may have been a chance finding include the absence of an imbalance in heart failure death in SAVOR, and the absence of a heart failure signal in the TECOS trial of another DPP4 inhibitor. Moreover, assuming that the 15 statistical tests (2 for the secondary outcomes and 13 for the other outcomes, including heart failure hospitalization) were independent, there was a 54% probability that this finding would have been significant at a nominal alpha level of 0.05 (ie, $[1-(1-0.05)]^{15}$), and a 10% chance it would have been significant at a nominal level of 0.007. No consensus on this question has been reached as of the time of this publication.[53]

Sodium-Glucose Linked Cotransporter 2 Inhibitors

Sodium-glucose linked cotransporter 2 (SGLT2) on the proximal convoluted tubule of the kidney normally reabsorbs 90% of the glucose from the glomerular filtrate along with sodium. SGLT2 inhibitors are molecules that can block this effect, resulting in a lowering of the renal threshold for glucose excretion to normal (ie, physiologic) levels and insulin-independent lowering of glucose levels.[53,54] As such, it acts as an osmotic diuretic. Additional effects (including modest reductions in blood pressure, weight, uric acid, and arterial stiffness; modest increases in hematocrit, glucagon, and ketone body levels; and renal protective effects including reduced glomerular filtration) suggest that it may have cardioprotective effects.[54–57] To date, 2 SGLT2 inhibitor cardiovascular outcomes trials have been reported.

Empagliflozin was assessed in 7020 people (mean age 63 years; 29% women) at high risk for a cardiovascular event in the EMPA REG outcomes trial (Empagliflozin, Cardiovascular Outcomes, and Mortality in Type 2 Diabetes).[58] Participants with type 2 diabetes and established cardiovascular disease were allocated randomly to receive empagliflozin (either 10 or 25 mg) or placebo in a 1:1:1 ratio. During a median follow-up period of 3.1 years, the incidence of the composite primary outcome of cardiovascular death, myocardial infarction, or stroke was 4.4% per year in the placebo group, and the hazard for this outcome in people allocated to empagliflozin (both groups combined) versus placebo was 0.86 (95% CI, 0.74–0.99). Notable for this trial was the observation that there may have been statistical heterogeneity in the 3 components of the primary outcome with a marked effect on cardiovascular death (HR, 0.62, 95% CI, 0.49–0.77) versus nonfatal myocardial infarction or stroke with HRs of 0.87 (95% CI, 0.70–1.09) and 1.24 (95% CI, 0.92–1.67), respectively.

Canagliflozin was assessed in 10,142 people (mean age 63 years; 36% women) at high risk for a cardiovascular event in the CANVAS trial (Canagliflozin Cardiovascular Assessment Study) program.[59] Participants with type 2 diabetes and established cardiovascular disease were allocated randomly to receive canagliflozin (either 100 or 300 mg) or placebo, with 1443 allocated to 300 mg. During a median follow-up period of 2.4 years the incidence of the composite primary outcome of cardiovascular death, myocardial infarction, or stroke in people allocated to placebo was 3.2% per year, and the hazard for this outcome in people allocated to canagliflozin (both doses combined) versus placebo was 0.86 (95% CI, 0.75–0.97). This trial also reported a doubling of the risk of amputations from 0.3% per year for placebo to 0.6% per year for canagliflozin, and an increase in volume depletion from 1.9% per year to 2.6% per year. Although not clearly seen in the EMPA REG outcomes trial, whether these safety signals are chance findings, specific to canagliflozin only or a property of SGLT2 inhibitors in general remains unclear. Unfortunately, data from the ongoing CANVAS trial were disclosed publicly in 2012, 3 years after the trial began.[59,60] This raises the possibility that the subsequent conduct of the trial and management of its participants may have changed in unexplained ways as a result of this disclosure and these changes may have affected the results in unmeasured and unanticipated ways.

The CANVAS program results are generally consistent with the results of the EMPA REG outcomes trial. Taken together, these 2 large trials strongly support the conclusion that SGLT2 inhibitors modestly reduce the composite cardiovascular outcome, while clearly reducing hospitalizations for heart failure and the progression of renal disease to a much greater and consistent extent. The time course during which these effects are evident in both these trials also suggest that the effect is fairly rapid and is mediated through renal and hemodynamic mechanisms rather than vascular remodeling or atherosclerosis. At the same time, the effect of these drugs on volume status highlights the importance of counseling individuals to temporarily stop the drug during intercurrent illnesses that cause volume depletion.

Table 4			
Ongoing cardiovascular outcomes trials of glucose-lowering drugs			
Drug Class	**Drug Being Tested**	**Outcomes Trial Acronym**	**Estimated n**
SGLT2 inhibitor	Dapagliflozin vs placebo	DECLARE	17,150
	Canagliflozin vs placebo	CREDENCE	4200
	Ertugliflozin vs placebo	VERTIS CV	3900
DPP4i	Linagliptin vs glimepiride	CAROLINA	6041
	Linagliptin vs placebo	CARMELINA	8300
GLP1 RA	Dulaglutide vs placebo	REWIND	9901
	Albiglutide vs placebo	HARMONY Outcomes	9400

Abbreviations: DPP4i, dipeptidyl peptidase 4 inhibitor; GLP1 RA, glucagon-like peptide receptor agonist; SGLT2, Sodium-glucose linked cotransporter 2.

SUMMARY

As recently as 20 years ago, there were essentially no randomized controlled trials of potentially cardiovascular protective therapies in people with type 2 diabetes. When viewed from that perspective, the recruitment of 123,757 people in the foregoing trials and the discovery of at least 4 agents (empagliflozin, canagliflozin, liraglutide, and semaglutide) that have cardioprotective properties represents a truly remarkable addition to the evidence for cardiovascular protection in people with type 2 diabetes (see **Fig. 2**). Moreover, the ongoing cardiovascular trials that are expected to report within the next few years will add to this evidence (**Table 4**). There is no question that both the primary analyses of these trials and their many subsidiary analyses have transformed diabetes from a largely eminence based specialty to one that is firmly evidence based. They have also provided evidence in support of particular glucose-lowering drugs when patients present with additional cardiovascular risk factors. These trials have not, however, provided all of the answers and there is much more to learn and much more to do. For example, evidence that diabetes can be prevented and clues that it may be put into remission raise hope that we can perhaps eliminate all cardiovascular disease in people with diabetes by making the epidemic go away. This clearly remains an aspirational goal but one for which ongoing research continues.

In the meantime, randomized controlled trials such as those described here will continue to challenge assumptions and create new approaches and paradigms that can be pursued to reduce and hopefully eliminate serious cardiovascular and other consequences in people with diabetes.

REFERENCES

1. American Diabetes Association. 2. Classification and diagnosis of diabetes. Diabetes Care 2017;40:S11–24.
2. Sarwar N, Gao P, Seshasai SR, et al. Diabetes mellitus, fasting blood glucose concentration, and risk of vascular disease: a collaborative meta-analysis of 102 prospective studies. Lancet 2010;375:2215–22.
3. Shah AD, Langenberg C, Rapsomaniki E, et al. Type 2 diabetes and incidence of cardiovascular diseases: a cohort study in 1.9 million people. Lancet Diabetes Endocrinol 2015;3:105–13.
4. Seshasai SR, Kaptoge S, Thompson A, et al. Diabetes mellitus, fasting glucose, and risk of cause-specific death. N Engl J Med 2011;364:829–41.

5. Emerging Risk Factors Collaboration, Di Angelantonio E, Kaptoge S, Wormser D, et al. Association of cardiometabolic multimorbidity with mortality. JAMA 2015; 314:52–60.
6. Cavender MA, Steg PG, Smith SC Jr, et al. Impact of diabetes mellitus on hospitalization for heart failure, cardiovascular events, and death: outcomes at 4 years from the Reduction of Atherothrombosis for Continued Health (REACH) Registry. Circulation 2015;132:923–31.
7. Gregg EW, Li Y, Wang J, et al. Changes in diabetes-related complications in the United States, 1990-2010. N Engl J Med 2014;370:1514–23.
8. Di AE, Gao P, Khan H, et al. Glycated hemoglobin measurement and prediction of cardiovascular disease. JAMA 2014;311:1225–33.
9. Brunner EJ, Shipley MJ, Witte DR, et al. Relation between blood glucose and coronary mortality over 33 years in the Whitehall Study. Diabetes Care 2006;29: 26–31.
10. Matsushita K, Blecker S, Pazin-Filho A, et al. The association of hemoglobin a1c with incident heart failure among people without diabetes: the Atherosclerosis Risk in Communities study. Diabetes 2010;59:2020–6.
11. Selvin E, Steffes MW, Zhu H, et al. Glycated hemoglobin, diabetes, and cardiovascular risk in nondiabetic adults. N Engl J Med 2010;362:800–11.
12. Gerstein HC, Swedberg K, Carlsson J, et al. The hemoglobin A1c level as a progressive risk factor for cardiovascular death, hospitalization for heart failure, or death in patients with chronic heart failure: an analysis of the Candesartan in Heart failure: Assessment of Reduction in Mortality and Morbidity (CHARM) program. Arch Intern Med 2008;168:1699–704.
13. Khaw KT, Wareham N, Bingham S, et al. Association of hemoglobin A1c with cardiovascular disease and mortality in adults: the European Prospective Investigation into Cancer in Norfolk. Ann Intern Med 2004;141:413–20.
14. Lawes CM, Parag V, Bennett DA, et al. Blood glucose and risk of cardiovascular disease in the Asia Pacific region. Diabetes Care 2004;27:2836–42.
15. Lind M, Olsson M, Rosengren A, et al. The relationship between glycaemic control and heart failure in 83,021 patients with type 2 diabetes. Diabetologia 2012; 55:2946–53.
16. Selvin E, Wattanakit K, Steffes MW, et al. HbA1c and peripheral arterial disease in diabetes: the Atherosclerosis Risk in Communities study. Diabetes Care 2006;29: 877–82.
17. Tancredi M, Rosengren A, Svensson AM, et al. Excess mortality among persons with type 2 diabetes. N Engl J Med 2015;373:1720–32.
18. Turnbull FM, Abraira C, Anderson RJ, et al. Intensive glucose control and macrovascular outcomes in type 2 diabetes. Diabetologia 2009;52:2288–98.
19. UK Prospective Diabetes Study (UKPDS) Group. Intensive blood-glucose control with sulphonylureas or insulin compared with conventional treatment and risk of complications in patients with type 2 diabetes (UKPDS 33). Lancet 1998;352: 837–53.
20. Action to Control Cardiovascular Risk in Diabetes Study Group, Gerstein HC, Miller ME, Byington RP, et al. Effects of intensive glucose lowering in type 2 diabetes. N Engl J Med 2008;358:2545–59.
21. Patel A, Macmahon S, Chalmers J, et al. Intensive blood glucose control and vascular outcomes in patients with type 2 diabetes. N Engl J Med 2008;358: 2560–72.
22. Duckworth W, Abraira C, Moritz T, et al. Glucose control and vascular complications in veterans with type 2 diabetes. N Engl J Med 2009;360:129–39.

23. Lachin JM. Point: intensive glycemic control and mortality in ACCORD–a chance finding? Diabetes Care 2010;33:2719–21.

24. Riddle MC, Ambrosius WT, Brillon DJ, et al. Epidemiologic relationships between A1C and all-cause mortality during a median 3.4-year follow-up of glycemic treatment in the ACCORD trial. Diabetes Care 2010;33:983–90.

25. American Diabetes Association. 6. Glycemic targets. Diabetes Care 2017;40:S48–56.

26. Frye RL, August P, Brooks MM, et al. A randomized trial of therapies for type 2 diabetes and coronary artery disease. N Engl J Med 2009;360:2503–15.

27. Gerstein HC, Bosch J, Dagenais GR, et al. Basal insulin and cardiovascular and other outcomes in dysglycemia. N Engl J Med 2012;367:319–28.

28. Marso SP, McGuire DK, Zinman B, et al. Design of DEVOTE (Trial comparing cardiovascular safety of insulin degludec vs insulin glargine in patients with type 2 diabetes at high risk of cardiovascular events) - DEVOTE 1. Am Heart J 2016;179:175–83.

29. Marso SP, McGuire DK, Zinman B, et al. Efficacy and safety of degludec versus glargine in type 2 diabetes. N Engl J Med 2017;377(8):723–32.

30. Raz I, Wilson PW, Strojek K, et al. Effects of prandial versus fasting glycemia on cardiovascular outcomes in type 2 diabetes: the HEART2D trial. Diabetes Care 2009;32:381–6.

31. UKPDS Study Group. Effect of intensive blood glucose control with metformin on complications in overweight patients with type 2 diabetes (UKPDS 34). Lancet 1998;352:854–65.

32. Marx N, Rosenstock J, Kahn SE, et al. Design and baseline characteristics of the CARdiovascular outcome trial of LINAgliptin versus glimepiride in type 2 diabetes (CAROLINA(R)). Diab Vasc Dis Res 2015;12:164–74.

33. McGuire DK, Inzucchi SE. New drugs for the treatment of diabetes mellitus: part I: thiazolidinediones and their evolving cardiovascular implications. Circulation 2008;117:440–9.

34. Schwartz AV, Vittinghoff E, Margolis KL, et al. Intensive glycemic control and thiazolidinedione use: effects on cortical and trabecular bone at the radius and tibia. Calcif Tissue Int 2013;92:477–86.

35. Punthakee Z, Almeras N, Despres JP, et al. Impact of rosiglitazone on body composition, hepatic fat, fatty acids, adipokines and glucose in persons with impaired fasting glucose or impaired glucose tolerance: a sub-study of the DREAM trial. Diabet Med 2014;31(9):1086–92.

36. Gerstein HC, Yusuf S, Bosch J, et al. Effect of rosiglitazone on the frequency of diabetes in patients with impaired glucose tolerance or impaired fasting glucose: a randomised controlled trial. Lancet 2006;368:1096–105.

37. DeFronzo RA, Tripathy D, Schwenke DC, et al. Pioglitazone for diabetes prevention in impaired glucose tolerance. N Engl J Med 2011;364:1104–15.

38. Gerstein HC, Yusuf S. Clinical outcomes trials and the cardiovascular effects of thiazolidinediones: implications for the evaluation of antidiabetic drugs. Am Heart J 2010;160:1–2.

39. Home PD, Pocock SJ, Beck-Nielsen H, et al. Rosiglitazone evaluated for cardiovascular outcomes in oral agent combination therapy for type 2 diabetes (RECORD): a multicentre, randomised, open-label trial. Lancet 2009;373:2125–35.

40. Singh S, Loke YK, Furberg CD. Long-term risk of cardiovascular events with rosiglitazone: a meta-analysis. JAMA 2007;298:1189–95.

41. Mahaffey KW, Hafley G, Dickerson S, et al. Results of a reevaluation of cardiovascular outcomes in the RECORD trial. Am Heart J 2013;166:240–9.
42. Punthakee Z, Bosch J, Dagenais G, et al. Design, history and results of the thiazolidinedione intervention with vitamin D evaluation (TIDE) randomised controlled trial. Diabetologia 2012;55:36–45.
43. Punthakee Z, Bosch J, Gerstein HC. Setting the record straight on TIDE: a lost opportunity for patients with diabetes. Diabetologia 2013;56(9):1884–7.
44. Holman RR, Haffner SM, McMurray JJ, et al. Effect of nateglinide on the incidence of diabetes and cardiovascular events. N Engl J Med 2010;362:1463–76.
45. Nauck MA, Meier JJ. The incretin effect in healthy individuals and those with type 2 diabetes: physiology, pathophysiology, and response to therapeutic interventions. Lancet Diabetes Endocrinol 2016;4:525–36.
46. Drucker DJ. The cardiovascular biology of glucagon-like peptide-1. Cell Metab 2016;24:15–30.
47. Meier JJ. GLP-1 receptor agonists for individualized treatment of type 2 diabetes mellitus. Nat Rev Endocrinol 2012;8:728–42.
48. Pfeffer MA, Claggett B, Diaz R, et al. Lixisenatide in patients with type 2 diabetes and acute coronary syndrome. N Engl J Med 2015;373:2247–57.
49. Marso SP, Daniels GH, Brown-Frandsen K, et al. Liraglutide and cardiovascular outcomes in type 2 diabetes. N Engl J Med 2016;375:311–22.
50. White WB, Cannon CP, Heller SR, et al. Alogliptin after acute coronary syndrome in patients with type 2 diabetes. N Engl J Med 2013;369:1327–35.
51. Green JB, Bethel MA, Armstrong PW, et al. Effect of sitagliptin on cardiovascular outcomes in type 2 diabetes. N Engl J Med 2015;373:232–42.
52. Scirica BM, Bhatt DL, Braunwald E, et al. Saxagliptin and cardiovascular outcomes in patients with type 2 diabetes mellitus. N Engl J Med 2013;369:1317–26.
53. Zaccardi F, Webb DR, Htike ZZ, et al. Efficacy and safety of sodium-glucose cotransporter-2 inhibitors in type 2 diabetes mellitus: systematic review and network meta-analysis. Diabetes Obes Metab 2016;18:783–94.
54. Monica Reddy RP, Inzucchi SE. SGLT2 inhibitors in the management of type 2 diabetes. Endocrine 2016;53:364–72.
55. Skrtic M, Cherney DZ. Sodium-glucose cotransporter-2 inhibition and the potential for renal protection in diabetic nephropathy. Curr Opin Nephrol Hypertens 2015;24:96–103.
56. Ferrannini E, Mark M, Mayoux E. CV protection in the EMPA-REG OUTCOME Trial: a "Thrifty Substrate" Hypothesis. Diabetes Care 2016;39:1108–14.
57. Mudaliar S, Alloju S, Henry RR. Can a shift in fuel energetics explain the beneficial cardiorenal outcomes in the EMPA-REG OUTCOME Study? A unifying hypothesis. Diabetes Care 2016;39:1115–22.
58. Zinman B, Wanner C, Lachin JM, et al. Empagliflozin, cardiovascular outcomes, and mortality in type 2 diabetes. N Engl J Med 2015;373:2117–28.
59. Neal B, Perkovic V, Mahaffey KW, et al. Canagliflozin and cardiovascular and renal events in type 2 diabetes. N Engl J Med 2017;377(7):644–57.
60. Neal B, Perkovic V, de Zeeuw D, et al. Rationale, design, and baseline characteristics of the canagliflozin cardiovascular assessment study (CANVAS)–a randomized placebo-controlled trial. Am Heart J 2013;166:217–23.e11.

Heart Failure

Epidemiology, Pathophysiology, and Management of Heart Failure in Diabetes Mellitus

Anders Jorsal, BSc, MD, PhD[a,b], Henrik Wiggers, BSc, MD, PhD, DMSc[a,b], John J.V. McMurray, MD, FRCP, FESC, FMedSci, FRSE[c,d],*

KEYWORDS

- Cardiac function • Cardiovascular events • Glucose lowering therapy • Glycemia
- Heart failure • Type 2 diabetes mellitus

KEY POINTS

- Heart failure is a common comorbidity in diabetes and patients with both conditions have a particularly poor prognosis.
- Most clinical outcome trials investigating the effects of glucose-lowering agents have excluded patients with heart failure.
- Glitazones and, possibly, some dipeptidyl peptidase-4 inhibitors, cause an increased risk of developing heart failure and deterioration in existing heart failure.
- One class of drugs, the sodium glucose cotransporter 2 inhibitors, reduce the risk of developing heart failure.

Disclosure Statement: A. Jorsal has served as a consultant for, and received lecture fees from, Novo Nordisk. H. Wiggers has been principal investigator or subinvestigator in studies involving the following pharmaceutical companies: MSD, Bayer, Daiichi-Sankyo, Novartis, Novo Nordisk, Sanofi-Aventis, and Pfizer. J.J.V. McMurray's employer has been paid for his role on executive/steering committees, data monitoring committees, and/or endpoint committees of trials funded by Abbvie, Amgen, AstraZeneca, Bayer, BMS, Cardiorentis, DalCor, GSK, Kidney Research UK, Merck, Oxford University, Pfizer, Resverlogix, Stealth Biotherapeutics, and Theracos.

[a] Department of Cardiology, Aarhus University Hospital, Palle Juul-Jensens Boulevard 99, 8200 Aarhus N, Denmark; [b] Department of Clinical Medicine, Aarhus University, Incuba Skejby, Building 2, Palle Juul-Jensens Boulevard 82, 8200 Aarhus N, Denmark; [c] BHF Cardiovascular Research Centre, Institute of Cardiovascular and Medical Sciences, University of Glasgow, 126 University Place, Glasgow G12 8TA, UK; [d] Queen Elizabeth University Hospital, 1345 Govan Road, Glasgow G51 4TF, UK
* Corresponding author. BHF Cardiovascular Research Centre, Institute of Cardiovascular and Medical Sciences, University of Glasgow, 126 University Place, Glasgow G12 8TA, UK.
E-mail address: JOHN.MCMURRAY@GLASGOW.AC.UK

Endocrinol Metab Clin N Am 47 (2018) 117–135
https://doi.org/10.1016/j.ecl.2017.10.007
0889-8529/18/

HEART FAILURE SYNDROME

Heart failure is a clinical syndrome characterized by symptoms and signs caused by structural or functional abnormalities of the heart. Typical symptoms are breathlessness, ankle swelling, and fatigue. Typical signs are increased jugular venous pressure, third heart sound, peripheral edema, and pulmonary crackles; however, the condition can be present in the absence of these findings. It is important to address the underlying cause of heart failure, because the specific etiology determines the choice of treatment. Common causes of heart failure are ischemic heart disease, dilated cardiomyopathies, valvular lesions, atrial fibrillation, and hypertension. The toxic impact of chemotherapy and high levels of alcohol consumption can also lead to systolic left ventricular failure.[1,2] Diabetes accelerates atherosclerosis and often leads to hypertension, but it is still debated whether diabetes causes a specific cardiomyopathy. Some data suggest that type 2 diabetes and hyperinsulinemia promote a "diabetic cardiomyopathy."[3]

The management of cardiovascular disease has undergone much change in recent years in general; notably, recent advances in the management of acute coronary syndromes have significantly reduced both short-term and long-term mortality.[4] This factor has led to increased survival, and thus, it could be argued, an increasing number of individuals with myocardial damage at risk of developing heart failure. The medical and device treatment of patients with established heart failure has also improved considerably, reducing both morbidity and mortality.[5–8] Both changes are thought to have led to an increase in prevalence of heart failure. Thus, heart failure has become one of the most common cardiovascular diseases in the Western world. Epidemiologic data show a prevalence of heart failure of 2%; among individuals older than 75 years, nearly 10% suffer from heart failure.[9] Notably, the prevalence is even higher in patients with diabetes.[10,11] Conversely, the prevalence of diabetes is very high in patients with heart failure with estimates of up to 40% in patients hospitalized with worsening symptoms.[12,13]

EPIDEMIOLOGY OF HEART FAILURE AND DIABETES

Compared with other cardiovascular events, observational data reveal a frequent occurrence of heart failure in patients with diabetes.[14,15] The *incidence* of hospital admission for heart failure in 65,619 patients with type 2 diabetes treated with insulin exceeded both myocardial infarction and stroke.[16] Heart failure also seems to be the most common complication in several clinical outcome trials, especially in patients with diabetes and nephropathy.[17,18] This circumstance is emphasized by the Irbesartan Diabetic Nephropathy Trial, in which hospitalization for heart failure was the most frequent cardiovascular event, despite exclusion of patients with heart failure at baseline.[17] The *prevalence* of heart failure in individuals with diabetes is also high, with 1 estimate of approximately 12%.[10] Furthermore, heart failure in diabetes is associated with very poor outcomes and very high health care expenses.[11,19] Once heart failure develops in individuals with diabetes mellitus, the outlook is grim, with as much as a 10-fold higher mortality, compared with people with diabetes without heart failure, and a 5-year survival rate of only 12.5%.[11] Although more recent data have shown a better prognosis with a 3-year mortality of 40%,[20] these findings highlight the clinical importance of the combination of heart failure and diabetes. Fortunately, the response to therapy for heart failure is similar in patients with and without diabetes,[21,22] and is standardized in evidence-based international guidelines.[1,2]

MANAGEMENT OF DIABETES MELLITUS IN HEART FAILURE

Although observational data suggest an association between lower glucose and less risk of macrovascular disease, randomized controlled trial data are generally not supportive.[23] For example, the UK Prospective Diabetes Study (UKPDS), which studied patients with newly diagnosed diabetes, showed a 16% lower risk of heart failure per 1% absolute lower hemoglobin A1c level.[24] Conversely, large-scale randomized controlled trials investigating the effect of more versus less intensive glycemic control, including the ACCORD (Action to Control Cardiovascular Risk in Diabetes), the ADVANCE (Action in Diabetes and Vascular Disease: Preterax and Diamicron Modified Release Controlled Evaluation), and the VADT (Veterans Affairs Diabetes Trial), did not report a reduced risk of heart failure,[25–27] and neither did extended follow-up of VADT show a reduction in new or worsening heart failure.[28] Indeed, some glucose-reducing agents are associated with either an increased risk of developing heart failure or caused further deterioration of existing heart failure.[29] This is a major concern, especially in light of the absence of hospital admissions for heart failure as a prespecified component of primary composite cardiovascular outcomes in most large-scale trials investigating glucose-lowering agents. Furthermore, the optimal level of glycemic control in heart failure is uncertain, with some evidence suggesting that tight glycemic control may be associated with poorer outcomes in heart failure, possibly because of a cardiovascular risk related to hypoglycemia.[30] Thus, how best to achieve glycemic control in patients with diabetes and heart failure remains an important and yet unanswered clinical question. We summarize the main findings from key clinical outcome trials, and discuss the potential mechanisms of benefit and harm of different glucose-lowering agents in heart failure.

PHYSICAL TRAINING AND WEIGHT LOSS

By reducing weight and blood pressure and perhaps by improving insulin sensitivity and other cardiovascular risk factors, regular exercise might be expected to reduce the risk of developing heart failure in patients with type 2 diabetes mellitus. However, in the 1 large prospective randomized trial testing this hypothesis, the Look-AHEAD (Action for Health in Diabetes) trial, carried out in 5145 overweight or obese adults with type 2 diabetes mellitus, an intensive lifestyle intervention promoting weight loss through decreased caloric intake and increased physical activity (intervention group) failed to improve cardiovascular outcomes compared with standard treatment. The primary outcome was a composite of death from cardiovascular causes, nonfatal myocardial infarction, nonfatal stroke, or hospitalization for angina during a maximum follow-up of 13.5 years and this was not reduced by the lifestyle intervention (hazard ratio [HR], 0.95; 95% confidence interval [CI], 0.83–1.09). However, there was a trend toward a reduction in episodes of heart failure (99 vs 119 episodes, respectively) but this was not significant (HR, 0.80; 95% CI, 0.61–1.04).[31]

In patients with established heart failure and diabetes, regular exercise is thought to be beneficial by helping to improve insulin sensitivity. By reducing blood pressure, cardiac hypertrophy, and left atrial volume, exercise and weight loss might be especially beneficial in patients with heart failure and preserved ejection fraction (HFpEF).[32] Two clinical trials provide data on the effects of exercise in patients with both diabetes and heart failure. One study in patients with heart failure and reduced ejection fraction (HFrEF) suggested that exercise improved ejection fraction but was too small to provide robust evidence (n = 42).[33] In the only large trial examining the effect of regular exercise on outcomes in heart failure, the HF-ACTION (Heart Failure: A Controlled Trial Investigating Outcomes of Exercise Training) trial, heart failure patients with and without diabetes (n = 2331) were randomized to aerobic exercise on top of usual care, or usual care alone, and exercise was shown to reduce the secondary composite endpoint of cardiovascular mortality or hospitalization owing to heart failure after adjustment for prognostic baseline variables (HR, 0.85; 95% CI, 0.74–0.99).[34] Importantly, there was no interaction between baseline diabetes status and the benefits of exercise training.[35] The patients in HF-ACTION had HFrEF, and it is unknown whether patients with diabetes and HFpEF might benefit from exercise. The only low-quality evidence comes from 1 small-randomized study of caloric restriction and exercise training in 100 severely obese HFpEF patients with (n = 35) and without (n = 65) diabetes, which suggested that these interventions led to both weight loss and improved functional capacity.[36]

ALPHA-GLUCOSIDASE INHIBITORS

Alpha-glucosidase inhibition lowers body weight and triglycerides. The efficacy and safety of 2 drugs in this class has recently been tested in randomized, placebo-controlled, clinical trials. In the first, the ABC (Alpha-glucosidase-inhibitor Blocks Cardiac Events in Patients with Myocardial Infarction and Impaired Glucose Tolerance) trial, patients with impaired glucose tolerance and coronary heart disease and an left ventricular ejection fraction (LVEF) of greater than 40% were randomized to placebo or voglibose. The original intent was to enroll approximately 3000 patients, but the trial was stopped early because an interim analysis of outcomes in the first 870 participants suggested a low probability of a positive outcome; that is, the trial was terminated for futility. Only 12 patients were hospitalized for heart failure during a follow-up period of 24 months.[37] The much larger ACE (Acarbose Cardiovascular Evaluation) trial randomized 6522 patients with coronary heart disease and impaired glucose tolerance to either acarbose or placebo. After a median follow-up of 5 years, there was no difference in the primary 5-point composite outcome of cardiovascular death, nonfatal myocardial infarction, nonfatal stroke, hospital admission for unstable angina, or hospital admission for heart failure (HR, 0.98; 95% CI, 0.86–1.11). There were 65 hospitalizations for heart failure in the acarbose group and 73 in the placebo group (HR, 0.89; 95% CI, 0.63–1.24).[38]

There are few data from studies conducted in patients with heart failure. A small, nonrandomized and underpowered study investigated the effect of 24 weeks of treatment with open-label voglibose on cardiovascular function in 30 patients with dilated cardiomyopathy and impaired glucose tolerance. Voglibose treatment was associated with reduced left ventricular dimensions, New York Heart Association functional classification, and plasma B-type natriuretic peptide (BNP) levels, compared with control subjects.[39] Clearly, the safety of alpha-glucosidase inhibitor treatment in patients with diabetes and chronic heart failure has not been adequately evaluated and should be, in light of its frequent use in Asian countries.

BIGUANIDES (METFORMIN)

There is a widely held view that metformin is cardioprotective, and proposed mechanisms of action include direct myocardial effects, and indirect effects related to weight loss and improved insulin sensitivity. The evidence for cardioprotection is, however, weak in general and nonexistent for heart failure in particular. The UKPDS randomized 753 overweight (>120% ideal bodyweight) patients with newly diagnosed type 2 diabetes and increased fasting plasma glucose (FPG; 6.1–15.0 mmol/L) despite 3 months of dietary intervention to conventional treatment, primarily with diet alone (n = 411), or an intensive blood glucose control approach with metformin, aiming for an FPG of less than 6 mmol/L (n = 342). The median follow-up was 10.7 years. There were few episodes of heart failure and these did not differ between treatment groups.[40] Long-term follow-up of UKPDS has been published recently, but heart failure was not reported.[41]

There is even less evidence about the potential actions of metformin in patients with established heart failure (as opposed to preventing incident heart failure). At present, the largest randomized study to evaluate the effect of metformin in heart failure patients randomized only 60 insulin-resistant subjects to treatment for 4 months. Metformin did not improve the primary endpoint of cardiopulmonary exercise capacity.[42]

Consequently, we have to rely on observational studies to examine the associations between metformin use and clinical outcomes in patients with heart failure, with the recognized and significant limitations of such studies. Metformin use seems to be associated with better outcomes than treatment with other glucose-lowering treatments in several observational studies. First, a Canadian cohort study examined outcomes in 1833 patients with diabetes and incident heart failure. The study demonstrated that use of metformin either as monotherapy or combined with a sulfonylurea was associated with a lower 1-year mortality compared with sulfonylurea treatment alone (HR, 0.83; 95% CI, 0.70–0.99).[43] The use of metformin in diabetic patients with heart failure has also been associated with better outcomes, including hospitalization for heart failure in several other cohort studies.[44–50] Although metformin use may be associated with both lower mortality and morbidity in heart failure, compared with other treatments, it is important to stress the limitations of observational studies, principally owing to confounding. For example, it is possible that the prescription of metformin is just a marker of less severe disease, but despite the lack of data from randomized trials, these observational analyses have led to the view that metformin is safe in heart failure in patients with an estimated glomerular filtration rate of greater than 30 mL/min/1.73m². However, it is also important to point out that metformin can potentially cause lactic acidosis, and should not be used in patients with severe disease, such as those who have become acutely decompensated or those with renal failure. Caution should also be exercised when administrating iodine contrast agents, during perioperative periods, and in situations with possible hypoxic states like respiratory failure, myocardial infarction, shock, or sepsis.

Ideally, a large randomized clinical trial is required to investigate the effects of metformin treatment on mortality and morbidity in heart failure patients, but 1 attempt to conduct such a trial failed because it seems that physicians did not accept that there was equipoise and preferred to prescribe metformin, rather than to randomize patients.[51]

SULFONYLUREAS

Sulfonylureas increase insulin release, thereby reducing blood glucose. However, the increases in insulin levels may cause hypoglycemia and weight gain. These actions could potentially exacerbate heart failure. The UGDP (University Group Diabetes Program) was the first large randomized trial in patients with type 2 diabetes mellitus conducted between 1961 and 1975. One treatment group received a fixed dose of the sulfonylurea tolbutamide (1.5 g/d in divided dose, regardless of plasma glucose response) and there were 2 insulin groups and a placebo group (a phenformin group was added later). An interim analysis of this trial in 1969 revealed a statistically significant excess of cardiovascular deaths in the tolbutamide arm, leading to premature discontinuation of this arm of the trial.[52] The number of heart failure events were not reported, only the number of patients receiving heart failure medication at any time after randomization (tolbutamide = 22 vs placebo = 13; P = .13), but the type of drug and doses were not reported.[53]

In the UKPDS, 3867 newly diagnosed patients with type 2 diabetes, who had FPG concentrations of 6.1 to 15.0 mmol/L despite 3 months treatment with diet, were randomly assigned to intensive treatment with a sulphonylurea (chlorpropamide, glibenclamide, or glipizide; n = 1234) or with insulin (n = 911), or conventional treatment with diet (n = 896). The aim in the intensive group was an FPG of less than 6 mmol/L. There were 48 new cases of heart failure in the sulfonylurea group compared with 62 in the conventional therapy group.[54]

As with metformin, the evaluation of the safety of sulfonylureas as a treatment for diabetes in patients with established heart failure has relied mainly on observational data. A retrospective cohort study of 16,417 patients with type 2 diabetes and heart failure found no evidence that mortality was higher in individuals treated with a sulfonylurea compared with other glucose-lowering drugs (HR, 0.99; 95% CI, 0.91–1.08).[44] However, follow-up in this study was limited to 1 year and treatment with sulfonylurea was compared with other glucose-lowering agents that in themselves may worsen heart failure, including insulin and thiazolidinedione. In another study, Eurich and colleagues[43] identified 1833 patients with incident heart failure who were treated with an oral glucose-lowering agent. The mean follow-up time was 2.5 years. Mortality, as well as the rate of hospitalization for heart failure, was higher in patients taking sulfonylurea monotherapy compared with metformin (metformin vs sulfonylurea; HR, 0.83; 95% CI, 0.70–0.99). A Danish registry study with more than 10,000 patients reported a similar finding.[48] Thus, the existing literature indicates that the safety of sulfonylureas in heart failure is uncertain, principally owing to the reliance on observational studies and lack of randomized controlled trials.

INSULIN

Insulin may have positive inotropic effects on myocardial tissue and improve other hemodynamic measures, but may also cause sodium retention, weight gain, and possibly edema, which are likely to be undesirable in heart failure. Sodium retention is dose dependent and present even in physiologic concentrations of insulin.[55] Fluid retention owing to insulin is usually mild, but it could potentially increase the severity of heart failure, and several case reports of new-onset heart failure in patients who started insulin treatment have been published. However, in the ORIGIN (Outcome Reduction With Initial Glargine Intervention) trial, 12,537 patients with impaired fasting glucose, impaired glucose tolerance, or type 2 diabetes and cardiovascular risk factors were randomized to insulin or standard care alone. Insulin had a neutral effect on the composite co-primary outcome including death from cardiovascular causes, nonfatal myocardial infarction, nonfatal stroke, cardiovascular revascularization procedures, or hospitalization for heart failure (HR, 1.04; 95% CI, 0.97–1.11).[56] There were 310 patients hospitalized with heart failure in the insulin group and 343 in the placebo group (HR, 0.90; 95% CI, 0.77–1.05). These findings are somewhat reassuring, but patients in the ORIGIN trial did not all have diabetes or had diabetes for a very short time, and the risk of heart failure increases with advancing age and duration of diabetes.

Only 1 small and short-term randomized clinical trial has evaluated the effect of insulin in patients with diabetes and established heart failure. This trial randomized 40 patients with type 2 diabetes, reduced left ventricular systolic function, and hemoglobin A1c levels of greater than 7.5% to optimized diabetes treatment including insulin use, or no optimization for 4 months. The primary outcome was defined as changes in left ventricular contractile reserve capacity from baseline to follow-up. The study showed no impairment of cardiac function and no patients were hospitalized for heart failure during the study period.[57] In contrast, in a variety of retrospective analyses of trials and in observational studies, treatment with insulin has been consistently associated with worse outcomes than no treatment with insulin. As with all observational studies, it is impossible to know whether these findings reflect "cause and effect" (ie, that insulin is harmful) or confounding, especially because insulin-treated patients are usually older with longer standing diabetes, more advanced cardiovascular and renal disease, and other adverse prognostic characteristics.[58–60] The bottom line is that the existing data available to the clinical community are insufficient to exculpate insulin from causing worse outcomes in patients with heart failure. If it proves necessary to start insulin in a patient with heart failure, it is important to monitor the patient for signs of fluid retention.

THIAZOLIDINEDIONES (GLITAZONES)

Thiazolidinediones (glitazones) enhance insulin sensitivity by increasing the efficiency of glucose transporters. However, these agents also cause weight gain, edema, and fractures. The mechanisms underlying edema are unknown, but may include activation of collecting duct sodium channels, and proximal tubular sodium channels, as well as peripheral arteriolar vasodilation.[61–63] The clinical manifestations are an essential part of the heart failure syndrome, and robust data suggest an increased risk of incident heart failure in patients with prediabetes as well as type 2 diabetes treated with a thiazolidinedione.[64] This was exemplified by the RECORD (Rosiglitazone Evaluated for Cardiac Outcomes and Regulation of Glycaemia in Diabetes) trial, in which 4447 patients with type 2 diabetes and dysglycemia on metformin or sulfonylurea monotherapy were randomized to either add-on rosiglitazone or a combination of metformin and sulfonylurea.[65] Patients were followed over an average period of 5.5 years, and rosiglitazone treatment was associated with a doubled risk of fatal or nonfatal heart failure events (61 vs 29; HR, 2.10; 95% CI, 1.35–3.27).[66] There are 3 large trials with pioglitazone in patients with diabetes and/or impaired glucose tolerance and these have shown a less striking increase in risk of heart failure (and a reduction in atherothrombotic events).[67–69]

There are few data from studies in patients with established heart failure. Only 2 small and short-term randomized clinical trials have investigated the effect of thiazolidinediones in heart failure patients with type 2 diabetes. The primary outcome was change in LVEF. There was no negative effect on left ventricular function in either study; however, thiazolidinedione treatments were associated with an increase in BNP, a marker of increased left ventricular wall stress and a predictor of adverse cardiovascular outcomes.[70,71] Dargie and colleagues[70] investigated the effect of rosiglitazone, compared with placebo, given for 52 weeks in 224 patients with type 2 diabetes and HFrEF. Rosiglitazone treatment was associated with a tendency toward an increased risk of all-cause mortality and hospitalization owing to heart failure (HR, 1.28; 95% CI, 0.51–3.21). Giles and colleagues[71] investigated the effect of pioglitazone in a similar way. In total, 300 patients with diabetes and HFrEF were randomized to 12 months of treatment with pioglitazone or glyburide (also known as glibenclamide); treatment with pioglitazone was associated with worsening heart failure symptoms as well as a greater number of hospitalizations for heart failure. The US Food and Drug Administration has given thiazolidinediones a black box warning in relation to use in acute or symptomatic chronic heart failure patients.[72]

INCRETIN THERAPIES

The incretins are a family of gut hormones produced by enteroendocrine cells. The 2 main molecules of interest are glucagon-like peptide-1 (GLP-1) and the gastric inhibitory hormone. GLP-1 is secreted in response to food intake; it decreases glucagon excretion and increases insulin levels.[73] The protease dipeptidyl peptidase-4 (DPP-4) rapidly decomposes native GLP-1. Pharmacologic inhibitors of DPP-4 and GLP-1 receptor agonists with longer bioavailability have been developed.[74]

DIPEPTIDYL PEPTIDASE-4 INHIBITORS

DPP-4 has several postulated substrates in addition to GLP-1, including BNP, erythropoietin, glucagon, vasoactive intestinal peptide, and vasostatin.[75] Thus, DPP-4 inhibition could affect pathways involving cardiac signaling, collagen turnover, and the sodium hydrogen exchanger in the renal proximal tubule.[76]

Clinical outcomes have been reported in 3 randomized controlled trials using of DPP-4 inhibitors. The SAVOR-TIMI 53 (Saxagliptin Assessment of vascular Outcomes Recorded in Patients with Diabetes Mellitus – Thrombolysis in Myocardial Infarction 53) trial was the first large-scale outcome trial to investigate the cardiovascular safety of a DPP-4 inhibitor in 16,492 patients with type 2 diabetes and either a high risk of cardiovascular disease or known cardiovascular disease. The trial did not show a decrease in the primary composite outcome of cardiovascular death, myocardial infarction, or ischemic stroke. Surprisingly, there was an increase in the risk of hospitalization for heart failure with saxagliptin, compared with placebo (289 vs 228 patients hospitalized, respectively; HR, 1.27; 95% CI, 1.07–1.51).[77] A subsequent analysis showed that the risk of heart failure was greatest among patients with an increased BNP, a history of heart failure, and chronic kidney disease.[78] Whether this completely unexpected finding reflected the play of chance, or, if real, was a DPP-4 inhibitor class effect (or even an issue for other incretin-based therapies including GLP-1 receptor agonists) or a drug-specific hazard was unknown at that point, but emphasized the importance of heart failure as an outcome in trials testing new therapies for diabetes. Therefore, the outcomes of subsequent trials with DPP4-inhibitors were eagerly awaited after SAVOR-TIMI 53. In the EXAMINE (Examination of Cardiovascular Outcomes with Alogliptin versus Standard of Care) trial, 5380 patients with type 2 diabetes and recent acute coronary syndrome were randomized to receive alogliptin or placebo. There was a nonsignificant trend to an increase in heart failure hospitalization with alogliptin compared with placebo (106 vs 89 cases, respectively; HR, 1.19; 95% CI, 0.90–1.58).[79] However, in TECOS (Trial to Evaluate Cardiovascular Outcomes after Treatment with Sitagliptin), no such risk was seen with sitagliptin. TECOS randomized 14,671 patients with type 2 diabetes and a history of major coronary artery disease, ischemic cerebrovascular disease, or atherosclerotic peripheral arterial disease to DPP-4 inhibitor therapy or placebo.[80] There were a similar number of patients hospitalized with heart failure in the sitagliptin group (228 cases) and placebo group (229 cases; HR, 1.00; 95% CI, 0.83–1.20). There were 2643 patients with heart failure at baseline in TECOS and the treatment effect in this subgroup was similar to that in the trial overall; however, the phenotype of patients with heart failure at baseline (and occurring after randomization) was not defined. Although TECOS may have been reassuring, none of these studies included a substantial number of patients with a diagnosis of heart failure at baseline, leaving uncertainty about the safety of DPP-4 inhibitors in patients with established heart failure. The US Food and Drug Administration has issued a safety communication concerning saxagliptin and alogliptin stating that health care professionals should consider discontinuing both drugs in patients who develop heart failure (http://www.fda.gov/Drugs/DrugSafety/ucm486096.htm).

As with the other blood glucose-lowering drugs discussed, there are few data on the use of DPP-4 inhibitors specifically in patients with established heart failure. The effects of alogliptin, saxagliptin, and sitagliptin on heart failure hospitalization in the subgroups of patients with prevalent heart failure at baseline in EXAMINE, SAVOR-TIMI 53 and TECOS are shown **Table 1**, but, as pointed out, the heart failure phenotype in these patients was not characterized. The VIVIDD (Vildagliptin in Ventricular Dysfunction Diabetes Trial) trial investigated the effect of vildagliptin on cardiac function in 254 patients with type 2 diabetes and HFrEF. The study met the primary endpoint of statistical noninferiority in terms of change in LVEF, and no difference in time to any first cardiovascular event between the 2 groups was observed (35 events in the vildagliptin group vs 31 in the placebo group). However, there were 11 deaths from any cause in the vildagliptin arm and 4 deaths in the placebo arm.[81] Although the study was not powered to evaluate hard endpoints, it highlights the uncertainty of DPP4-inhibitor use in patients with chronic heart failure.

GLUCAGON-LIKE PEPTIDE-1 RECEPTOR AGONISTS

The effect of GLP-1 receptor agonists on glucose lowering and weight loss exceeds the effects of DPP4-inhibitors. Substances can be divided in to 2 groups according to their structural basis (exendin or GLP-1 related) and their half-life:

I. *Short acting (terminal half-life of <24 hours)/exendin-4 based: exenatide;*
II. *Long acting (terminal half-life of >24 hours)/exendin-4 based: extended duration exenatide;*
III. *Short-acting (terminal half-life of <24 hours)/GLP-1 based: lixisenatide, liraglutide; and*
IV. *Long-acting (terminal half-life of >24 hours)/GLP-1 based: dulaglutide, albiglutide, and semaglutide.*

The effect of the short-acting GLP-1 analogue lixisenatide on cardiovascular outcomes was tested in the ELIXA (Evaluation of Lixisenatide in Acute Coronary Syndrome) trial. Patients with type 2 diabetes and an acute coronary syndrome (n = 6068) within 15 to 180 days were randomized to receive lixisenatide or placebo in addition to standard of care. Lixisenatide had a neutral effect on the primary and secondary outcomes, including hospitalization for heart failure (122 vs 127 patients hospitalized; HR, 0.96; 95% CI, 0.75–1.23).[82] The effect of the longer acting GLP-1 analogue liraglutide was tested in the LEADER (Liraglutide Effect and Action in Diabetes: Evaluation of Cardiovascular Outcome Results) trial. LEADER included patients (n = 9340) with type 2 diabetes and established cardiovascular disease or cardiovascular risk factors, and 14% of patients in LEADER had a history of New York Heart Association functional class II or III heart failure at enrollment (probably a mixture of HFrEF and HFpEF).[83] Liraglutide decreased the risk of the primary composite endpoint (HR, 0.87; 95% CI, 0.78–0.97) as well as cardiovascular and all-cause mortality; there was also a nominally statistically significant reduction in myocardial infarction. The risk of heart failure hospitalization, however, did not differ between groups (218 vs 248 patients hospitalized; HR, 0.87; 95% CI, 0.73–1.05).[84] In the subgroup of 11305 patients with heart failure at baseline the treatment effect of liraglutide was consistent with that observed in the trial overall; however, the phenotype of patients with heart failure at baseline (and occurring after randomization) was not defined.

Table 1
Outcomes with glucose-lowering agents in relation to heart failure

	PROactive	RECORD	EXAMINE	SAVOR-TIMI 53	TECOS	ELIXA	LEADER	SUSTAIN-6	EXSCEL	EMPA-REG OUTCOME	CANVAS	ACE
Year of completion	2005	2009	2013	2013	2015	2015	2016	2016	2017	2015	2017	2017
Drug studied	Pioglitazone	Rosiglitazone	Alogliptin	Saxagliptin	Sitagliptin	Lixisenatide	Liraglutide	Semaglutide	Exenatide	Empagliflozin	Canagliflozin	Acarbose
Class	TZD	TZD	DPP-4 I	DPP-4 I	DPP-4 I	GLP-1 RA	GLP-1 RA	GLP-1 RA	GLP-1 RA	SGLT2-i	SGLT2-i	α-Glucosidase inhibitor
Participants (n)	5238	4447	5380	16,492	14,671	6068	9340	3297	14,752	7020	10,142	6522
Trial duration (median)	2.9 y[b]	5.5 y[b]	1.5 y	2.1 y	3.0 y	2.1 y	3.8 y	2.1 y	3.2 y	3.1 y	3.6 y[b]	5.0 y
Prevalent HF % (n)	N/A	N/A	28 (1501)	13 (2105)	18 (2643)	22.4 (1358)	18 (1667)[a]	23.6 (777)	16.2 (2389)	10 (706)	14.4 (1461)	3.7 (243)
Treatment effects on HF hospitalization in overall group and in those with prevalent HF												
HR overall (95% CI)	1.41 (1.10–1.80)	2.10 (1.35–3.27)	1.19 (0.9–1.58)	1.27 (1.07–1.51)	1.00 (0.83–1.19)	0.96 (0.75–1.23)	0.87 (0.73–1.05)	1.11 (0.77–1.61)	0.94 (0.78–1.13)	0.65 (0.50–0.85)	0.67 (0.52–0.87)	0.89 (0.63–1.24)
HR for prevalent HF (95% CI)	N/A	N/A	1.00 (0.71–1.42)	1.21 (0.99–1.58)	1.03 (0.77–1.36)	0.93 (0.66–1.30)	0.95 (0.71–1.28)	NR	NR	0.75 (0.48–1.19)	NR	NR

Abbreviations: DPP-4 I, dipeptidyl peptidase-4 inhibitor; GLP-1 RA, glucagon-like peptide-1 analogue; HF, heart failure; HR, hazard ratio; N/A, not applicable; SGLT2-i, sodium glucose cotransporter-2 inhibitor; TZD, thiazolidinedione.

[a] Fourteen percent (1305) were in New York Heart Association functional classes II and III and 18% (1667) were in New York Heart Association functional classes I through III.

[b] Mean.

Consistent with these findings, a very long-acting GLP-1 agonist, semaglutide, was shown in SUSTAIN-6 (Trial to Evaluate Cardiovascular and Other Long-term Outcomes with Semaglutide in Subjects with Type 2 Diabetes) (n = 3297) to reduce the same combined primary cardiovascular endpoint (HR, 0.74; 95% CI, 0.58–0.95) although without a statistically significant effect on mortality or myocardial infarction (but with a reduction in stroke). Semaglutide did not reduce the risk of heart failure hospitalization (HR, 1.11; 95% CI, 0.77–1.61).[85]

Most recently, the EXSCEL (Exenatide Study of Cardiovascular Event Lowering Trial) trial tested an alternative long-acting GLP-1 receptor agonist, with a different structural basis than liraglutide and semaglutide, but similar to that of lixisenatide (exenatide and lixisenatide are exendin-4 based). In EXSCEL, 14752 patients were randomized equally to exenatide once weekly or placebo. There was a trend to a reduction in the primary composite endpoint of cardiovascular death, nonfatal myocardial infarction, or nonfatal stroke with exenatide (HR, 0.91; 95% CI, 0.83–1.00; P = .061 for superiority) and a nominally statistically significant reduction in all-cause death. There were 219 patients hospitalized with heart failure in the exenatide group and 231 in the placebo group (HR, 0.94; 95% CI, 0.78–1.13).[86] In keeping with all other large cardiovascular outcome trials in patients with diabetes, none of these trials reported data on LVEF.

Once again, there are few data about the effects of GLP-1 receptor agonists in patients with established heart failure. The effects of lixisenatide and liraglutide on heart failure hospitalization in the subgroups of patients with prevalent heart failure at baseline in ELIXA and LEADER are shown **Table 1**, but, as pointed out, the heart failure phenotype in these patients was not characterized. The FIGHT (Functional Impact of GLP-1 for Heart Failure Treatment)[87] trial and the LIVE (Effect of Liraglutide on Left Ventricular Function in Stable Chronic Heart Failure Patients)[88] study investigated the effects of liraglutide in more than 500 patients with HFrEF. Neither of these studies showed an effect on LVEF, but they raised concerns about the safety of liraglutide in patients with HFrEF.[87,88] In LIVE, liraglutide increased heart rate by 7 beats per minute compared with placebo and there were more serious cardiac events (composite of death or hospitalization for any cardiovascular event). A total of 12 patients in the treatment group and 3 patients in the placebo group experienced a serious cardiac event (HR, 3.9; 95% CI, 1.1–13.8). The FIGHT study reported a trend toward more serious cardiac events in liraglutide-treated patients. This was notable for the combined endpoint of death or rehospitalization owing to heart failure (liraglutide = 72 and placebo = 57; HR, 1.30; 95% CI, 0.92–1.83).[87] Although not powered to evaluate clinical outcomes, the results of these 2 studies demonstrate why outcome trials with diabetes drugs are needed specifically in patients with heart failure—it cannot be assumed that treatments will have the same safety profile in patients with heart failure as in those without. Furthermore, the effect of treatments may be very different in patients with HFrEF compared with HFpEF.

SODIUM GLUCOSE COTRANSPORT 2 RECEPTOR INHIBITORS

Sodium glucose cotransport 2 receptor (SGLT2) is a low-affinity, high-capacity sodium glucose cotransporter thought to be exclusively located in the renal proximal tubule. SGLT2 is responsible for 90% of glucose reabsorption, and inhibition induces a decrease in blood glucose owing to glycosuria. Secondary effects of SGLT2 inhibition include a modest diuretic effect, weight loss, lowering of blood pressure, and reduced levels of uric acid and triglycerides.[89] The first cardiovascular outcome trial with a SGLT2 inhibitor to report, the EMPA-REG OUTCOME (Empagliflozin, Cardiovascular

Outcomes, and Mortality in Type 2 Diabetes trial), included 7020 patients with type 2 diabetes and known cardiovascular disease. EMPA-REG OUTCOME showed a significant reduction in the primary composite outcome of cardiovascular death, nonfatal myocardial infarction or nonfatal stroke with empagliflozin (HR, 0.86; 95% CI, 0.74–0.99; $P = .04$ for superiority). This treatment benefit was mainly owing to a relative risk reduction of 38% in death from cardiovascular causes (HR, 0.62; 95% CI, 0.49–0.77). There was also a 35% relative risk reduction in hospitalization for heart failure (HR, 0.65; 95% CI, 0.50–0.85) with empagliflozin compared with placebo.[90] It is noteworthy that this effect was independent of baseline treatment with anticongestive medication and consistent in the subgroup of patients with heart failure at baseline (n = 706, again, without the phenotype defined). The findings from EMPA-REG OUTCOME have been supported by the CANVAS Program (CANagliflozin cardioVascular Assessment Study program), which consisted of 2 trials enrolling 10,142 participants with type 2 diabetes and either established cardiovascular disease or with cardiovascular risk factors, randomized to receive canagliflozin or placebo. Overall, the findings of CANVAS were broadly similar to EMPA-REG OUTCOME with a 14% relative risk reduction in the same primary outcome in the canagliflozin group (HR, 0.86; 95% CI, 0.75–0.97; $P = .02$ for superiority). Although there was not a statistically significant reduction in cardiovascular mortality, there was a 33% relative risk reduction in hospitalization for heart failure (HR, 0.67; 95% CI, 0.52–0.87), similar to that seen in EMPA-REG OUTCOME. The benefit of canagliflozin seemed to be consistent in the subgroup of 1461 patients with heart failure at baseline (not phenotyped) and possibly greater in participants treated with a diuretic at baseline.[91] The mechanism or mechanisms by which SGLT-2 inhibitors reduce heart failure hospitalization are unknown; however, natriuresis and blood pressure reduction may be important, leading to a reduction in preload and afterload. Other suggestions include an improvement in myocardial metabolism as a result of the mild ketonemia caused by SGLT-2 inhibition (damaged myocardium may use ketones as an alternative or more metabolically efficient substrate) and a possible inhibition of sodium–hydrogen exchange in cardiomyocytes (potentially reducing intracellular calcium accumulation and risk of arrhythmias).

There are no substantial completed trials in patients with established heart failure, so, to date we must rely on the subgroup analyses from EMPA-REG OUTCOME and CANVAS. The effects of empagliflozin on heart failure hospitalization in the subgroup of patients with prevalent heart failure at baseline in EMPA-REG OUTCOME is shown **Table 1**, but, as pointed out, the heart failure phenotype in these patients was not characterized. Fortunately, 3 large randomized outcome trials in patients with heart failure are underway. Two of these, with empagliflozin and dapagliflozin, are in patients with HFrEF (NCT03036124 and NCT03057977) and one, with empagliflozin, in HFpEF (NCT03057951).

OTHER GLUCOSE LOWERING DRUGS
Nateglinide

The meglitinides ("glinides") bind to an ATP-dependent K^+ channel on the membrane of pancreatic beta cells in a similar manner to sulfonylureas and lead to a short-term increase secretion of insulin. The safety of nateglinide - in addition to lifestyle modification - was evaluated in the Nateglinide and Valsartan in Impaired Glucose Tolerance Outcomes Research (NAVIGATOR) trial.[92] In total, 9306 participants with impaired glucose tolerance and either cardiovascular disease or cardiovascular risk factors received nateglinide (up to 60 mg three times daily) or placebo, in a 2-by-2 factorial design with valsartan or placebo. Patients were followed for a median of 5.0 years and one co-primary outcomes was a composite of death from cardiovascular causes, nonfatal myocardial infarction, nonfatal stroke, or hospitalization for heart failure. Nateglinide did not reduce the incidence of the composite endpoint, and although hospitalizations for heart failure were numerically fewer, this reduction was not statistically significant (nateglinide = 85 vs. placebo = 100, HR, 0.85; 95% CI, 0.64–1.14).[93]

Bromocriptine

Bromocriptine-QR (a quick-release formulation of bromocriptine mesylate), a dopamine D2 receptor agonist, is a US Food and Drug Administration–approved treatment for type 2 diabetes mellitus. Taken in the morning, bromocriptine-QR is thought to cause an increase in central dopaminergic tone at the time of day it normally peaks in healthy individuals (this circadian peak linked to preservation and/or induction of normal insulin sensitivity and glucose metabolism). A total of 3,095 patients with type 2 diabetes were randomized 2:1 to bromocriptine-QR or placebo in conjunction with the patient's usual diabetes therapy in a 52-week evaluation of cardiovascular and overall safety.[94,95] As part of this assessment there was a pre-specified analysis of a composite cardiovascular endpoint of myocardial infarction, stroke, coronary revascularization, and hospitalization for angina or congestive heart failure, evaluated using modified intent-to-treat analysis.[94,95] Fewer people experienced this end point in the bromocriptine-QR group compared with the placebo group: 37 (1.8%) vs. 32 (3.2%), respectively, HR 0.60 (95% CI 0.35–0.96). Subsequently, a composite including death from cardiovascular causes was reported: 39 (1.9%) 33 (3.2%), respectively, HR 0.61 (0.38 to 0.97).[94,95] There were 9 patients (0.4%) hospitalized for heart failure in the bromocriptine-QR group and 6 (0.6%) in the placebo group.

SUMMARY AND INTERPRETATION

It is only in the past few years that, after decades of use, we are beginning to obtain evidence on the cardiovascular effects of glucose lowering drugs, although these recent data only apply to the newer agents and not to established therapies such as metformin and sulphonylureas. Notably, 1 class of treatment, the thiazolidinediones (glitazones) clearly increase the risk of developing heart failure and worsening of heart failure in patients with the syndrome. There is a similar concern about at least some DPP-4 inhibitors. Although GLP-1 receptor agonists do not seem to increase the risk of developing heart failure, their safety and efficacy in patients with established heart failure is uncertain. Uniquely among all glucose-lowering therapies, the SGLT-2 inhibitors reduce the incidence of heart failure in patients with type 2 diabetes and their safety and efficacy in patients with established heart failure are being extensively assessed in 3 new large mortality and morbidity outcome trials, setting a new benchmark for evaluation of the effects of new diabetes drugs on cardiovascular outcomes.

What can we conclude on the basis of the currently available evidence? **Table 1** summarizes what we know about outcomes with glucose-lowering agents in relation to heart failure. Clearly, at present, it is not possible to make firm evidence-based recommendations about any treatment for diabetes in patients with HFrEF or HFpEF. Our tentative conclusions from the available data are that the SGLT-2 inhibitors seem to be the class of treatment least likely to be harmful and thiazolidinediones should be avoided.

REFERENCES

1. Ponikowski P, Voors AA, Anker SD, et al, Authors/Task Force Members, Document Reviewers. 2016 ESC guidelines for the diagnosis and treatment of acute and chronic heart failure: the Task Force for the diagnosis and treatment of acute and chronic heart failure of the European Society of Cardiology (ESC). Developed with the special contribution of the Heart Failure Association (HFA) of the ESC. Eur J Heart Fail 2016;18(8):891–975.
2. Yancy CW, Jessup M, Bozkurt B, et al. 2017 ACC/AHA/HFSA focused update of the 2013 ACCF/AHA guideline for the management of heart failure: a report of the American College of Cardiology/American Heart Association Task Force on clinical practice guidelines and the Heart Failure Society of America. J Card Fail 2017;23(8):628–51.
3. Jia G, DeMarco VG, Sowers JR. Insulin resistance and hyperinsulinaemia in diabetic cardiomyopathy. Nat Rev Endocrinol 2016;12(3):144–53.
4. Schmidt M, Jacobsen JB, Lash TL, et al. 25 year trends in first time hospitalisation for acute myocardial infarction, subsequent short and long term mortality, and the prognostic impact of sex and comorbidity: a Danish nationwide cohort study. BMJ 2012;344:e356.
5. CONSENSUS Trial Study Group. Effects of enalapril on mortality in severe congestive heart failure. Results of the Cooperative North Scandinavian Enalapril Survival Study (CONSENSUS). N Engl J Med 1987;316(23):1429–35.
6. SOLVD Investigators, Yusuf S, Pitt B, Davis CE, et al. Effect of enalapril on survival in patients with reduced left ventricular ejection fractions and congestive heart failure. N Engl J Med 1991;325(5):293–302.
7. Effect of metoprolol CR/XL in chronic heart failure: metoprolol CR/XL randomised intervention trial in congestive heart failure (MERIT-HF). Lancet 1999;353(9169):2001–7.
8. Pitt B, Zannad F, Remme WJ, et al. The effect of spironolactone on morbidity and mortality in patients with severe heart failure. Randomized Aldactone Evaluation Study Investigators. N Engl J Med 1999;341(10):709–17.
9. Redfield MM, Jacobsen SJ, Burnett JC Jr, et al. Burden of systolic and diastolic ventricular dysfunction in the community: appreciating the scope of the heart failure epidemic. JAMA 2003;289(2):194–202.
10. Nichols GA, Hillier TA, Erbey JR, et al. Congestive heart failure in type 2 diabetes: prevalence, incidence, and risk factors. Diabetes Care 2001;24(9):1614–9.
11. Bertoni AG, Hundley WG, Massing MW, et al. Heart failure prevalence, incidence, and mortality in the elderly with diabetes. Diabetes Care 2004;27(3):699–703.
12. Sarma S, Mentz RJ, Kwasny MJ, et al. Association between diabetes mellitus and post-discharge outcomes in patients hospitalized with heart failure: findings from the EVEREST trial. Eur J Heart Fail 2013;15(2):194–202.
13. Maggioni AP, Greene SJ, Fonarow GC, et al. Effect of aliskiren on post-discharge outcomes among diabetic and non-diabetic patients hospitalized for heart failure: insights from the ASTRONAUT trial. Eur Heart J 2013;34(40):3117–27.
14. Kannel WB, McGee DL. Diabetes and cardiovascular disease. The Framingham study. JAMA 1979;241(19):2035–8.
15. Nichols GA, Gullion CM, Koro CE, et al. The incidence of congestive heart failure in type 2 diabetes: an update. Diabetes Care 2004;27(8):1879–84.
16. Juhaeri J, Gao S, Dai WS. Incidence rates of heart failure, stroke, and acute myocardial infarction among Type 2 diabetic patients using insulin glargine and other insulin. Pharmacoepidemiol Drug Saf 2009;18(6):497–503.

17. Berl T, Hunsicker LG, Lewis JB, et al. Cardiovascular outcomes in the Irbesartan Diabetic Nephropathy Trial of patients with type 2 diabetes and overt nephropathy. Ann Intern Med 2003;138(7):542–9.

18. Carr AA, Kowey PR, Devereux RB, et al. Hospitalizations for new heart failure among subjects with diabetes mellitus in the RENAAL and LIFE studies. Am J Cardiol 2005;96(11):1530–6.

19. De Groote P, Lamblin N, Mouquet F, et al. Impact of diabetes mellitus on long-term survival in patients with congestive heart failure. Eur Heart J 2004;25(8): 656–62.

20. Cubbon RM, Adams B, Rajwani A, et al. Diabetes mellitus is associated with adverse prognosis in chronic heart failure of ischaemic and non-ischaemic aetiology. Diab Vasc Dis Res 2013;10(4):330–6.

21. Gustafsson I, Torp-Pedersen C, Kober L, et al. Effect of the angiotensin-converting enzyme inhibitor trandolapril on mortality and morbidity in diabetic patients with left ventricular dysfunction after acute myocardial infarction. Trace Study Group. J Am Coll Cardiol 1999;34(1):83–9.

22. Haas SJ, Vos T, Gilbert RE, et al. Are beta-blockers as efficacious in patients with diabetes mellitus as in patients without diabetes mellitus who have chronic heart failure? A meta-analysis of large-scale clinical trials. Am Heart J 2003;146(5): 848–53.

23. Brown A, Reynolds LR, Bruemmer D. Intensive glycemic control and cardiovascular disease: an update. Nat Rev Cardiol 2010;7(7):369–75.

24. Stratton IM, Adler AI, Neil HA, et al. Association of glycaemia with macrovascular and microvascular complications of type 2 diabetes (UKPDS 35): prospective observational study. BMJ 2000;321(7258):405–12.

25. ACCORD Study Group, Cushman WC, Evans GW, Byington RP, et al. Effects of intensive blood-pressure control in type 2 diabetes mellitus. N Engl J Med 2010;362(17):1575–85.

26. ADVANCE Collaborative Group, Patel A, MacMahon S, Chalmers J, et al. Intensive blood glucose control and vascular outcomes in patients with type 2 diabetes. N Engl J Med 2008;358(24):2560–72.

27. Duckworth W, Abraira C, Moritz T, et al. Glucose control and vascular complications in veterans with type 2 diabetes. N Engl J Med 2009;360(2):129–39.

28. Hayward RA, Reaven PD, Wiitala WL, et al. Follow-up of glycemic control and cardiovascular outcomes in type 2 diabetes. N Engl J Med 2015;372(23):2197–206.

29. Gilbert RE, Krum H. Heart failure in diabetes: effects of anti-hyperglycaemic drug therapy. Lancet 2015;385(9982):2107–17.

30. Eshaghian S, Horwich TB, Fonarow GC. An unexpected inverse relationship between HbA1c levels and mortality in patients with diabetes and advanced systolic heart failure. Am Heart J 2006;151(1):91.

31. Look AHEAD Research Group, Wing RR, Bolin P, Brancati FL, et al. Cardiovascular effects of intensive lifestyle intervention in type 2 diabetes. N Engl J Med 2013; 369(2):145–54.

32. Sundstrom J, Bruze G, Ottosson J, et al. Weight loss and heart failure: a nationwide study of gastric bypass surgery versus intensive lifestyle treatment. Circulation 2017;135(17):1577–85.

33. Miche E, Herrmann G, Nowak M, et al. Effect of an exercise training program on endothelial dysfunction in diabetic and non-diabetic patients with severe chronic heart failure. Clin Res Cardiol 2006;95(Suppl 1):i117–24.

34. O'Connor CM, Whellan DJ, Lee KL, et al. Efficacy and safety of exercise training in patients with chronic heart failure: HF-ACTION randomized controlled trial. JAMA 2009;301(14):1439–50.

35. Banks AZ, Mentz RJ, Stebbins A, et al. Response to exercise training and outcomes in patients with heart failure and diabetes mellitus: insights from the HF-ACTION trial. J Card Fail 2016;22(7):485–91.

36. Kitzman DW, Brubaker P, Morgan T, et al. Effect of caloric restriction or aerobic exercise training on peak oxygen consumption and quality of life in obese older patients with heart failure with preserved ejection fraction: a randomized clinical trial. JAMA 2016;315(1):36–46.

37. Asakura M, Kim J, Asanuma H, et al. Does treatment of impaired glucose tolerance improve cardiovascular outcomes in patients with previous myocardial infarction? Cardiovasc Drugs Ther 2017. [Epub ahead of print].

38. Holman RR, Coleman RL, Chan JCN, et al. Effects of acarbose on cardiovascular and diabetes outcomes in patients with coronary heart disease and impaired glucose tolerance (ACE): a randomised, double-blind, placebo-controlled trial. Lancet Diabetes Endocrinol 2017. https://doi.org/10.1016/S2213-8587(17)30309-1.

39. Kim J, Nakatani S, Hashimura K, et al. Abnormal glucose tolerance contributes to the progression of chronic heart failure in patients with dilated cardiomyopathy. Hypertens Res 2006;29(10):775–82.

40. Effect of intensive blood-glucose control with metformin on complications in overweight patients with type 2 diabetes (UKPDS 34). UK Prospective Diabetes Study (UKPDS) Group. Lancet 1998;352(9131):854–65.

41. Holman RR, Paul SK, Bethel MA, et al. 10-year follow-up of intensive glucose control in type 2 diabetes. N Engl J Med 2008;359(15):1577–89.

42. Wong AK, Symon R, AlZadjali MA, et al. The effect of metformin on insulin resistance and exercise parameters in patients with heart failure. Eur J Heart Fail 2012;14(11):1303–10.

43. Eurich DT, Majumdar SR, McAlister FA, et al. Improved clinical outcomes associated with metformin in patients with diabetes and heart failure. Diabetes Care 2005;28(10):2345–51.

44. Masoudi FA, Inzucchi SE, Wang Y, et al. Thiazolidinediones, metformin, and outcomes in older patients with diabetes and heart failure: an observational study. Circulation 2005;111(5):583–90.

45. MacDonald MR, Eurich DT, Majumdar SR, et al. Treatment of type 2 diabetes and outcomes in patients with heart failure: a nested case-control study from the U.K. General practice research database. Diabetes Care 2010;33(6):1213–8.

46. Evans JM, Doney AS, AlZadjali MA, et al. Effect of Metformin on mortality in patients with heart failure and type 2 diabetes mellitus. Am J Cardiol 2010;106(7):1006–10.

47. Roussel R, Travert F, Pasquet B, et al. Metformin use and mortality among patients with diabetes and atherothrombosis. Arch Intern Med 2010;170(21):1892–9.

48. Andersson C, Olesen JB, Hansen PR, et al. Metformin treatment is associated with a low risk of mortality in diabetic patients with heart failure: a retrospective nationwide cohort study. Diabetologia 2010;53(12):2546–53.

49. Aguilar D, Chan W, Bozkurt B, et al. Metformin use and mortality in ambulatory patients with diabetes and heart failure. Circ Heart Fail 2011;4(1):53–8.

50. Eurich DT, Weir DL, Majumdar SR, et al. Comparative safety and effectiveness of metformin in patients with diabetes mellitus and heart failure: systematic review

of observational studies involving 34,000 patients. Circ Heart Fail 2013;6(3): 395–402.

51. Eurich DT, Tsuyuki RT, Majumdar SR, et al. Metformin treatment in diabetes and heart failure: when academic equipoise meets clinical reality. Trials 2009;10:12.

52. Meinert CL, Knatterud GL, Prout TE, et al. A study of the effects of hypoglycemic agents on vascular complications in patients with adult-onset diabetes. II. Mortality results. Diabetes 1970;19(Suppl):789–830.

53. A study of the effects of hypoglycemia agents on vascular complications in patients with adult-onset diabetes. VI. Supplementary report on nonfatal events in patients treated with tolbutamide. Diabetes 1976;25(12):1129–53.

54. Intensive blood-glucose control with sulphonylureas or insulin compared with conventional treatment and risk of complications in patients with type 2 diabetes (UKPDS 33). UK Prospective Diabetes Study (UKPDS) Group. Lancet 1998; 352(9131):837–53.

55. Skott P, Hother-Nielsen O, Bruun NE, et al. Effects of insulin on kidney function and sodium excretion in healthy subjects. Diabetologia 1989;32(9):694–9.

56. ORIGIN Trial Investigators, Gerstein HC, Bosch J, Dagenais GR, et al. Basal insulin and cardiovascular and other outcomes in dysglycemia. N Engl J Med 2012;367(4):319–28.

57. Nielsen R, Wiggers H, Thomsen HH, et al. Effect of tighter glycemic control on cardiac function, exercise capacity, and muscle strength in heart failure patients with type 2 diabetes: a randomized study. BMJ Open Diabetes Res Care 2016; 4(1):e000202.

58. Domanski M, Krause-Steinrauf H, Deedwania P, et al. The effect of diabetes on outcomes of patients with advanced heart failure in the BEST trial. J Am Coll Cardiol 2003;42(5):914–22.

59. Smooke S, Horwich TB, Fonarow GC. Insulin-treated diabetes is associated with a marked increase in mortality in patients with advanced heart failure. Am Heart J 2005;149(1):168–74.

60. Pocock SJ, Wang D, Pfeffer MA, et al. Predictors of mortality and morbidity in patients with chronic heart failure. Eur Heart J 2006;27(1):65–75.

61. Guan Y, Hao C, Cha DR, et al. Thiazolidinediones expand body fluid volume through PPARgamma stimulation of ENaC-mediated renal salt absorption. Nat Med 2005;11(8):861–6.

62. Endo Y, Suzuki M, Yamada H, et al. Thiazolidinediones enhance sodium-coupled bicarbonate absorption from renal proximal tubules via PPARgamma-dependent nongenomic signaling. Cell Metab 2011;13(5):550–61.

63. Emoto M, Fukuda N, Nakamori Y, et al. Plasma concentrations of vascular endothelial growth factor are associated with peripheral oedema in patients treated with thiazolidinedione. Diabetologia 2006;49(9):2217–8.

64. Lago RM, Singh PP, Nesto RW. Congestive heart failure and cardiovascular death in patients with prediabetes and type 2 diabetes given thiazolidinediones: a meta-analysis of randomised clinical trials. Lancet 2007;370(9593):1129–36.

65. Home PD, Pocock SJ, Beck-Nielsen H, et al. Rosiglitazone evaluated for cardiovascular outcomes in oral agent combination therapy for type 2 diabetes (RECORD): a multicentre, randomised, open-label trial. Lancet 2009;373(9681): 2125–35.

66. Komajda M, McMurray JJ, Beck-Nielsen H, et al. Heart failure events with rosiglitazone in type 2 diabetes: data from the RECORD clinical trial. Eur Heart J 2010; 31(7):824–31.

67. Dormandy JA, Charbonnel B, Eckland DJ, et al. Secondary prevention of macro-vascular events in patients with type 2 diabetes in the PROactive Study (PRO-spective pioglitAzone Clinical Trial In macroVascular Events): a randomised controlled trial. Lancet 2005;366(9493):1279–89.
68. Kernan WN, Viscoli CM, Furie KL, et al. Pioglitazone after ischemic stroke or transient ischemic attack. N Engl J Med 2016;374(14):1321–31.
69. Vaccaro O, Masulli M, Nicolucci A, et al. Effects on the incidence of cardiovascular events of the addition of pioglitazone versus sulfonylureas in patients with type 2 diabetes inadequately controlled with metformin (TOSCA.IT): a randomised, multicentre trial. Lancet Diabetes Endocrinol 2017. https://doi.org/10.1016/S2213-8587(17)30317-0.
70. Dargie HJ, Hildebrandt PR, Riegger GA, et al. A randomized, placebo-controlled trial assessing the effects of rosiglitazone on echocardiographic function and cardiac status in type 2 diabetic patients with New York Heart Association Functional Class I or II Heart Failure. J Am Coll Cardiol 2007;49(16):1696–704.
71. Giles TD, Elkayam U, Bhattacharya M, et al. Comparison of pioglitazone vs glyburide in early heart failure: insights from a randomized controlled study of patients with type 2 diabetes and mild cardiac disease. Congest Heart Fail 2010; 16(3):111–7.
72. Nesto RW, Bell D, Bonow RO, et al. Thiazolidinedione use, fluid retention, and congestive heart failure: a consensus statement from the American Heart Association and American Diabetes Association. October 7, 2003. Circulation 2003; 108(23):2941–8.
73. Drucker DJ. The biology of incretin hormones. Cell Metab 2006;3(3):153–65.
74. Madsbad S, Schmitz O, Ranstam J, et al, NN2211-1310 International Study Group. Improved glycemic control with no weight increase in patients with type 2 diabetes after once-daily treatment with the long-acting glucagon-like peptide 1 analog liraglutide (NN2211): a 12-week, double-blind, randomized, controlled trial. Diabetes Care 2004;27(6):1335–42.
75. Mulvihill EE, Drucker DJ. Pharmacology, physiology, and mechanisms of action of dipeptidyl peptidase-4 inhibitors. Endocr Rev 2014;35(6):992–1019.
76. Hocher B, Reichetzeder C, Alter ML. Renal and cardiac effects of DPP4 inhibitors–from preclinical development to clinical research. Kidney Blood Press Res 2012;36(1):65–84.
77. Scirica BM, Bhatt DL, Braunwald E, et al. Saxagliptin and cardiovascular outcomes in patients with type 2 diabetes mellitus. N Engl J Med 2013;369(14): 1317–26.
78. Scirica BM, Braunwald E, Raz I, et al. Heart failure, saxagliptin, and diabetes mellitus: observations from the SAVOR-TIMI 53 randomized trial. Circulation 2014; 130(18):1579–88.
79. White WB, Cannon CP, Heller SR, et al. Alogliptin after acute coronary syndrome in patients with type 2 diabetes. N Engl J Med 2013;369(14):1327–35.
80. Green JB, Bethel MA, Armstrong PW, et al. Effect of sitagliptin on cardiovascular outcomes in type 2 diabetes. N Engl J Med 2015;373(3):232–42.
81. McMurray JJ, Ponikowksi P, Bolli GB, et al. Effects of vildagliptin on ventricular function in patients with type 2 diabetes mellitus and heart failure. a randomized placebo-controlled trial. JACC Heart Fail 2017. https://doi.org/10.1016/j.jchf.2017.08.004.
82. Pfeffer MA, Claggett B, Diaz R, et al. Lixisenatide in patients with type 2 diabetes and acute coronary syndrome. N Engl J Med 2015;373(23):2247–57.

83. Marso SP, Poulter NR, Nissen SE, et al. Design of the liraglutide effect and action in diabetes: evaluation of cardiovascular outcome results (LEADER) trial. Am Heart J 2013;166(5):823–30.e5.
84. Marso SP, Daniels GH, Brown-Frandsen K, et al. Liraglutide and cardiovascular outcomes in type 2 diabetes. N Engl J Med 2016;375(4):311–22.
85. Marso SP, Bain SC, Consoli A, et al. Semaglutide and Cardiovascular outcomes in patients with type 2 diabetes. N Engl J Med 2016;375(19):1834–44.
86. Holman RR, Bethel MA, Mentz RJ, et al. Effects of once-weekly exenatide on cardiovascular outcomes in type 2 diabetes. N Engl J Med 2017;377(13):1228–39.
87. Margulies KB, Hernandez AF, Redfield MM, et al. Effects of liraglutide on clinical stability among patients with advanced heart failure and reduced ejection fraction: a randomized clinical trial. JAMA 2016;316(5):500–8.
88. Jorsal A, Kistorp C, Holmager P, et al. Effect of liraglutide, a glucagon-like peptide-1 analogue, on left ventricular function in stable chronic heart failure patients with and without diabetes (LIVE): a multicentre, double-blind, randomised, placebo-controlled trial. Eur J Heart Fail 2017;19(1):69–77.
89. Marx N, McGuire DK. Sodium-glucose cotransporter-2 inhibition for the reduction of cardiovascular events in high-risk patients with diabetes mellitus. Eur Heart J 2016;37(42):3192–200.
90. Zinman B, Wanner C, Lachin JM, et al. Empagliflozin, Cardiovascular outcomes, and mortality in type 2 diabetes. N Engl J Med 2015;373(22):2117–28.
91. Neal B, Perkovic V, Mahaffey KW, et al. Canagliflozin and cardiovascular and renal events in type 2 diabetes. N Engl J Med 2017;377(7):644–57.
92. Califf RM, Boolell M, Haffner SM, et al. Prevention of diabetes and cardiovascular disease in patients with impaired glucose tolerance: rationale and design of the Nateglinide And Valsartan in Impaired Glucose Tolerance Outcomes Research (NAVIGATOR) Trial. Am Heart J 2008;156(4):623–32.
93. NAVIGATOR Study Group, Holman RR, Haffner SM, et al. Effect of nateglinide on the incidence of diabetes and cardiovascular events. N Engl J Med 2010;362(16):1463–76.
94. Gaziano JM, Cincotta AH, O'Connor CM, et al. Randomized clinical trial of quick-release bromocriptine among patients with type 2 diabetes on overall safety and cardiovascular outcomes. Diabetes Care 2010;33(7):1503–8.
95. Gaziano JM, Cincotta AH, Vinik A, et al. Effect of bromocriptine-QR (a quick-release formulation of bromocriptine mesylate) on major adverse cardiovascular events in type 2 diabetes subjects. J Am Heart Assoc 2012;1(5):e002279.

Personalizing Glucose-Lowering Therapy in Patients with Type 2 Diabetes and Cardiovascular Disease

Silvio E. Inzucchi, MD

KEYWORDS

- Glucose-lowering therapy • Type 2 diabetes • Cardiovascular disease

KEY POINTS

- Type 2 diabetes is a complex disease with a pathogenesis that is multidimensional.
- Personalized therapy in the patient with established cardiovascular disease (CVD) involves the control of hyperglycemia and the management of other frequently coexisting atherosclerosis risk factors.
- The treating clinician should first determine the optimal hemoglobin A1c target for the individual, based on a variety of patient and disease characteristics.
- The intensiveness of glycemic control may need to be tempered in the setting of overt CVD, particularly when there is a need to use agents associated with hypoglycemia.
- Recently, several specific glucose-lowering agents have been demonstrated to improve cardiovascular outcomes and may be favored in type 2 diabetes patients with coexisting CVD.

BACKGROUND

Over the past 2 decades, the variety of glucose-lowering agents available for treating type 2 diabetes mellitus (T2DM) has increased substantially. As a result, the management of patients with this condition is becoming increasingly complex, with many more choices now available (alone and in combination) to improve glycemic control. Owing to its low cost, absence of significant long-term adverse consequences, and possible inherent cardiovascular (CV) benefit, metformin is endorsed as the best initial therapy by most prevailing treatment guidelines, including the joint position statement from the American Diabetes Association (ADA) and the European Association for the Study of Diabetes (EASD).[1,2] Beyond metformin monotherapy, however, there remains

Disclosure: Dr S.E. Inzucchi discloses that he has served on clinical trial steering or executive committees for Boehringer Ingelheim, AstraZeneca, Novo Nordisk, Sanofi/Lexicon, Daiichi Sankyo, and Eisai (TIMI) and on a data monitoring committee for Intarcia. He has also been an advisor to Janssen and VTV Therapeutics.
Yale Endocrinology, Fitkin 106, Box 208020, New Haven, CT 06520-8020, USA
E-mail address: silvio.inzucchi@yale.edu

Endocrinol Metab Clin N Am 47 (2018) 137–152
https://doi.org/10.1016/j.ecl.2017.10.011
0889-8529/18/© 2017 Elsevier Inc. All rights reserved.

substantial debate regarding the optimal drug (or even drug class) to use for individuals needing additional reduction in hemoglobin A1c (HbA1c). When the most recent version of the ADA-EASD position statement was published in early 2015, there were few clear distinguishing features related to long-term outcomes to favor one category over another.[2] Specifically from the vantage point of CV disease (CVD), such as myocardial infarction (MI), stroke, CV death, and heart failure, there was considerable clinical equipoise regarding the best next step after metformin. Consequently, prevailing recommendations were not highly prescriptive; clinicians were simply advised to choose subsequent agents based mainly the avoidance of adverse effects while taking into account the financial constraints of patients and/or health systems. Since 2015, however, the results from several major CV outcome trials involving diabetes medications have been released.[3] These data are now allowing for a more refined approach to the management of T2DM, incorporating evidence-based strategies in antihyperglycemic therapy, particularly in patients with heart disease.

This article reviews the individualization of T2DM therapy in the patient with preexisting CVD. First, the calibration of glycemic targets in this population will be described, followed by a discussion of the approach to choosing actual glucose-lowering drugs. Neither is necessarily a straightforward undertaking and should continue to be based on multiple interrelated patient and disease factors. The emerging CV benefits of certain glucose-lowering medications and the need to harness these effects to optimize patient outcomes will be emphasized.

CALIBRATING GLYCEMIC TARGETS IN THE PATIENT WITH CARDIOVASCULAR DISEASE: HOW LOW TO GO

With a change in the diagnostic criteria in 2010, the HbA1c test is now accepted as a screening tool for diabetes.[4] If confirmed on a second occasion, or if paired with an elevated fasting plasma glucose (>126 mg/dL or 7 mmol/L), an HbA1c of greater than or equal to 6.5% is now considered diagnostic of diabetes. Unless very early on in the disease course, it is difficult to uniformly lower the HbA1c to this level once the diagnosis is established. Accordingly, most treatment guidelines suggest that the general HbA1c target be less than or equal to 7.0%, although some latitude is allowed to individualize this based on a variety of patient and disease characteristics. For example, younger and healthier patients may be targeted at less than 6.5%, as explicitly advised by the American Association of Clinical Endocrinologists[5] and inferred by the ADA-EASD position statement.[1,2] The goal here is to mitigate the long-term risk for diabetic microvascular complications, such as retinopathy and kidney disease. In contrast, in older patients, especially in those with preexisting heart disease, the target can be modulated to 7.0% to 7.5%, or even slightly higher, toward the 8.0% range. Moreover, in patients of advanced age who are infirm with multiple comorbidities or in those with a propensity for severe hypoglycemic reactions and who require insulin therapy, even higher targets are reasonable (8.0%–8.5%).

In the original trials to demonstrate a benefit from glucose-lowering (the Diabetes Control and Complications Trial[6] involving patients with type 1 diabetes [T1DM] and the United Kingdom Prospective Diabetes Study [UKPDS][7] involving recently diagnosed individuals with T2DM), participants randomized to the more intensive therapy arms actually achieved an HbA1c of 7.0% to 7.5%. In these studies, most of the benefit from intensive therapy seemed to be on microvascular complications but without substantive effects on macrovascular complications, such as those related to atherosclerosis. Importantly, the latter is the major cause of morbidity, mortality, and excess health care expenditures in this disease. Subsequent large trials

(ACCORD [Action to Control Cardiovascular Risk in Diabetes],[8] ADVANCE [Action in Diabetes and Vascular Disease: Preterax and Diamicron MR Controlled Evaluation],[9] and VADT [Veterans Affairs Diabetes Trial][10]) were designed to determine if even more stringent glycemic control could improve CVD risk, with attempts to lower HbA1c to less than 6.0% to 6.5%. First, these studies were not successful in achieving glycemic targets as tight as initially intended. Second, although very modest further benefits on microvascular complications were demonstrated, no major advantage from a CV standpoint could be demonstrated. In fact, the ACCORD trial, involving older patients at high CV risk, an increase in CV mortality was observed in the more intensive arm. The precise explanation for this finding has remained elusive but may relate to increased hypoglycemia or simply the increased treatment burden required by these patients, many of whom were placed on multiple daily insulin injections in conjunction with 2 to 3 other glucose-lowering agents. ACCORD provides some caution concerning the benefits of overly aggressive HbA1c targets in a CV population, which may be particularly vulnerable to the deleterious aspects of rigorous glucose control.

Such trials have curbed the initial enthusiasm for tight glycemic management in every patient with T2DM. Their findings are also buttressed by epidemiologic data that now suggest that an optimal HbA1c in older patients with T2DM may be approximately 7.5%. The specific target for an individual patient should also account for other clinical factors, as seen in **Fig. 1**, which describes the various patient and disease characteristics used to modulate the intensiveness of glycemic control efforts. Not considered in this figure, yet a concept of significant importance, is that targeting lower HbA1c levels becomes riskier when drugs that possess intrinsic hypoglycemia risk, such as sulfonylureas and insulin, are used. This is in contrast to metformin, thiazolidinediones (TZDs), and certain newer categories of medications that do not predispose to hypoglycemia, allowing glucose levels to be controlled more safely. These include dipeptidyl peptidase (DPP)-4 inhibitors, glucagon-like peptide (GLP)-1 receptor agonists (RAs), and sodium-glucose cotransporter (SGLT)-2 inhibitors.

There is also a growing consensus that optimization of glucose-lowering therapy may be more about the specific pharmacologic strategy used as opposed to the precise HbA1c achieved.[3] Such a notion lies in stark contrast to the conventional paradigm regarding diabetes treatment and microvascular disease prevention in which evidence points to a tight correlation between mean glucose concentration achieved and risk reduction, irrespective of treatment modality. That CV risk is improved more by drug strategy than the degree of HbA1c-lowering is borne out by further analyses from recent positive CV outcome trials in T2DM, most of which have not shown major separations in HbA1c between groups assigned to the investigational agent versus placebo combined with standard of care. They have shown a general lack of correlation between HbA1c and the CV benefits in active therapy patients. Accordingly, the prior glucocentricity in dealing with patients with T2DM and CVD may require a reassessment.

GLUCOSE-LOWERING STRATEGIES IN PATIENTS WITH TYPE 2 DIABETES MELLITUS AND CARDIOVASCULAR DISEASE: WHICH DRUG FOR WHICH PATIENT?

Over the past 2 decades, there has been a 6-fold increase in the available categories of glucose-lowering drugs. These advances are in part due in part to the growing understanding of the pathogenesis of T2DM, now known to involve multiple abnormalities in several organ systems, including skeletal muscle (insulin resistance), the endocrine pancreas (relative insulin deficiency and failure of the suppression of glucagon secretion), the liver (increased glucose production), adipocytes (increased lipolysis and abnormal adipokine biology), the intestines (altered physiology of incretin

Approach to the management of hyperglycemia

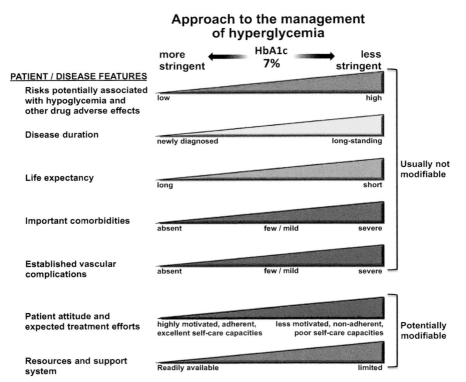

Fig. 1. Individualizing HbA1c targets in patients with T2DM. The elements of decision-making used to determine the intensiveness of glycemic lowering efforts are listed. Greater concerns within a particular domain are represented by an increasing height of the colored ramp. Situations toward the left justify more stringent efforts to lower HbA1c, whereas those toward the right necessitate less stringent efforts. In the patient with established CVD, overly intensive HbA1c targets may be risky, especially when using glucose-lowering agents that place the patient at risk of hypoglycemia. An HbA1c target in the 7.0% to 7.5% range may be reasonable in these circumstances. This scale is not designed to be applied rigidly but to be used as a broad construct to help guide clinical care. (*From* Inzucchi SE, Bergenstal RM, Buse JB, et al. Management of Hyperglycemia in type 2 diabetes, 2015: a patient-centered approach: update to a position statement of the American Diabetes Association and the European Association for the Study of Diabetes. Diabetes Care 2015;38(1):140–9, with permission.)

hormones, eg, GLP-1), and the kidney (relative decreased urinary excretion of glucose), among others. There are now 12 individual medication classes available in the United States, most represented by more than one compound, each with generic and trade names, and most now also available in combination products. Clearly, the management of this disease has become a complicated enterprise. The artful navigation through this expanding pharmacopeia is particularly important for clinicians treating T2DM patients who have CVD, given that some agents may present unique risks, whereas others possess key benefits in this population.

Table 1 lists currently available glucose-lowering medication classes approved in the United States for use in T2DM, along with their benefits and risks relating to the CV system. The optimal initial choice for most patients with CVD remains metformin, widely viewed as foundation therapy by most professional organizations. This designation is based on longstanding and worldwide experience, unsurpassed efficacy, and a

Table 1
Advantages and disadvantages related to the CV system of the main glucose-lowering drugs for type 2 diabetes

Drug Category	CV Advantages	CV Disadvantages
Biguanides Metformin	• Reduced hyperglycemia • Hypoglycemia risk not increased • No weight gain • Decreased MI, MACE in small trials • Increased CV mortality in observational studies	• Increased risk of lactic acidosis (advanced CKD, severe HF)
Sulfonylureas Glyburide Glipizide Glimepiride	• Reduced hyperglycemia	• Hypoglycemia • Weight gain • Blunt ischemic preconditioning • Increased CV mortality in observational studies
TZDs Pioglitazone Rosiglitazone	• Reduced hyperglycemia • Hypoglycemia risk not increased • Reduced insulin resistance, hyperinsulinemia • Reduced TG, increases HDL-C • Antiinflammatory effects • No hypoglycemia • Decreased MACE (pioglitazone)	• Increased risk of HF • Edema • Weight gain
DPP-4 Inhibitors Sitagliptin Saxagliptin Alogliptin Linagliptin	• Reduced hyperglycemia • Hypoglycemia risk not increased • No weight gain • ? Direct and indirect (via GLP-1) effects on myocardium	• Increased risk of HF (saxagliptin)
GLP-1 Receptor Agonists Exenatide Liraglutide Albiglutide Lixisenatide Semaglutide	• Reduced hyperglycemia • Hypoglycemia risk not increased • Weight loss • Reduced BP • ? Direct effects on myocardium • Decreased MACE (liraglutide, semaglutide) • Decreased CV mortality (liraglutide) • Decreased albuminuria progression (liraglutide, semaglutide)	• Increased pulse rate
SGLT-2 Inhibitors Canagliflozin Dapagliflozin Empagliflozin Ertugliflozin	• Reduced hyperglycemia • Hypoglycemia risk not increased • Weight loss • Reduced BP • Reduced TG, increases HDL-C • Decreased MACE (empagliflozin, canagliflozin) • Decreased CV mortality (empagliflozin) • Decreased HF hospitalization (empagliflozin, canagliflozin) • Decreased CKD progression (empagliflozin, canagliflozin)	• Risk of dehydration, hypovolemia • Increased LDL-C • Increased risk of amputations (canagliflozin) • Increased risk of DKA
Insulin Various	• Reduced hyperglycemia • Antiinflammatory effects	• Hypoglycemia • Weight gain • Increased hyperinsulinemia (?mitogenic effects)

Abbreviations: ?, uncertain evidence; BP, blood pressure; CKD, chronic kidney disease; DKA, diabetic ketoacidosis; HF, heart failure; HDL-C, high-density lipoprotein cholesterol; LDL-C, low-density lipoprotein cholesterol; MACE, major adverse cardiovascular events; TG, triglycerides.

well-established safety profile. Also, several early studies pointed to a CV benefit from this biguanide. After metformin, however, there remains no broad consensus regarding the best next agent to use for patients requiring additional glucose-lowering. According to the 2015 ADA-EASD position statement,[2] reiterated in the annual updated ADA *Standards of Care*,[11] the choice in combination therapy must be individualized, based on a variety of patient and disease characteristics. A convenient framework for recalling the specific areas of individualization is provided in **Table 2**, personalizing therapy using the "6-Ps" of decision-making: pathophysiology, potency, precautions, perks, practicalities, and price. Each of these domains should be considered whenever additional glucose lowering is being considered beyond metformin in the patient with T2DM. This is particularly important in the individual with established CVD.

Pathophysiology

In contrast to the relatively straightforward pathogenesis of T1DM (autoimmune destruction of insulin-producing beta cells within the endocrine pancreas), that of T2DM is more complex, as previously described.[12] Importantly, these metabolic defects coexist and the typical patient exhibits multiple abnormalities. Unfortunately, and, in general, outside of the research setting, reliable tools are not widely available to precisely assess the degree to which each of these pathophysiological abnormalities are contributing to hyperglycemia and/or which can be ameliorated pharmacologically. Not surprisingly, current treatment guidelines actually provide little guidance on how to match drug therapy to pathobiology at the level of the individual patient. However, there are some key exceptions which, although uncommon, should be recognized. Also, even in more routine T2DM patients, clinical features can sometimes help guide drug selection.

Obesity is linked to insulin resistance. Therefore, the more obese patient, especially if accompanied by several features of the metabolic syndrome (eg, central adiposity, acanthosis nigricans, hypertension, hypertriglyceridemia, low high-density lipoprotein cholesterol concentrations, hyperuricemia, and/or history of gout), history of CVD, and polycystic ovary disease in women, should do well with agents that improve insulin sensitivity, such as biguanides (eg, metformin) or TZDs (eg, pioglitazone). Actual studies, however, have

Table 2	
The 6 Ps to be considered when personalizing diabetes therapies	
1 Pathophysiology	• Assess insulin-resistance vs insulin-deficiency as the predominate phenotype • Recognize the stage of disease • Discern fasting vs postprandial hyperglycemia • Rule out secondary forms of diabetes
2 Potency	• Determine the distance from patient's HbA1c target • Acknowledge the HbA1c-reducing potency of each drug or drug category
3 Precautions	• Recognize contraindications • Discuss side effects, their likelihood and potential impact on the patient
4 Perks	• Consider a drug's additional evidence-based benefits (ie, weight loss, BP reduction, improved CVD outcomes, improved CKD outcomes)
5 Practicalities	• Tablets vs injections • Determine frequency of administration • Consider requirements for and frequency of blood glucose and other monitoring
6 Price	• Branded vs generic • Consider insurance formulary restrictions

demonstrated that metformin indeed works equally well irrespective of body mass index.[13] For TZDs, a metaanalysis has demonstrated modestly greater HbA1c-lowering in obese than in nonobese patients.[14] (Interestingly, this class' most notable side effect of weight gain presents an interesting paradox). In contrast, leaner individuals with T2DM usually express a greater degree of insulin deficiency, and may experience more benefit from sulfonylureas or insulin. These concepts, although logical, have not been specifically tested in clinical trials.[15] Accordingly, the consideration of the relative balance between insulin resistance and insulin deficiency may be at the present time an academic exercise.

Perhaps more important, the stage of disease should be incorporated in decision-making because individuals with long-standing diabetes tend to have more severe deficiency in insulin secretion and typically more commonly will require the institution of insulin therapy.

Temporal glycemic patterns may also be used to help steer drug choice. Patients with mainly fasting hyperglycemia tend to do very well with metformin because the prime driver of fasting glucose is hepatic glucose production, the specific target of this biguanide drug. Those with predominately postprandial hyperglycemia may do best with drugs that target this, such as incretin-based therapies (particularly shorter-acting GLP-1 RAs) or even the uncommonly used alpha-glucosidase inhibitors. It should be noted that most diabetes medications have some effects on both fasting and postprandial glucose, so most drugs chosen will ameliorate both to at least some degree. One obvious exception, in insulin-users, is that prandial-dosed rapid-acting analogues (lispro, aspart, glulisine) target solely postprandial glucose, whereas basal insulin analogues (glargine, detemir, degludec) mainly address fasting glucose concentrations.

Actually, most drugs approved for use in T2DM will reduce HbA1c in most patients to whom they are prescribed.[1,2,11] There are certain circumstances, however, in which careful consideration of the specific pathogenesis of a patient's diabetes is more important for successful management. This group includes the less common forms of the disease that may present as T2DM because they emerge in adults but actually exhibit unique mechanistic features.[16] For example, special caution is needed in the lean individual, especially when severe or labile glycemic control is demonstrated, or when there is a family history of T1DM, or coexisting autoimmune afflictions, such as primary hypothyroidism from Hashimoto disease or hyperthyroidism due to Graves disease, Addison disease, inflammatory arthritides, inflammatory bowel disease, vitiligo, alopecia areata, or pernicious anemia. These individuals frequently have latent autoimmune diabetes of adulthood (LADA), which is, essentially, a later-onset form of T1DM.[17] These patients may be identified by measuring elevated titers of islet-cell antibodies, such as antiglutamic acid decarboxylase (GAD). In general, these individuals progress to insulin therapy rapidly and titration of multiple oral agents is usually (but not always) ineffective.

Other conditions that must be identified for optimal management are those that belong in the category of secondary diabetes; that is, hyperglycemic states associated with other conditions or in which the pathogenesis is distinct from traditional T2DM.[16] One of the most common is that associated with pancreatic disease (eg, chronic pancreatitis, hemochromatosis, or following pancreatic surgery) in which severe (or even absolute) insulin deficiency is present, requiring multiple daily injections of insulin, as is used in T1DM.

Various endocrinopathies may exacerbate insulin resistance or deficiency or both. They are treated differently insofar as identification of the underlying disease and its ultimate treatment usually improves glycemia and sometimes cures the diabetes. Examples include hyperthyroidism, Cushing syndrome, acromegaly, pheochromocytoma, and rare neuroendocrine neoplasms of the pancreas, such as glucagonoma or somatostatinoma.

Many drugs have also been linked to diabetes,[16] such as glucocorticoids, thiazides, beta-adrenergic antagonists, antipsychotics, phenytoin, nicotinic acid, and cyclosporine and related compounds, as well as newer immune-based oncologic therapies known as check-point inhibitors, which have been reported to induce autoimmune diabetes requiring insulin therapy.[18]

A long list of genetic syndromes, including genetic defects of either insulin sensitivity or beta cell function have also been associated with diabetes,[14] but most are beyond the scope of this article. Of these, maturity onset diabetes of youth or MODY deserves special mention because of the specific therapy for the most common form, MODY-3.[19] Patients with MODY are typically diagnosed before the fourth decade of life, exhibit an autosomal dominant inheritance pattern, with deficient but not absent insulin secretion, and do not have pancreatic autoantibodies. MODY-3 patients (due to mutation in the hepatocyte nuclear factor-1α gene) tend to respond very well to sulfonylureas, at least early on in the disease course, because these quickly correct their subnormal pancreatic insulin secretion.

In summary, an initial assessment of the pathogenesis of diabetes should be undertaken in all patients because this information may help guide optimal glucose-lowering drug choice. However, there are no specific additional concerns in this regard as related to the patient with CVD.

Potency

With perhaps the exception of insulin, most drugs have an expected efficacy range of somewhere between 0.5% and 1.5%, greater when baseline HbA1c is very high (eg, >9% to 10%).[1,2,10] Certain drug classes, however, such as DPP-4 inhibitors, SGLT-2 inhibitors, alpha-glucosidase inhibitors, binding resins, and dopamine agonists tend to cluster on the lower end of this efficacy range with HbA1c reductions of 0.5% to less than 1.0%. Other categories, such as sulfonylureas, metformin, TZDs, and GLP-1 RAs, tend to decrease HbA1c more, typically in the 1.0% to 1.5% range. It should be noted, however, that sulfonylureas, although initially resulting in a strong treatment effect, may begin to lose potency after 6 to 12 months owing to further decrements in beta-cell function in the face of the stimulation of insulin secretion. Insulin, when titrated aggressively has no specific ceiling per se. However, in clinical trials involving comparisons of injectable agents, basal insulin seems to reduce HbA1c to a similar degree as GLP-1 RAs. Moreover, the addition of a GLP-1 RA to baseline basal insulin has been demonstrated to be as effective as adding 3 injections of mealtime rapid-acting insulin.[20]

Although there is some evidence that TZDs work better in the obese (as previously noted) and in women,[14] clinical trials that have assessed the relative glucose-lowering with other diabetes drugs across subgroups have generally failed to find any clinically significantly greater effect in specific patient types.[15] The main exception is the nearly universal finding that any glucose-lowering medication will reduce HbA1c to a greater extent in those in whom, as noted above, the baseline HbA1c is higher.[21]

In summary, the current HbA1c level and target (and, therefore, the HbA1c-lowering needs of the patient) help the clinician determine which glucose-lowering regimen to use. For example, in the patient on metformin with an HbA1c of 10.5% whose target is 7.0%, a DPP-4 inhibitor would not typically be the first choice.

Precautions

Each class of diabetes medication has specific side effects (see **Table 1**), some of which are more important in those with CVD.[1,2,11] Optimal management of T2DM should consider these and avoid use of certain drugs in patients in whom there may be a contraindication, who are predisposed to certain toxicities, or who are anticipated to tolerate specific adverse effects poorly.

Gastrointestinal symptoms, for example, predominate with metformin (mainly diarrhea), GLP-1 RAs (nausea, vomiting, diarrhea), and alpha-glucosidase inhibitors (flatulence, diarrhea).[1,11,22,23] These categories may be best avoided in patients with baseline intestinal diseases or frequent digestive complaints. Specifically, in those with gastroparesis, GLP-1 RAs should not be prescribed given their mechanism of action to slow gastric emptying. Metformin is also contraindicated in those with advanced renal disease (glomerular filtration rate [GFR] <30 mL/min) and used with caution and perhaps at a reduced dose in those with a GFR of 30 to 45 mL per minute or other risk factors for lactic acidosis (severe liver disease, alcoholism, baseline metabolic acidosis).

Hypoglycemia is the main adverse consequence of insulin and sulfonylurea therapy and, to a lesser extent, with shorter-acting insulin secretagogues, known as the glinides.[1,11] This may be of particular concern in patients who have already demonstrated a propensity to hypoglycemia or in those with risk factors for hypoglycemia, such as advanced age, irregular meal schedules, inconsistent adherence to therapy, and/or decreased kidney function. The latter is due to the metabolism and pharmacokinetics of certain sulfonylureas (eg, glyburide) but also that insulin is renally excreted so that any drug that increases insulin supply will tend to produce hypoglycemia more when GFR is reduced, especially less than 30 mL per minute. Weight gain is another concern with both insulin and sulfonylureas, as well as TZDs (ie, pioglitazone). This may be particularly problematic in those who are already obese and are being advised to lose weight. Also, sulfonylurea drugs may impair ischemic preconditioning, a self-protecting mechanism of cardiomyocytes to reduce their oxygen requirements under ischemic conditions, although most of the data in this area stem from animal models. Of course, at times (especially with insulin), such therapy is absolutely necessary and should not be avoided merely because of the possibility of adverse consequences, which can be managed with proper patient education.

There are additional concerns with TZDs, including fluid retention, edema, and an increased risk of heart failure.[1,11] Accordingly, they are contraindicated in patients with clinical heart failure and may need to be avoided in those with significant known left ventricular dysfunction, even if not yet symptomatic. This class also seems to increase the risk of bone fractures and should probably not be used in those with preexisting osteoporosis or at high risk for fracture. Finally, pioglitazone has been associated with an increased risk of bladder cancer, although the largest and longest prospective study did not confirm this. Nonetheless, the prescribing labels in most countries still advise against using TZD in those with a history of or even at high risk (undiagnosed hematuria, prior cyclophosphamide therapy, pelvic irradiation) for this neoplasm.

With SGLT-2 inhibitors, polyuria, urinary frequency, and genitourinary infections (especially candida vaginitis in women and balanitis in men) are the predominating adverse consequences.[2,11,24,25] Accordingly, men already symptomatic from benign prostatic hypertrophy or those with baseline incontinence, tendency toward severe urinary tract infections, or recurrent genital yeast infections may not optimal candidates for this class of medication. Recently, an increase in lower extremity amputation rates has been observed with canagliflozin, a drug which also seems to increase fracture rates.[21] Therefore, this SGLT-2 inhibitor should probably be avoided in those with peripheral arterial disease or history of prior amputations or foot ulcerations. Notably, to date, these adverse effects have not been reported with the 2 other members of this class available in the United States: dapagliflozin and empagliflozin. In the EMPA-REG OUTCOME trial, amputation rates were similar between the 2 randomized groups.[26]

DPP-4 inhibitors are among the best tolerated of glucose-lowering drugs but likely increase the risk of pancreatitis to a small degree and should be avoided in patients with such a history. The same caveat is described in the prescribing label for the other incretin-based therapy, the GLP-1 RAs, although large trials to date have not confirmed such a link. Certain GLP-1 RAs have been linked to an increased risk of gall bladder events, specifically cholecystitis (liraglutide)[22] and retinopathy (semaglutide),[23] and these newer concerns should at least be considered before prescribing these.

Colesevelam and bromocriptine are rarely used but the former promotes constipation and the latter has a variety of nonspecific side effects, including dizziness, nausea, and fatigue.[1] Patients with similar baseline symptoms are not optimal candidates for these corresponding classes. Finally, the rarely used injectable amylin mimetic, pramlintide, like GLP-1 RAs, slows gastric emptying and may induce nausea and vomiting.[1] These adverse effects should be kept in mind when this medication is being considered.

"Perks"

As with adverse effects, most drug categories (or drugs) have specific nonglycemic benefits[1,2,11]; that is, "perks" (or perquisites) of therapy (see **Table 1**). Some of these are of particular and growing importance in those with CVD.

Weight loss, for example, is experienced by most patients treated with either GLP-1 RAs or SGLT-2 inhibitors. Both of these drug classes also result in modest blood pressure lowering, particularly the latter category, with reductions of 4 mm systolic and 2 mm diastolic. Lipid lowering effects are also seen with some agents. For example, pioglitazone, a TZD, has a triglyceride-lowering effect. These added benefits may obviously be incorporated into treatment decision-making.

Metformin may reduce adverse CV events. In a substudy of the UKPDS, randomization to metformin in overweight patients was associated with a 39% reduction in the risk of MI compared with the control group managed with diet alone.[27] There was a trend toward fewer MIs when compared with the intensively managed group that was assigned to sulfonylurea or insulin, but the difference was not statistically significant. There were significantly fewer strokes in the metformin versus sulfonylurea or insulin group, however. Two subsequent studies seemed to confirm this benefit of metformin, with similar risk reductions. All of these trials were comparatively small, however, and all transpired in the era before statins. In larger, observational studies, treatment with metformin has been associated with reduction in CV mortality compared with sulfonylureas. Of course, even the most carefully controlled of these retrospective studies likely possess some residual confounding by indication; they should be considered hypothesis-generating but not conclusive. Accordingly, although metformin may have some CV benefit, the data are far from robust.

The TZD saga is more complex. Initially, this drug class was hoped to reduce CV events because they reduced insulin resistance, which itself is an independent CV risk factor. However, a metaanalysis of rosiglitazone trials suggested that this drug might increase the risk of myocardial ischemic events.[28] A large randomized CV outcome trial, RECORD (Rosiglitazone Evaluated for Cardiovascular Outcomes in Oral Agent Combination Therapy for Type 2 Diabetes), however, subsequently demonstrated neutrality for this TZD on major adverse CV events (MACE) in 4447 T2DM subjects using metformin or sulfonylureas.[29] In contrast, in PROactive (Prospective Pioglitazone Clinical Trial In Macrovascular Events), another TZD, pioglitazone, was associated with a 16% reduction in the risk of a MACE in 5238 subjects with T2DM and established macrovascular disease.[30] More recently, in the IRIS (Insulin Resistance Intervention after Stroke) trial, pioglitazone therapy resulted in 24% fewer fatal or nonfatal strokes and MIs in 3876 insulin-resistant but nondiabetic subjects with recent prior stroke or transient ischemic attack.[31] Accordingly, this TZD is now recognized as having significant atherosclerotic properties, which could be of obvious importance in patients with overt CVD.

In 2013 to 2017, a series of large CV outcome trials involving specific newer T2DM medications were reported. These had been developed in response to the 2008 guidance to industry from the US Food and Drug Administration, requesting the demonstration of CV safety for all new glucose-lowering agents.[32] The first four such trials, three involving DPP-4 inhibitors (saxagliptin,[33] alogliptin,[34] sitagliptin[35]) and one involving a GLP-1 RA (lixisenatide[36]) demonstrated neutrality and, therefore, safety for MACE. In the SAVOR-TIMI (Saxagliptin Assessment of Vascular Outcomes Recorded in Patients with Diabetes Mellitus–Thrombolysis in Myocardial Infarction) trial, saxagliptin was associated with a 27% increase in the risk for hospitalization for heart failure, although an explanation for this has remained elusive.[33]

After this initial somewhat disappointing series of trials, since 2015, 4 others have demonstrated an actual CV benefit. These results should be considered when designing a glucose-lowering regimen for patients with CVD. Two trials involved SGLT-2 inhibitors: empagliflozin in EMPA-REG OUTCOME[20] and canagliflozin in the CANVAS (Canagliflozin Cardiovascular Assessment Study)[21] program; both were associated with a 14% relative risk reduction in MACE. The behavior of the components of MACE were different between the trials, with CV mortality (−38%) driving the MACE reduction and the all-cause mortality reduction (−32%) with empagliflozin, but not significantly with canagliflozin. Both drugs were associated with major reductions in heart failure hospitalization (−35% and −33%, respectively), as well as in the progression of chronic kidney disease (CKD; −39% and −40%, respectively).[24,37] As previously mentioned, in CANVAS, canagliflozin was associated with a doubling of lower limb amputations, the mechanisms for which remain unknown but which partially counterbalances the CV benefits.[25] EMPA-REG OUTCOME studied only subjects with overt CVD, whereas about one-third of the CANVAS subjects had CV risk factors only (ie, a primary prevention cohort). Notably, the MACE effect in the latter group was neutral, although other outcomes have not yet been reported by subgroups.[25]

Two GLP-1 RA trials have also shown a CV benefit. In the first, LEADER (Liraglutide Effect and Action in Diabetes: Evaluation of Cardiovascular Outcome Results), liraglutide was associated a 13% relative risk reduction in MACE, including a 22% reduction in CV mortality (and 15% fewer all cause deaths) but no reduction in heart failure hospitalization.[22] In SUSTAIN-6 (Trial to Evaluate Cardiovascular and Other Long-Term Outcomes with Semaglutide in Subjects with Type 2 Diabetes), the investigational GLP-1 RA, semaglutide, resulted in a 26% reduction in MACE, driven mainly by a 62% reduction in stroke, and no effect on either CV mortality or heart failure outcomes.[23] Progression of renal disease was reduced in both these trials, driven by reductions in the progression to macroalbuminuria. In contrast, the renal benefits with both SGLT-2 inhibitor trials previously described included significant reductions in worsening renal function. In both LEADER and SUSTAIN-6, about 20% of participants had only CV risk factors. In both studies, the hazard ratio for MACE was neutral, suggesting no benefit unless CVD is already established. Finally, the fourth and most recent GLP-1 RA CV outcome trial to report, EXSCEL (Exenatide Study of Cardiovascular Event Lowering), involving the long-acting version of exenatide (once weekly), showed a neutral effect on MACE.[38]

Emerging data from 5 of these trials (IRIS, EMPA-REG OUTCOME, CANVAS, LEADER, and SUSTAIN-6)[22–25,31] should now be incorporated into decision-making about glucose-lowering drug choices after metformin monotherapy when CVD coexists with T2DM.

Practicalities

The additional requirements of therapy with certain agents, such as home glucose monitoring or laboratory monitoring, should also be considered. To prescribe metformin and sulfonylureas, for example, at least annual monitoring of kidney function is necessary. For the safe implementation of sulfonylurea or insulin therapy, home glucose monitoring is also important. These drugs should, therefore, not be considered in patients unable or unwilling to undergo such testing or monitoring.

Price

The cost of diabetes medications has increased dramatically over the past decade especially for insulin analogues, with therapy with some agents costing several hundred dollars per month.[39] Depending on insurance coverage, in some circumstances a patient may simply not be able to afford a certain product. Accordingly, generic formularies may need to be favored. Currently, generically available drugs include all sulfonylureas, metformin, and pioglitazone. Also available at affordable prices through certain national retailers, at prices less than 10% of those of branded analogues, are the human insulins, neutral protamine Hagedorn (NPH) and regular insulin.

Practical Application to the Patient with Cardiovascular Disease

Metformin is standard therapy and may have CV benefits, as previously noted. After metformin, additional glucose-lowering agents should include one or more of the following agents: an SGLT-2 inhibitor, empagliflozin or canagliflozin; the GLP-1 RA, liraglutide (or, conceivably, semaglutide, when available); and the TZD, pioglitazone. The differential effects of these therapies on body weight should be recognized and considered. Based on the CANVAS program's results, there is the additional new concern regarding amputations with canagliflozin. This issue, as well as the more potent effect of empagliflozin on CV death, may make it the SGLT-2 inhibitor with the preferred benefit to risk ratio. Also, of course, left ventricular function should be documented to be normal before prescribing pioglitazone in the context of known CVD, information that should be readily available because most patients will have already undergone echocardiography at some point during their evaluation for coronary and/or cerebrovascular complications.

Should the specific type of CVD channel a patient toward 1 of these agents? The evidence points to pioglitazone as a potentially preferred choice for stroke survivors, and either an evidence-based GLP-1 RA or SGLT-2 inhibitor in those with ischemic heart disease (ie, status post MI, acute coronary syndrome, coronary artery bypass grafting, or percutaneous coronary intervention), with the specific drug chosen based on the prevailing evidence from the literature. To date, the only GLP-1 RA marketed in the United States to be proven effective in reducing MACE is liraglutide. As for SGLT-2 inhibitors, it seems that empagliflozin may provide the best benefit to risk ratio. Moreover, in the specific context of an individual with CVD with heart failure, the optimal choice may be an SGLT-2 inhibitor, given the nature of the benefits demonstrated in both EMPA-REG OUTCOME and CANVAS. The coexistence of CKD in the CVD patient might also favor an SGLT-2 inhibitor, given the benefits on renal functional outcomes in this class. Ongoing studies with SGLT-2 inhibitors focused on patients with heart failure and CKD, including both diabetic and nondiabetic individuals, should further elucidate the overall effectiveness of these drugs on long-term outcomes.

Finally, in the patient with primarily peripheral arterial disease, either a GLP-1 RA or an SGLT-2 inhibitor is indicated. However, canagliflozin should be avoided, given the amputation signal from CANVAS. Although no signal for any increased amputation risk was reported in EMPA-REG OUTCOME, if the patient has advanced disease, especially if he or she has already undergone amputations, it is reasonable to avoid the SGLT-2 inhibitor drug class entirely until more safety data are available.

In the patient with ischemic heart disease and/or heart failure, it is also important to avoid hypoglycemia because these events, especially when severe, will activate the sympathetic nervous system. They are also associated with mortality, although a precise cause and effect relationship remains uncertain. Accordingly, if hyperglycemia can be adequately controlled without resorting to sulfonylureas, meglitinides, or insulin, this is preferred.

Fig. 2 shows a proposed glucose-lowering strategy in patients with T2DM who also have CVD, based on the recent clinical trial evidence of CV benefits from certain drugs or drug categories.

SUMMARY

T2DM is a complex disease with a pathogenesis that is multidimensional. Personalized therapy in the patient with established CVD involves the control of hyperglycemia and the management of other frequently coexisting atherosclerosis risk factors. The treating clinician should first determine the optimal HbA1c target for the individual, based on a variety of patient and disease characteristics. The intensiveness of glycemic control may need to be tempered in the setting of overt CVD, particularly when there is a need to use agents associated with hypoglycemia. The specific glucose-lowering strategy should then be

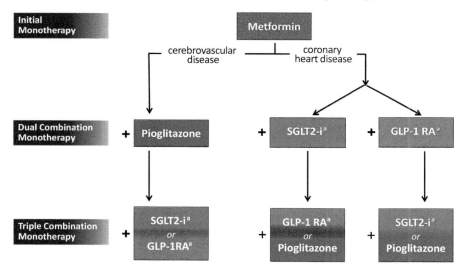

Fig. 2. Proposed glucose-lowering strategy in T2DM patients with CVD, favoring agents demonstrated to improve CV outcomes. Proposed algorithm for the treatment of T2DM in the patient with established CVD after metformin monotherapy is no longer adequate to control blood glucose concentrations. Several evidence-based therapies to reduce CV complications are now available. In dual combination therapy, pioglitazone may be preferred in those with cerebrovascular disease (PROactive, IRIS) but cannot be used when heart failure is present. For coronary heart disease patients, choose a drug shown to reduce CV events from either the SGLT-2 inhibitor or the GLP-1 RA classes. As of this writing, empagliflozin and liraglutide may be preferred because both reduced MACE and CV mortality in their respective trials (EMPA-REG OUTCOME and LEADER). Canagliflozin may be used if empagliflozin is not available; however, the former has been associated with increased amputation risk and did not reduce CV mortality in CANVAS. An SGLT-2 inhibitor may be favored when heart failure is present. Note that there is no evidence for additional CV benefits in patients beyond dual therapy (eg, in triple combination therapy). The drug combination recommendations proposed by this algorithm assume that the benefits will be additive. [a] Use specific agents from these classes which have been demonstrated to improve CV outcomes in large randomized outcome trial. i, inhibitor.

considered, typically beginning with lifestyle changes and metformin. When this no longer controls glucose levels adequately, additional therapies are warranted, with many treatment options now available, each with a specific mechanism of action, and certain advantages and disadvantages. In the context of CVD, evidence-based glucose-lowering therapies should be favored. These now include specific drugs from the following classes: SGLT-2 inhibitors, GLP-1 RAs, and TZDs. Treatment guidelines will likely soon be updated in favor of these choices to improve CV outcomes in high-risk patients.

REFERENCES

1. Inzucchi SE, Bergenstal RM, Buse JB, et al. Management of hyperglycemia in type 2 diabetes: a patient-centered approach. Position Statement of the American Diabetes Association (ADA) and the European Association for the Study of Diabetes (EASD). Diabetes Care 2012;35:1364–79.
2. Inzucchi SE, Bergenstal RM, Buse JB, et al. Management of hyperglycemia in type 2 diabetes, 2015: a patient-centered approach. Update to a position statement of the American Diabetes Association (ADA) and the European Association for the Study of Diabetes (EASD). Diabetes Care 2015;38:140–9.
3. Ismail-Beigi F, Moghissi E, Kosiborod M, et al. Shifting paradigms in medical management of type 2 diabetes: reflections on recent cardiovascular safety trials. J Gen Intern Med 2017. https://doi.org/10.1007/s11606-017-4061-7.
4. Inzucchi SE. Clinical practice. Diagnosis of diabetes. N Engl J Med 2012;367:542–50.
5. Available at: https://www.aace.com/publications/algorithm. Accessed October 15, 2017.
6. The Diabetes Control and Complications Trial Research Group. The effect of intensive treatment of diabetes on the development and progression of long-term complications in insulin-dependent diabetes mellitus. N Engl J Med 1993;329:977–86.
7. UK Prospective Diabetes Study (UKPDS) Group. Intensive blood-glucose control with sulphonylureas or insulin compared with conventional treatment and risk of complications in patients with type 2 diabetes (UKPDS 33). Lancet 1998;352:837–53.
8. Gerstein HC, Miller ME, Byington RP, et al. Effects of intensive glucose lowering in type 2 diabetes. N Engl J Med 2008;358:2545–59.
9. The ADVANCE Collaborative Group. Intensive blood glucose control and vascular outcomes in patients with type 2 diabetes. N Engl J Med 2008;358:2560–72.
10. Duckworth W, Abraira C, Moritz T, et al. Glucose control and vascular complications in Veterans Affairs Diabetes Trial with type 2 diabetes. N Engl J Med 2009;360:129–39.
11. American Diabetes Association. Standards of medical care in diabetes–2017. Diabetes Care 2017;40:S1–135.
12. Defronzo RA. From the triumvirate to the ominous octet: a new paradigm for the treatment of type 2 diabetes mellitus. Diabetes 2009;58:773–95.
13. Donnelly LA, Doney AS, Hattersley AT, et al. The effect of obesity on glycaemic response to metformin or sulphonylureas in Type 2 diabetes. Diabet Med 2006;23:128–33.
14. Flory JH, Small DS, Cassano PA, et al. Comparative effectiveness of oral diabetes drug combinations in reducing glycosylated hemoglobin. J Comp Eff Res 2014;3:29–39.

15. Cantrell RA, Alatorre CI, Davis EJ, et al. A review of treatment response in type 2 diabetes: assessing the role of patient heterogeneity. Diabetes Obes Metab 2010;12:845–57.

16. American Diabetes Association. Classification and diagnosis of diabetes. Diabetes Care 2016;39(Suppl 1):S13–22.

17. Laugesen E, Østergaard JA, Leslie RD. Latent autoimmune diabetes of the adult: current knowledge and uncertainty. Diabet Med 2015;32:843–52.

18. Hughes J, Vudattu N, Sznol M, et al. Precipitation of autoimmune diabetes with anti-PD-1. Diabetes Care 2015;38:e55–7.

19. Fajans SS, Bell GI. History, genetics, pathophysiology, and clinical decision making. Diabetes Care 2011;34:1878–84.

20. Eng C, Kramer CK, Zinman B, et al. Glucagon-like peptide-1 receptor agonist and basal insulin combination treatment for the management of type 2 diabetes: a systematic review and meta-analysis. Lancet 2014;384:2228–34.

21. Bloomgarden ZT, Dodis R, Viscoli CM, et al. Lower baseline glycemia reduces apparent oral agent glucose-lowering efficacy: a meta-regression analysis. Diabetes Care 2006;29:2137–9.

22. Marso SP, Daniels GH, Brown-Frandsen K, et al. Liraglutide and cardiovascular outcomes in type 2 diabetes. N Engl J Med 2016;375:311–22.

23. Marso SP, Bain SC, Consoli A, et al. Semaglutide and cardiovascular outcomes in patients with type 2 diabetes. N Engl J Med 2016;375:1834–44.

24. Zinman B, Wanner C, Lachin JM, et al. Empagliflozin, cardiovascular outcomes, and mortality in type 2 diabetes. N Engl J Med 2015;373:2117–28.

25. Neal B, Perkovic V, Mahaffey KW, et al. Canagliflozin and cardiovascular and renal events in type 2 diabetes. N Engl J Med 2017;377:644–57.

26. Inzucchi SE, Iliev H, Pfarr E, et al. Empagliflozin and assessment of lower-limb amputations in the EMPA-REG OUTCOME trial. Diabetes Care 2017. [Epub ahead of print].

27. UK Prospective Diabetes Study (UKPDS) Group. Effect of intensive blood-glucose control with metformin on complications in overweight patients with type 2 diabetes (UKPDS 34). Lancet 1998;352:854–65.

28. Nissen SE, Wolski K. Effect of rosiglitazone on the risk of myocardial infarction and death from cardiovascular causes. N Engl J Med 2007;356:2457–71.

29. Home PD, Pocock SJ, Beck-Nielsen H, et al. Rosiglitazone evaluated for cardiovascular outcomes in oral agent combination therapy for type 2 diabetes (RECORD): a multicentre, randomised, open-label trial. Lancet 2009;373:2125–35.

30. Dormandy JA, Charbonnel B, Eckland DJ, et al. Secondary prevention of macrovascular events in patients with type 2 diabetes in the PROactive Study (PROspective pioglitAzone Clinical Trial In macroVascular Events): a randomised controlled trial. Lancet 2005;366:1279–89.

31. Kernan WN, Viscoli CM, Furie KL, et al. Pioglitazone after Ischemic Stroke or Transient Ischemic Attack. N Engl J Med 2016;374:1321–31.

32. Available at: https://www.fda.gov/downloads/Drugs/.../Guidances/ucm071627.pdf. Accessed October 15, 2017.

33. Scirica BM, Bhatt DL, Braunwald E, et al. Saxagliptin and cardiovascular outcomes in patients with type 2 diabetes mellitus. N Engl J Med 2013;369:1317–26.

34. White WB, Cannon CP, Heller SR, et al. Alogliptin after acute coronary syndrome in patients with type 2 diabetes. The EXAMINE Trial. N Engl J Med 2013;369:1327–35.

35. Green JB, Bethel MA, Armstrong PW, et al, TECOS Study Group. Effect of sitagliptin on cardiovascular outcomes in type 2 diabetes. N Engl J Med 2015;373:232–42.

36. Pfeffer MA, Claggett B, Diaz R, et al. Lixisenatide in patients with type 2 diabetes and acute coronary syndrome. N Engl J Med 2015;373:2247–57.

37. Wanner C, Inzucchi SE, Lachin JM, et al. Empagliflozin and progression of kidney disease in type 2 diabetes. N Engl J Med 2016;375:323–34.

38. Holman RR, Bethel MA, Mentz RJ, et al. Effects of once-weekly exenatide on cardiovascular outcomes in type 2 diabetes. N Engl J Med 2017;377:1228–39.

39. Lipska KJ, Ross JS, Van Houten HK, et al. Use and out-of-pocket costs of insulin for type 2 diabetes mellitus from 2000 to 2010. JAMA 2014;311:2331–3.

Managing Dyslipidemia in Type 2 Diabetes

Adam J. Nelson, BMedSc, MBBS, Simon K. Rochelau, BMBS,
Stephen J. Nicholls, MBBS, PhD, FRACP*

KEYWORDS

- Diabetes • Dyslipidemia • Triglycerides • LDL • Statin

KEY POINTS

- Despite significant improvements in the treatment of T2DM, patients continue to suffer a reduction in life expectancy, more than half of which is attributable to atherosclerotic cardiovascular disease.
- Although some of this risk remains unexplained and a focus of ongoing research, mitigating traditional and modifiable factors remains a central tenet in the management of these patients.
- Dyslipidemia is one such focus, yet contemporary data show that treatment efforts continue to disappoint.
- Established therapies of statins and ezetimibe remain the cornerstone of dyslipidemia treatment however, in patients with persistent residual risk, bile acid sequestrants, fibrates, and ultimately PCSK-9 inhibitors need to be considered.

Cardiovascular disease (CVD) is the most frequent cause of morbidity and mortality among individuals with diabetes (type 2 diabetes mellitus [T2DM]). The presence of T2DM is associated with a two- to four-fold increased risk for CVD and has been variably identified as a coronary artery disease risk-equivalent in prevention guidelines.[1] The increasing incidence of T2DM, 20% by 2035 in developed nations,[2] in parallel with the spread of abdominal obesity, is likely to result in commensurate growth in the burden of atherosclerotic CVD (ASCVD). Accordingly there is considerable interest in evaluating ways to mitigate risk in these patients at a population and individual patient level. Aggressive management of traditional risk factors, such as dyslipidemia, remains an essential part of this strategy.

Disclosure: Dr S.J. Nicholls has received research support from AstraZeneca, Amgen, Anthera, Eli Lilly, Novartis, Cerenis, The Medicines Company, Resverlogix, InfraReDx, Roche, SanofiRegeneron and LipoScience and is a consultant for AstraZeneca, Eli Lilly, Anthera, Omthera, Merck, Takeda, Resverlogix, Sanofi-Regeneron, CSL Behring, Esperion, Boehringer Ingelheim.
South Australian Health and Medical Research Institute, PO Box 11060, Adelaide, SA 5001, Australia
* Corresponding author.
E-mail address: Stephen.nicholls@sahmri.com

Endocrinol Metab Clin N Am 47 (2018) 153–173
https://doi.org/10.1016/j.ecl.2017.10.004
0889-8529/18/© 2017 Elsevier Inc. All rights reserved.

DIABETES AND CARDIOVASCULAR RISK

Although the last 20 years has seen a narrowing in the excess CVD risk associated with T2DM, contemporary data continue to show these individuals remain at substantially higher risk than their counterparts without diabetes.[3–5] Diabetes is believed to shorten the lifespan of a 50-year-old person by approximately 6 years, more than half of which is caused by vascular disease.[6,7] The excess CVD risk in patients with T2DM is caused by a poorly understood interaction between nonmodifiable factors, such as age, gender, and genetics, with more traditional risk factors that include hypertension, dyslipidemia, and smoking. Although hyperglycemia is undoubtedly contributory, intensive glycemic control seems to reduce morbidity and microvascular complications, yet there is an underwhelming impact on atherosclerotic CV mortality.[8–10] Recently, this has driven a shift away from a glucocentric approach to one focused on modifiable risk factors, such as dyslipidemia.

PREVALENCE AND RISK OF DYSLIPIDEMIA IN TYPE 2 DIABETES

Some form of lipid abnormality is found in up to 85% of patients with diabetes.[11] The spectrum of qualitative and quantitative change in lipids and lipoproteins is influenced by comorbid obesity, hyperinsulinemia, and insulin resistance. Although there exists a classic phenotype, a variety of lipid abnormalities are observed. Moreover it is unlikely one sole feature of the complex phenotype is responsible for the dyslipidemic risk; however, each of the associated abnormalities has established CVD risk.

Low-Density Lipoprotein Cholesterol

Somewhat counterintuitively, elevated low-density lipoprotein cholesterol (LDL-C) seems to be no more prevalent in patients with diabetes than age-matched control subjects. Data from the United States National Health and Nutritional Examination Survey from 1999 to 2000 revealed that 25.3% of patients with diabetes had an LDL-C of greater than 100 mg/dL, which was similar (24.3%) to that of the general population. Notwithstanding this, absolute levels of LDL-C and more potently the percentage reduction of LDL-C tightly correlated with ASCVD in the unselected[12] and diabetic populations.[13] Total LDL-C may, however, be a coarse, potentially misleading parameter in diabetes because there seems to be a critical shift in LDL-C composition to more numerous, small-density LDL-C particles (sdLDLp) associated with greater ASCVD risk.[14]

Triglycerides

Plasma triglycerides (TG) of patients with T2DM are significantly increased as evidenced by the Framingham study where 19% of male sufferers had levels greater than the 90% centile compared with 9% of their counterparts without diabetes. Numerically in the UK Prospective Diabetes Study mean TG levels were up to 50% higher than the normal population. Genome-wide association studies implicate an independent, causal role of TG in CVD even after accounting for associated effects of LDL-C and high-density lipoprotein cholesterol (HDL-C).[15] This is described at a clinical[16] and subclinical atherosclerotic level.[17] Of particular interest, nonfasting TG, probably reflective of the atherogenic TG remnants, is a stronger predictor of CVD events than fasting TG levels.

High-Density Lipoprotein Cholesterol

Levels of HDL-C are frequently and often markedly reduced in patients with T2DM. Patients with diabetes in the Heart Protection Study were two-fold more likely to have an HDL-C level less than the 10th centile compared with patients without diabetes (21% vs 12%). The association of low levels of HDL-C with ASCVD has been variably shown across different cohorts and trials clinically[18,19] and subclinically.[20] Pharmacologic attempts to raise,[21] or studies evaluating genetic mutations associated with an increase in levels,[22] have not yet readily conferred mortality reduction. Whether HDL-C levels instead represent a coarse marker for HDL-C function or other players, such as ApoA-1 level, remains the basis of ongoing study.

Described in some form as early as the 1990s, the term "atherogenic dyslipidemia" was given to the combination of increased TG, reduced HDL-C, and increased quantity of sdLDLp. This term at times has been used interchangeably with "diabetic dyslipidemia": however, in its purest form it has its basis in insulin resistance and the metabolic syndrome, both of which frequently coexist with prediabetic or diabetic states. The exact prevalence of this lipid phenotype in diabetes is not known because there is no uniformly accepted definition and it is significantly affected by comorbidity profile and treatment status. The most contemporary data come from the FIELD study evaluating the primary prevention role of fibrates in patients with diabetes already treated with a statin.[23] In this trial, 38% of subjects had the combination of both elevated TG (>66 mg/dL) and low HDL-C (<39.8 mg/dL for males and <49.9 mg/dL for females).

PATHOPHYSIOLOGY OF DYSLIPIDEMIA

The underlying pathophysiology generating the milieu of lipid and lipoprotein abnormalities in insulin resistance is detailed and incompletely understood. Hyperglycemia is clearly associated with diabetic dyslipidemia[24]; however, that cannot fully explain the breadth of abnormalities. The core features of the phenotype are underpinned by insulin resistance and result in abnormal metabolism and quantity of TG rich lipoproteins (TRLs) derived either from the intestine (as chylomicrons) or the liver (as very-low-density lipoprotein [VLDL]). A full description of the abnormalities is outside the scope of this review; however, it is worth highlighting some key points. Brief structure of lipid types is seen in **Fig. 1**.

Triglyceride-Rich Lipoproteins Species

Insulin resistance is associated with increased levels of serum insulin and results in impaired regulation of circulating lipoprotein and glucose levels. Impaired insulin feedback at the adipocyte results in defective suppression of intracellular hydrolysis of TG with the release of free fatty acids into the circulation. These fatty acids reach the liver and stimulate the secretion of apolipoprotein B (apoB)-100, which scaffolds with TG to

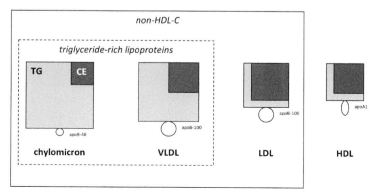

Fig. 1. Broad classification and relative composition of lipid. CE, cholesteryl ester; TG, triglyceride.

form the VLDL, a TRL. Excess fatty acids seen in the insulin resistant state seem to remove the negative feedback, which would usually result in apoB-100 degradation, hence there is an overproduction of VLDL. Kinetic studies using radioisotopes show VLDL catabolism is reduced in T2DM mainly because of a reduction in lipoprotein lipase activity and via increased apoprotein-CIII (a known inhibitor of lipoprotein lipase) expression, which has been tightly linked to impaired VLDL clearance in insulin-resistant individuals.[25]

Adding to the TRL pool is the development of chylomicrons. These are TRLs that are generated from intestinal absorption of fatty acids, which in turn undergo re-esterification back to TG before being scaffolded with apoB-48. In insulin resistant states there is impaired negative feedback and thus apoB-48 secretion is unimpeded generating larger numbers of chylomicrons. In addition to increased production, reduced activity of lipoprotein lipase results in less chylomicron hydrolysis/catabolism. Furthermore the reuptake of chylomicrons at a hepatic level, usually driven by insulin signaling, is blunted in insulin-resistant mice leading to increased plasma transit time.

Small-Density Low-Density Lipoprotein Particles and High-Density Lipoprotein

When HDL and VLDL are exposed to cholesteryl ester transfer protein, TG within VLDL is exchanged for cholesterol ester within HDL. This interaction results in TG-rich VLDL remnant particles and TG-rich cholesterol-depleted HDL particles. These HDL particles are less functional and more likely to be catabolized, nullifying any of HDL's anti-inflammatory, antioxidant effects.

Furthermore, cholesteryl ester transfer protein activity in the presence of VLDL causes transfer of TG to LDL in exchange for cholesterol ester. The TG-rich LDL undergoes hydrolysis by hepatic lipase, which results in lipid-depleted sdLDLp. This means that at any given LDL-C concentration there are more LDL particles present in an individual with insulin resistance compared with those with normal density LDL-C, hence the overall measure of LDL-C may be misleading in T2DM.[26] These particles are more prone to oxidation and more readily adhere and invade the arterial wall when compared with their larger, more buoyant precursor.[27]

MANAGEMENT OF DIABETIC DYSLIPIDEMIA

Effective management of dyslipidemia in diabetes requires a comprehensive approach including lifestyle measures and pharmacologic intervention. There are several consensus guidelines available for review in the European and American literature (**Table 1**). All recommend at least moderate-intensity statin in patients with diabetes older than 40 although differ with regards to treatment targets and recommendations for step up or second-line therapy. With more recent data available, particularly with nonstatin alternatives, a review of the current options available for management of dyslipidemia is presented.

Nonpharmacologic Management

Diet

Diet is a key aspect of mitigating metabolic derangements in patients with diabetes. This review is focused on lipid profile; however, dietary intervention clearly has several other key sequelae, such as weight loss and glycemic control, and is modified by several factors including genetics, the microbiome, and baseline lipid phenotype. A recent meta-analysis attempted to evaluate the effects of different types of diet on glycemic control and lipid profile.[28] In total 16 studies of 3073 patients were included for quantitative analysis because they were randomized and their follow-up was greater

Table 1
Summary of the most recent published guidelines for dyslipidemia in diabetes

Society	Cohort	Recommendation	Goal	Second Line
AHA/ACC (2013 & 2016)	Established ASCVD	High intensity statin	50% LDL reduction (or LDL <70 mg/dL)	Consider ezetimibe or replace with PCSK9 inhibitor
	DM 40–75 yo and estimated 10 y ASCVD >7.5% with Cardiovascular risk calculator or high risk features (retinopathy, CKD, albuminuria, elevated Lp(a), subclinical athero)	High intensity statin	50% LDL reduction (or LDL 70–189 mg/dL) or non-HDL-C <130 mg/dL	Consider ezetimibe or bile acid sequestrant
	DM 40–75 yo and estimated 10 y ASCVD <7.5% with Cardiovascular risk calculator and no high risk features (retinopathy, CKD, albuminuria, elevated Lp(a), subclinical athero)	Moderate intensity statin	30% LDL reduction (or LDL <100 mg/dL) or non-HDL-C <130 mg/dL	Consider high intensity statin
	DM <40 or >75 yo or LDL <70 mg/dL	Consider statin based on risk-benefit profile	—	—

(continued on next page)

Table 1
(continued)

Society	Cohort	Recommendation	Goal	Second Line
ADA (2015)	Established ASCVD	High intensity statin	LDL-C <70 mg/dL	—
	>75 yo:			
	With ASCVD RF	High intensity	LDL-C <100 mg/dL or 30% reduction from baseline	—
	Without ASCVD RF	Moderate or high intensity		—
	40–75 yo:			
	With ASCVD RF	High intensity statin	LDL-C <100 mg/dL or 30% reduction from baseline	—
	Without ASCVD RF	Moderate intensity statin		—
	<40 yo:			
	With ASCVD RF	Moderate or high intensity statin	LDL-C <100 mg/dL or 30% reduction from baseline	
	Without ASCVD RF	Lifestyle		
ESC/EAS (2016)	Established CVD or CKD	Statin up to highest recommended dose or highest tolerable to reach goal	LDL-C <70 mg/dL Non-HDLC <100 mg/dL apoB <80 mg/dL	Consider ezetimibe (level B) or bile acid sequestrant (level C) or PCSK-9 (level C)
	>40 yo and have one or more CVD risk factors or target organ damage			
	No risk factors and/or evidence of target organ damage	Statin up to highest recommended dose or highest tolerable to reach goal	LDLC <100 mg/dL Non-HDLC <130 mg/dL apoB <100 mg/dL	Consider ezetimibe (level B) or bile acid sequestrant (level C) or PCSK-9 (level C)

'ASCVD RFs' = LDL-C >100, hypertension, smoking, overweight/obesity, FHx of premature ASCVD; *Estimated 10 year risk* = Pooled equations utilizing age, sex, race, total cholesterol, systolic blood pressure, blood pressure medications, diabetes status and smoking status; *High-intensity* [i.e. atorvastatin 80 mg/day (40 mg/day if 80 mg not tolerated) and rosuvastatin 20–40 mg/day]; *Moderate-intensity* [i.e. atorvastatin 10–20 mg/day, rosuvastatin 5–10 mg/day, simvastatin 20–40 mg/day].

Abbreviations: ADA, American Diabetes Association; AHA/ACC, American Heart Association and American College of Cardiology; ESC/EAS, European Society of Cardiology and European Atherosclerosis Society.

Data from Stone NJ, Robinson J, Lichtenstein AH, et al. 2013 ACC/AHA guideline on the treatment of blood cholesterol to reduce atherosclerotic cardiovascular risk in adults: a report of the American College of Cardiology/American Heart Association Task Force on Practice Guidelines. Circulation 2014;129(25 Suppl 2):S1–45; and Lloyd-Jones DM, Morris PB, Ballantyne CM, et al. 2016 ACC expert consensus decision pathway on the role of non-statin therapies for LDL-cholesterol lowering in the management of atherosclerotic cardiovascular disease risk: a report of the American College of Cardiology Task Force on Clinical Expert Consensus Documents. J Am Coll Cardiol 2016;68(1):92–125.

than 6 months. Using a variety of control groups there were nine studies comparing a low-carbohydrate diet, four studies comparing a Mediterranean diet, three studies comparing a low glycemic index diet, and two comparing a high-protein diet.

- Low-carbohydrate diet: generally restricts carbohydrate intake to 20 to 60 g/d. The low-carbohydrate diets increased HDL-C by 10% with no significant reduction in LDL-C or TG.
- Low glycemic index diet: although variably defined within each of the three trials, these diets had between 3 and 14 less glycemic index points compared with the control diet. Analysis of these trials showed a marginal increase in HDL by 5%; however, there was no significant difference compared with control diets for either LDL-C or TG.
- Mediterranean diet: generally rich in olive oil, legumes, unrefined cereals, fruit, and vegetables; low in meat; and with moderate contents of dairy products, fish, and wine. In meta-analysis, the Mediterranean diet significantly reduced TG by 9% and increased HDL-C by 5%; however, there was no significant reduction in LDL.
- High-protein diet: generally require 20% to 30% or more of the total daily calories to come from proteins. The two high-protein diets included in the meta-analysis together had no appreciable effect on any lipid parameter.

Although the optimal diet to prevent CVD among patients with diabetes remains controversial, any recommendations ought to be individualized and centered on sustainability of any proposed dietary change.

Lifestyle: diet, exercise, and weight loss

More than three out of every four adults with diabetes are at least overweight,[29] and nearly half of individuals with diabetes are obese.[30] Insulin resistance is tightly linked with obesity, although when measured coarsely by body mass index (BMI) alone, does not explain all of the association. It may be rather than generalized obesity (measured with BMI), it is the metabolically active, visceral or ectopic fat depots that are playing significant roles. Nevertheless weight reduction has consistently been shown to improve insulin sensitivity suggesting it is perhaps not weight loss alone, but the direct effects on metabolic pathways via increasing improved insulin signal transduction, improved secretory processes, and reduced rates of hepatic glucose production.[31] All weight-loss studies are confounded by mode of intervention and the inability to dissect out causal association from downstream processes; however, there has been an unconvincing effect on CV risk factors or events.

A recent meta-analysis of overweight patients with T2DM demonstrated that most lifestyle interventions do not result in sustained weight loss and at least 5% weight loss was required to observe any, if only modest improvements in lipid profile.[32] The largest randomized trial included in the analysis, Look-AHEAD, ran from 2001 to 2012 and evaluated whether long-term weight reduction would reduce CV morbidity and mortality in overweight patients (BMI >25 kg/m^2) with T2DM.[33] Half of the 5000 subjects randomized to the intensive lifestyle intervention were reviewed weekly for the first year and then 1 to 2 monthly thereafter to maintain a goal 7% weight loss. Most were prescribed meal replacements and were encouraged, via a pedometer, to meet a goal of greater than 175 min/wk of activity. At median follow-up of 9.6 years, although there was improvement in several parameters including blood pressure, hemoglobin (Hb) A$_{1c}$, and lipid profile, this did not translate to reduced CV events and thus the trial was ceased early. Compared with counseling alone, there was modest overall incremental benefit including 6% more weight loss, mean reduction in TG of

5.8 mg/dL, subtle 1.7 mg/dL increase in HDL, and no significant change in LDL when adjusted for medication use.[34,35] Furthermore, it would seem unlikely this degree of intensive support could be provided in real-world care to maintain the weight loss long term.

Despite the unimpressive effect on lipid profile, weight-loss via any means remains a central tenet in the care of the overweight individual with diabetes with established benefit on glycemic control and improvement in insulin sensitivity.

Physical exercise

Only a paucity of exercise intervention studies is robust enough to include in a meta-analysis; however of those, there is established benefit for HbA_{1c}, blood pressure, and weight loss. Irrespective of exercise modality (aerobic, resistance, or combined), and when controlled for other confounders, there does not seem to be any significant, reproducible, and independent effect of exercise on LDL-C, HDL-C, or TG.[36,37]

Pharmacologic Management

Statins

Competitive 3-hydroxy-3-methylglutaryl-coenzyme A (HMG-CoA) reductase inhibitors, or statins, have become the cornerstone of treatment of dyslipidemia. Blocking HMG-CoA results in a reduction in intrahepatic cholesterol, which leads to an increase in LDL receptor turnover and LDL uptake by the liver, thus reducing the circulating levels of LDL between 30% and 50% from baseline. The fundamental role of LDL-C in atherogenesis has been well recognized, and the utility of statins in reducing CVD risk is established through numerous large clinical trials and meta-analyses. The role of statins for the management of dyslipidemia among patients with diabetes has also been established. The Heart Protection Study randomized 5963 subjects with T2DM to either simvastatin or placebo, which resulted in a 39 mg/dL reduction in LDL compared with placebo and a reduction in Major Adverse Cardiac Event (MACE) of 22%.[38] CARDS (Collaborative Atorvastatin Diabetes Study) randomized 2838 patients with T2DM and an LDL less than 160 mg/dL to low-dose atorvastatin over a median follow-up of 4 years.[39] Although there was a significant 37% reduction in MACE ($P = .0001$), the mortality end point did not reach significance at -27% ($P = .0569$). A large meta-analysis that included more than 18,000 patients with diabetes treated with statin monotherapy showed a 9% reduction in all-cause mortality and a 21% reduction in the incidence of MACE per mmol/L reduction in LDL, a similar finding for those without diabetes.[13]

Furthermore, among all participants with diabetes, the proportional reduction in major vascular events per mmol/L reduction in LDL cholesterol was similar irrespective of other comorbidities and baseline LDL. Additional reductions in LDL cholesterol with more intensive therapy either through higher doses or more potent statins has also been shown to further reduce the incidence of major vascular events with no significant interaction from diabetes status.[40] Therefore, the established relationship between reducing LDL cholesterol and risk reduction remains proportional and holds true among patients with diabetes. Despite the small effect on glucose metabolism raising HbA_{1c} on average 0.12%,[41] the safety and efficacy of statin therapy among patients with diabetes make it an obvious first-line choice in the treatment of dyslipidemia.

Ezetimibe

Ezetimibe targets the Niemann-Pick C1-like 1 (NPC1L1) protein, which results in reduced absorption of cholesterol from the intestine.[42] The decrease in absorbed cholesterol causes the liver to use more circulating cholesterol, thus reducing the plasma concentration. Several phase III trials in unselected patients with and without established disease have shown ezetimibe reduces LDL cholesterol levels by an additional 23% to 24%, on average.[43]

IMPROVE-IT (IMProved Reduction of Outcomes: Vytorin Efficacy International Trial) was by far the largest randomized controlled trial comparing ezetimibe and simvastatin with simvastatin and placebo among 18,144 patients post acute coronary syndrome.[44] The intervention arm overall observed a 24% reduction in LDL-C (70 mg/dL vs 53 mg/dL) and a modest overall 2% reduction in CV events.

Approximately one-quarter of all subjects in each arm had comorbid diabetes in which a prespecified subgroup analysis was performed demonstrating a 14% relative reduction in events for those receiving ezetimibe therapy. When stratified into those with and without diabetes, it was those with diabetes (40% vs 45.5%; hazard ratio, 0.86; confidence interval, 0.78–0.94) that benefitted significantly more than those without diabetes (30.2% vs 30.8%; hazard ratio, 0.98; confidence interval, 0.91–1.04), for the primary end point. Clearly this is a subgroup and there were differences in baseline population; however, there are some additional data to support this benefit in patients with diabetes.

An evolving body of data now supports ezetimibe's capacity not only in lowering LDL-C but also modifying other aspects of lipid profile. In the ESD (Ezetimibe and Simvastatin in Dyslipidemia) trial, the addition of ezetimibe to simvastatin in subjects who failed to reach their LDL goal with statin alone observed a further reduction in LDL-C of 31% and total cholesterol of 22% but also reduced apoB levels by 20%.[45] Another small clinical trial evaluating the addition of ezetimibe to weight loss compared with weight loss alone showed reduced plasma levels of apoB-100 and a significant increase in its catabolism. Furthermore, there was a decrease in intrahepatic TG independent of weight loss changes observed in both arms.

It is possible the reductions in LDL-C and non-HDL-C are observed to greater extent in those with diabetes because animal models of hyperglycemia and insulin resistance seem to not only drive cholesterol absorption in the setting of statin use, at least in part mediated by upregulation of ezetimibe's target, NPC1L1.[46,47] Not only does ezetimibe therefore have a role in patients not at LDL target or intolerant of statins, there is increasing interest in its application as upfront dual therapy to mitigate these diabetes-specific pathways.

Fibrates
Fibrates are agonists of the peroxisome proliferator receptors selective for the α receptor and have been shown to reduce TG by up to 30% and increase HDL by 10%.[48] Fibrates reduce TG substrate availability in the liver by stimulating peroxisomal and mitochondrial β-oxidation, which in turn decreases secretion of VLDL.[48] Furthermore, they promote intravascular lipolysis of TRLs by inducing LPL expression and inhibiting apoC-III expression.[49] The two largest trials in this space are FIELD (Fenofibrate Intervention and Event Lowering in Diabetes) and ACCORD (Action to Control Cardiovascular Risk in Diabetes) Lipid.

The FIELD trial compared fenofibrate therapy with placebo in 9795 subjects and found a significant reduction in nonfatal myocardial infarction (MI) and coronary revascularization among individuals with diabetes taking fenofibrate.[50] Statin use was variable and ultimately higher in the placebo arm. At mean follow-up of 5 years, there was no difference between the two groups when looking at the composite end point of CV death, MI, stroke, and need for coronary or carotid revascularization. Of note, in a prespecified subgroup of subjects with elevated TG (>89 mg/dL) and low HDL (<43 mg/dL) there was a significant relative risk reduction in the composite end point of 27% ($P = .005$).

The ACCORD Lipid study compared 5518 patients who in addition to statin therapy received either fenofibrate or placebo.[51] Overall the trial failed to show any benefit in the composite of fatal CV events, nonfatal MI, or nonfatal stroke; however, as seen in the FIELD trial, a subgroup of patients with the highest TG and lowest HDL experienced a 29% relative risk reduction (17.3% vs 12.4%). To interrogate this subgroup, the largest meta-analysis found fibrates reduced vascular events by 25% in subjects with elevated TGs alone (n = 7389), 29% of subjects with both elevated TG and low HDL (n = 5068), and by 16% in those with low HDL only (n = 15,303).[52] There was, however, no benefit in those without high TG or reduced HDL levels (n = 9872). These analyses translated to the inclusion of fibrates as add-on therapy for patients with elevated TG (>89 mg/dL) and reduced HDL (<35 mg/dL) with surveillance for rhabdomyolysis, which is observed slightly more with gemfibrozil than other fibrates.[53]

Niacin
Niacin, a nicotinic acid derivative and B3 complex vitamin, inhibits lipolysis in adipose tissue thereby reducing supply of free fatty acid to the liver. This in turn results in reduced hepatic output of VLDL and the subsequent production of LDL.[54] Because of a reduction in TG, there is a qualitative shift in LDL from sdLDLp to larger LDL. Separately, administration of niacin results in increased secretion and delayed catabolism of apoA-I, which likely explains the observed elevation in HDL-C.[49]

Niacin has been shown to decrease TG and HDL by up to 30% and reduce LDL-C and lipoprotein(a) levels by between 15% and 30%, respectively.[49] Although there was early enthusiasm for niacin in smaller clinical trials, more recent and large-scale studies in a statin era have been less convincing. There have been no dedicated trials enrolling patients with diabetes; however, AIM HIGH and HPS-2 Thrive, the two largest studies, included 34% and 32% patients with diabetes, respectively. There was no interaction with the overall outcome in this diabetic subgroup. The AIM HIGH trial randomized 3414 patients who were already on simvastatin and ezetimibe to receive either placebo or niacin.[55] Despite an increase in HDL by 15% over 3 years, there was no improvement in the primary end point of death or CV events. Of note, a secondary analysis of 522 patients (15.3% of the trial) with the highest TG (>188 mg/dL) and lowest HDL levels (<32 mg/dL) experienced fewer CV events (hazard ratio, 0.74; P = .07).[56]

In the HPS-2 THRIVE trial, more than 25,000 patients with vascular disease and controlled LDL-C on statin therapy were randomized to receive either niacin (and prostaglandin D_2 inhibitor laropiprant to mitigate the side effect of flushing) or placebo.[57] Despite a 20% reduction in LDL-C and a mean increase in HDL-C of 17%, there was no reduction in the CV end points over 4 years of follow-up. Furthermore, there were side effects from niacin therapy including significant worsening of diabetic control among patients with diabetes (3.7%) and gastrointestinal upset (1%). In view of its lack of outcome efficacy and potential harm, niacin has subsequently been removed from the American guidelines and is not approved for administration in Europe.

Bile acid sequestrants
The administration of bile acid sequestrants depletes the endogenous bile acid pool thus stimulating an increase in bile acid synthesis from cholesterol, which in turn upregulates LDL receptor expression, thus removing LDL from the plasma circulation. At the maximum dose of cholestyramine (resin), colestipol (resin), or colesevelam (synthetic), a reduction in LDL-C of 18% to 25% has been observed. There are, however, no major effects on HDL levels and potentially some tendency to increase TGs. All of this comes with significant gastrointestinal effects of flatulence, nausea, dyspepsia,

and drug interactions. The widespread use of statins has demonstrated a more robust reduction in LDL with less side effects and therefore has largely replaced use of bile acid sequestrants as first-line therapy.

Of interest, the depletion of bile acids with a sequestrant also results in the upregulation of HMG-CoA reductase and thus there is the potential for a synergistic reduction in LDL when combined with statin therapy. To date there have been no studies with CV end points as the primary outcome for combined statin and bile acid therapy despite several small trials demonstrating similar LDL-C reductions compared with high-dose statin therapy alone.[58] Without CV outcome trials, bile acid sequestrants remain an option for statin-intolerant patients either as monotherapy or potentially in addition to ezetimibe where there was some additional LDL-lowering efficacy without adverse effects in a small clinical trial.[59]

Omega-3 fatty acids

Omega-3 fatty acids (OM3FA) can be used at pharmacologic doses (2-4 g/d) to lower TGs up to 45%.[60] The underlying mechanism remains unclear; however, it may be related to their ability to interact with peroxisome proliferator receptors selective for the α receptor in addition to reduced secretion of apoB. There has been conflicting outcome data on OM3FA supplementation; however, the most recent and largest meta-analysis included more than 63,000 subjects from 20 primary and secondary prevention trials and reported no overall effect of OM3FA on a composite of CV events or mortality.[61] Two key randomized placebo-controlled trials each with 8000 or more subjects (Reduction of Cardiovascular Events with EPA-Intervention Trial [REDUCE-IT] and Outcomes Study to Assess STatin Residual Risk Reduction with EpaNova in HiGh CV Risk PatienTs with Hypertriglyceridemia [STRENGTH]) are studying the potential benefits of OM3FA on CVD outcomes with elevated TGs. Of particular interest in the diabetic sphere is the ASCEND study, which is evaluating whether aspirin and/or OM3FA will reduce CV events in 15,000 subjects with diabetes without established disease. Follow-up is now complete with results anticipated in 2018.

PCSK-9 inhibitors

PCSK9 serine protease is a protein primarily synthesized and secreted from the liver and is involved in cholesterol homeostasis by binding to the LDL receptor and triggering its degradation. Antibodies have been created that interfere with PCSK9 and thus prevent binding to the LDL-receptor, which in turn allows the receptor to be recycled to the cell surface and thus remove additional LDL from the plasma. Sattar and colleagues[62] recently performed a random-effects, patient-level meta-analysis of randomized controlled trials comparing evolocumab, placebo, and ezetimibe on lipid parameters in DM (n = 413) or without DM (n = 2119). In subjects with DM, the PCSK9 inhibitor reduced LDL by 60% versus placebo and 39% versus ezetimibe, which was similar to that observed in the non-DM cohort (69% and 40%, respectively). Of particular interest, however, is the effect of these agents on other aspects of the lipid profile including a 31% reduction in lipoprotein(a), an agent recently elevated to causal status in mendelian randomization studies. This phenomenon, in addition to a 55% reduction in overall non–HDL-C, has not been seen in statin treatment alone.

The FOURIER (Further Cardiovascular Outcomes Research with PCSK9 Inhibition in Subjects with Elevated Risk) trial was designed to evaluate whether both these changes and impressive LDL reduction would translate into improved CV outcomes.[63] The study was a randomized double-blind trial that looked at the addition of evolocumab or placebo to statin therapy in more than 27,000 patients with atherosclerotic disease and LDL levels greater than 70 mg/dL. After a median follow-up of just over

2 years, a 59% reduction in LDL brought the LDL median of 92 mg/dL to 30 mg/dL and was associated with a 15% reduction in the primary end point of CV death, MI, stroke, unstable angina, or revascularization; however, it did not reach statistical significance for mortality. Notwithstanding this was a short trial and it is expected longer follow-up may provide this outcome. A prespecified subgroup analysis of patients with diabetes in the FOURIER trial, currently in press, reports similar reductions in LDL and overall MACE compared with their counterparts without diabetes.[64] Given their baseline higher risk, however, patients with diabetes seem to derive a greater absolute risk reduction from PCSK-9 inhibition without any signal for harm. Presently available only to familial dyslipidemia, cost-benefit analyses may dictate who and how patients can receive this presently expensive therapy.

DISCUSSION

Despite significant improvements in the treatment of T2DM, patients continue to suffer a reduction in life expectancy, more than half of which is attributable to atherosclerotic CVD. Although some of this risk remains unexplained and a focus of ongoing research, mitigating traditional and modifiable factors remains a central tenet in the management of these patients. Dyslipidemia is one such focus, yet contemporary data show that treatment efforts continue to disappoint (**Table 2**). Recent randomized controlled trial data show that up to one in five patients with diabetes with established coronary disease are not on statin therapy[62] and of those who were treated in another cross-sectional population study, up to 50% did not reach prespecified LDL treatment goals.[65]

The presence and nature of dyslipidemia in diabetes is often established some years earlier by insulin resistance and hyperglycemia. It is therefore likely that these patients may respond to aggressive risk factor management before the onset of established metabolic derangement. Endocrinologists and primary care physicians need to prioritize dyslipidemia alongside glycemic control in managing these patients, particularly before an established diabetes diagnosis. Initiation of lipid-lowering therapy after the clinical manifestation of ASCVD represents a missed opportunity to retard the disease process at the most optimal time.

To make inroads into atherosclerotic disease event rates in patients with diabetes, interventions need to be timely, targeted, and their effects evaluated. This includes, but is not limited to the following suggestions:

- Prioritizing treatment of modifiable CV risk factors, such as dyslipidemia, with equal importance of glucose-lowering therapy
- Regular reiteration of dietary and lifestyle advice to obtain weight loss
- Increased awareness of risk stratification and potentially, embarking on a lower threshold for treatment in patients who have borderline risk
- Regular reassessment of LDL to guide statin up-titration
- Early recognition of the need for nonstatin alternatives, such as ezetimibe or bile acid sequestrants if LDL remains elevated
- Consideration of fibrates when TG is raised or HDL is reduced.
- Explore beyond normal LDL levels into non–HDL-C to further risk stratify those patients

In 2014, close to 30 million Americans, or 10% of the population, had either type I or type II diabetes. Today, of those who reach theirs 60s, more than half will die from ASCVD or its complications.[7] The early stratification and mitigation of evolving and traditional risk factors in these individuals needs to become a priority for family

Table 2
Summary of randomized trials for each of the main agents which included a significant number of patients with diabetes

Agent	Outcome Trial	Intervention	Cohort	Follow up	Outcome
Statins	Heart Protection Study (HPS)[37]	Simvastatin 40 mg vs. placebo	n = 5963 Age 40–80 y AND Type 2 DM AND TC >135 mg/dL	Median: 5 y	LDL: ↓39 mg/dL (-31%) $P<.001$ HDL: ↑0.4 mg/dL (+1%), $P = NS$ TG: ↓27 mg/dL (-13%), $P<.001$ MACE: ↓22% ($P<.0001$, CI 13–30%)
	Collaborative Atorvastatin Diabetes Study (CARDS)[38]	Atorvastatin 10 mg vs. placebo	n = 2838 Age 40–75 y AND Type 2 DM AND LDL <160 mg/dL AND TG <531 mg/dL	Median: 4 y	LDL ↓46 mg/dL (-40%) $P<.001$ HDL: ↑0.8 mg/dL (+1%), $P<.001$ TG: ↓35 mg/dL (-19%), $P<.001$ MACE: ↓37% ($P<.0001$, CI 17–52%)
Ezetimibe	IMProved Reduction of Outcomes: Vytorin Efficacy Intervention Trial (IMPROVE IT)[44]	Simvastatin 40 mg and ezetimibe 10 mg vs. simvastatin 40 mg	n = 18,144 10 d post ACS AND LDL 50–100 mg/dL • 27% of cohort diabetic	Median 6 y	LDL: ↓17 mg/dL (-24%), $P = <.001$ HDL: ↑0.7 mg/dL (+1%), $P<.001$ TG: ↓14 mg/dL (-11%), $P<.001$ MACE: ↓6% ($P<.016$, CI 0.89-0.99) • DM pre-specified group: MACE ↓14%, HR 0.86, CI 0.78–0.94)

(continued on next page)

Table 2
(*continued*)

Agent	Outcome Trial	Intervention	Cohort	Follow up	Outcome
Fibrates	Fenofibrate Intervention and Event Lowering in Diabetes (FIELD)[50]	Fenofibrate 200 mg daily vs. placebo	n = 9795, Age 50–75 y AND Type 2 DM AND TC 115–250 mg/dL AND Naïve to lipid lowering therapy	Median: 5 y	LDL: ↓15 mg/dL (-12%), P = <.05; HDL: ↑1.9 mg/dL (+5%), P<.05; TG: ↓48 mg/dL (-29%), P<.05; Major coronary event: ↓11% (P = .16, CI 0.75–1.05); • Post hoc subgroup: ↑TG and ↓HDL, major coronary event ↓27% (P = .0005, CI 9–42%)
	Action to Control Cardiovascular Risk in Diabetes (ACCORD) Lipid[51]	Fenofibrate 160 mg vs. placebo (in addition to simvastatin background)	n = 5518, Type 2 DM with A1c >7.5% AND Age 40–79 y AND LDL 60–180 mg/dL AND HDL <55 mg/dL AND TG <750 mg/dL	Median: 5 y	LDL: ↓1.1 mg/dL (-4%), P = .16; HDL: ↑0.7 mg/dL (+1.7%), P<.01; TG: ↓23 mg/dL (-13.5%), P<.0001; MACE: ↓8%, HR 0.92, CI 0.79–1.08, P = .32; • In pre-specified ↑TG and ↓HDL subgroup, MACE ↓31% (P = .005)

Niacin	Atherothrombosis Intervention in Metabolic Syndrome with Low HDL/High Triglycerides: Impact on Global Health Outcomes (AIM HIGH)[55]	Niacin 1500–2000 mg/d vs. placebo. On background of simvastatin +/- ezetimibe	n = 3414. Age >45 y AND Established CVD AND LDL 40–80 mg/dL • 34% of cohort diabetic	Mean: 3 y	LDL: ↓3.1 mg/dL (-6%), P<.001; HDL: ↑5 mg/dL (+14%), P<.001; TG: ↓32 mg/dL (-19%), P<.001; MACE: ↑1.2%, HR 1.02, CI 0.87–1.21, P = .8 • In pre-specified diabetic cohort, no interaction with primary endpoint.
	The Heart Protection Study 2–Treatment of HDL to Reduce the Incidence of Vascular Events (HPS-2 Thrive)[57]	Extended release niacin-laropiprant vs. placebo. On background of statin-based LDL therapy	N = 25,673. Age 50 to 80 y. Established CVD OR DM with symptomatic coronary disease • 32% of cohort diabetic	Median 4 y	LDL: ↓10 mg/dL (-16%); HDL: ↑6 mg/dL (+14%); TG: ↓33 mg/dL (% not given); Worsening of diabetic control (3.7%); MACE: ↓4%, HR 0.96, CI 0.9–1.03, P = .29 • In pre-specified diabetic cohort, no interaction with primary endpoint.

(continued on next page)

Table 2
(continued)

Agent	Outcome Trial	Intervention	Cohort	Follow up	Outcome
PCSK-9 inhibitors	Further Cardiovascular Outcomes Research with PCSK9 Inhibition in Subjects with Elevated Risk (FOURIER)[63,64]	Evolocumab vs. placebo On background of statin-based LDL therapy	N = 27,564 Age 40–85 y Established CVD AND LDL >70 mg/dL • 40% of cohort diabetic	Median 2 y	LDL: ↓56 mg/dL (-59%), P<.001 HDL: ↑3.5 mg/dL (+8.1%), P<.001 TG: ↓21 mg/dL (-15.5%), P<.001 Non-HDL C-51.6% MACE: 15%, HR 0.85 CI 0.79–0.92, P<.001 • Pre-specified diabetic cohort, HR 0.83, CI 0.75–0.93, P = .0008)
Bile acid sequestrants	NO CVOT				
OM3FA	NO CVOT. Await Reduction of Cardiovascular Events with EPA-Intervention Trial (REDUCE-IT) and Outcomes Study to Assess STatin Residual Risk Reduction with EpaNova in HiGh CV Risk PatienTs with Hypertriglyceridemia (STRENGTH)				

Abbreviations: CVD, cardiovascular disease; CVOT, Cardiovascular Outcome Trial; DM, diabetes mellitus; HDL, high-density lipoprotein; LDL, low-density lipoprotein; MACE, major atherosclerotic cardiovascular events; TC, total cholesterol; TG, triglycerides.
Data from Refs.[37,38,44,50,51,55,57,63,64]

physicians and specialists. The established therapies of statins and ezetimibe remain the cornerstone of dyslipidemia treatment. However, in patients with persistent residual risk, bile acid sequestrants, fibrates, and ultimately PCSK-9 inhibitors need to be considered.

REFERENCES

1. Haffner SM, Lehto S, Ronnemaa T, et al. Mortality from coronary heart disease in subjects with type 2 diabetes and in nondiabetic subjects with and without prior myocardial infarction. N Engl J Med 1998;339:229–34.
2. Guariguata L, Whiting DR, Hambleton I, et al. Global estimates of diabetes prevalence for 2013 and projections for 2035. Diabetes Res Clin Pract 2014;103: 137–49.
3. Faerch K, Carstensen B, Almdal TP, et al. Improved survival among patients with complicated type 2 diabetes in Denmark: a prospective study (2002-2010). J Clin Endocrinol Metab 2014;99:E642–6.
4. Rawshani A, Rawshani A, Franzen S, et al. Mortality and cardiovascular disease in type 1 and type 2 diabetes. N Engl J Med 2017;376:1407–18.
5. Tancredi M, Rosengren A, Svensson AM, et al. Excess mortality among persons with type 2 diabetes. N Engl J Med 2015;373:1720–32.
6. Almdal T, Scharling H, Jensen JS, et al. The independent effect of type 2 diabetes mellitus on ischemic heart disease, stroke, and death: a population-based study of 13,000 men and women with 20 years of follow-up. Arch Intern Med 2004;164: 1422–6.
7. Rao Kondapally Seshasai S, Kaptoge S, Thompson A, et al, Emerging Risk Factors Collaboration. Diabetes mellitus, fasting glucose, and risk of cause-specific death. N Engl J Med 2011;364:829–41.
8. Action to Control Cardiovascular Risk in Diabetes Study Group, Gerstein HC, Miller ME, Byington RP, et al. Effects of intensive glucose lowering in type 2 diabetes. N Engl J Med 2008;358:2545–59.
9. Duckworth W, Abraira C, Moritz T, et al, VADT Investigators. Glucose control and vascular complications in veterans with type 2 diabetes. N Engl J Med 2009;360: 129–39.
10. ADVANCE Collaborative Group, Patel A, MacMahon S, Chalmers J, et al. Intensive blood glucose control and vascular outcomes in patients with type 2 diabetes. N Engl J Med 2008;358:2560–72.
11. Doucet J, Le Floch JP, Bauduceau B, et al, SFD/SFGG Intergroup. GERODIAB: glycaemic control and 5-year morbidity/mortality of type 2 diabetic patients aged 70 years and older: 1. Description of the population at inclusion. Diabetes Metab 2012;38:523–30.
12. Scherer DJ, Nelson AJ, Psaltis PJ, et al. Targeting low-density lipoprotein cholesterol with PCSK9 inhibitors. Intern Med J 2017;47(8):856–65.
13. Cholesterol Treatment Trialists' (CTT) Collaborators, Kearney PM, Blackwell L, Collins R, et al. Efficacy of cholesterol-lowering therapy in 18,686 people with diabetes in 14 randomised trials of statins: a meta-analysis. Lancet 2008;371: 117–25.
14. Malave H, Castro M, Burkle J, et al. Evaluation of low-density lipoprotein particle number distribution in patients with type 2 diabetes mellitus with low-density lipoprotein cholesterol <50 mg/dl and non-high-density lipoprotein cholesterol <80 mg/dl. Am J Cardiol 2012;110:662–5.

15. Do R, Willer CJ, Schmidt EM, et al. Common variants associated with plasma tri-glycerides and risk for coronary artery disease. Nat Genet 2013;45:1345–52.

16. Voight BF, Peloso GM, Orho-Melander M, et al. Plasma HDL cholesterol and risk of myocardial infarction: a mendelian randomisation study. Lancet 2012;380: 572–80.

17. Pollin TI, Damcott CM, Shen H, et al. A null mutation in human APOC3 confers a favorable plasma lipid profile and apparent cardioprotection. Science 2008;322: 1702–5.

18. Boekholdt SM, Arsenault BJ, Hovingh GK, et al. Levels and changes of HDL cholesterol and apolipoprotein A-I in relation to risk of cardiovascular events among statin-treated patients: a meta-analysis. Circulation 2013;128:1504–12.

19. Gordon T, Castelli WP, Hjortland MC, et al. High density lipoprotein as a protective factor against coronary heart disease. The Framingham Study. Am J Med 1977; 62:707–14.

20. Nicholls SJ, Tuzcu EM, Sipahi I, et al. Statins, high-density lipoprotein cholesterol, and regression of coronary atherosclerosis. JAMA 2007;297:499–508.

21. Lincoff AM, Nicholls SJ, Riesmeyer JS, et al, ACCELERATE Investigators. Evac-etrapib and cardiovascular outcomes in high-risk vascular disease. N Engl J Med 2017;376:1933–42.

22. Sirtori CR, Calabresi L, Franceschini G, et al. Cardiovascular status of carriers of the apolipoprotein A-I(Milano) mutant: the Limone sul Garda study. Circulation 2001;103:1949–54.

23. Scott R, Donoghoe M, Watts GF, et al, FIELD Study Investigators. Impact of meta-bolic syndrome and its components on cardiovascular disease event rates in 4900 patients with type 2 diabetes assigned to placebo in the FIELD randomised trial. Cardiovasc Diabetol 2011;10:102.

24. Khan HA, Sobki SH, Khan SA. Association between glycaemic control and serum lipids profile in type 2 diabetic patients: HbA1c predicts dyslipidaemia. Clin Exp Med 2007;7:24–9.

25. Taskinen MR, Adiels M, Westerbacka J, et al. Dual metabolic defects are required to produce hypertriglyceridemia in obese subjects. Arterioscler Thromb Vasc Biol 2011;31:2144–50.

26. Goff DC Jr, Gerstein HC, Ginsberg HN, et al, ACCORD Study Group. Prevention of cardiovascular disease in persons with type 2 diabetes mellitus: current knowl-edge and rationale for the Action to Control Cardiovascular Risk in Diabetes (ACCORD) trial. Am J Cardiol 2007;99:4i–20i.

27. Krentz AJ. Lipoprotein abnormalities and their consequences for patients with type 2 diabetes. Diabetes Obes Metab 2003;5(Suppl 1):S19–27.

28. Ajala O, English P, Pinkney J. Systematic review and meta-analysis of different di-etary approaches to the management of type 2 diabetes. Am J Clin Nutr 2013;97: 505–16.

29. Ali MK, Bullard KM, Saaddine JB, et al. Achievement of goals in U.S. diabetes care, 1999-2010. N Engl J Med 2013;368:1613–24.

30. Nguyen NT, Nguyen XM, Lane J, et al. Relationship between obesity and dia-betes in a US adult population: findings from the National Health and Nutrition Ex-amination Survey, 1999-2006. Obes Surg 2011;21:351–5.

31. Henry RR, Wallace P, Olefsky JM. Effects of weight loss on mechanisms of hyper-glycemia in obese non-insulin-dependent diabetes mellitus. Diabetes 1986;35: 990–8.

32. Franz MJ, Boucher JL, Rutten-Ramos S, et al. Lifestyle weight-loss intervention outcomes in overweight and obese adults with type 2 diabetes: a systematic

review and meta-analysis of randomized clinical trials. J Acad Nutr Diet 2015;115: 1447–63.

33. Look AHEAD Research Group, Pi-Sunyer X, Blackburn G, Brancati FL, et al. Reduction in weight and cardiovascular disease risk factors in individuals with type 2 diabetes: one-year results of the look AHEAD trial. Diabetes Care 2007; 30:1374–83.

34. Look AHEAD Research Group, Wing RR. Long-term effects of a lifestyle intervention on weight and cardiovascular risk factors in individuals with type 2 diabetes mellitus: four-year results of the Look AHEAD trial. Arch Intern Med 2010;170: 1566–75.

35. Look AHEAD Research Group, Wing RR, Bolin P, Brancati FL, et al. Cardiovascular effects of intensive lifestyle intervention in type 2 diabetes. N Engl J Med 2013; 369:145–54.

36. Chudyk A, Petrella RJ. Effects of exercise on cardiovascular risk factors in type 2 diabetes: a meta-analysis. Diabetes Care 2011;34:1228–37.

37. Hayashino Y, Jackson JL, Fukumori N, et al. Effects of supervised exercise on lipid profiles and blood pressure control in people with type 2 diabetes mellitus: a meta-analysis of randomized controlled trials. Diabetes Res Clin Pract 2012;98: 349–60.

38. Collins R, Armitage J, Parish S, et al, Heart Protection Study Collaborative Group. MRC/BHF Heart Protection Study of cholesterol-lowering with simvastatin in 5963 people with diabetes: a randomised placebo-controlled trial. Lancet 2003;361: 2005–16.

39. Colhoun HM, Betteridge DJ, Durrington PN, et al, CARDS Investigators. Primary prevention of cardiovascular disease with atorvastatin in type 2 diabetes in the Collaborative Atorvastatin Diabetes Study (CARDS): multicentre randomised placebo-controlled trial. Lancet 2004;364:685–96.

40. Cholesterol Treatment Trialists' (CTT) Collaboration, Baigent C, Blackwell L, Emberson J, et al. Efficacy and safety of more intensive lowering of LDL cholesterol: a meta-analysis of data from 170,000 participants in 26 randomised trials. Lancet 2010;376:1670–81.

41. Erqou S, Lee CT, Adler A. Intensive glycemic control and the risk of heart failure in patients with type 2 diabetes. Am Heart J 2012;163:e35 [author reply: e37].

42. Sudhop T, Lutjohann D, Kodal A, et al. Inhibition of intestinal cholesterol absorption by ezetimibe in humans. Circulation 2002;106:1943–8.

43. Morrone D, Weintraub WS, Toth PP, et al. Lipid-altering efficacy of ezetimibe plus statin and statin monotherapy and identification of factors associated with treatment response: a pooled analysis of over 21,000 subjects from 27 clinical trials. Atherosclerosis 2012;223:251–61.

44. Cannon CP, Blazing MA, Giugliano RP, et al, IMPROVE-IT Investigators. Ezetimibe added to statin therapy after acute coronary syndromes. N Engl J Med 2015;372:2387–97.

45. Ruggenenti P, Cattaneo D, Rota S, et al, Ezetimibe and Simvastatin in Dyslipidemia of Diabetes (ESD) Study Group. Effects of combined ezetimibe and simvastatin therapy as compared with simvastatin alone in patients with type 2 diabetes: a prospective randomized double-blind clinical trial. Diabetes Care 2010;33:1954–6.

46. Lally S, Owens D, Tomkin GH. Genes that affect cholesterol synthesis, cholesterol absorption, and chylomicron assembly: the relationship between the liver and intestine in control and streptozotosin diabetic rats. Metabolism 2007;56:430–8.

47. Ravid Z, Bendayan M, Delvin E, et al. Modulation of intestinal cholesterol absorption by high glucose levels: impact on cholesterol transporters, regulatory enzymes, and transcription factors. Am J Physiol Gastrointest Liver Physiol 2008; 295:G873–85.

48. Staels B, Dallongeville J, Auwerx J, et al. Mechanism of action of fibrates on lipid and lipoprotein metabolism. Circulation 1998;98:2088–93.

49. Chapman MJ, Redfern JS, McGovern ME, et al. Niacin and fibrates in atherogenic dyslipidemia: pharmacotherapy to reduce cardiovascular risk. Pharmacol Ther 2010;126:314–45.

50. Keech A, Simes RJ, Barter P, et al, FIELD Study Investigators. Effects of long-term fenofibrate therapy on cardiovascular events in 9795 people with type 2 diabetes mellitus (the FIELD study): randomised controlled trial. Lancet 2005;366: 1849–61.

51. ACCORD Study Group, Ginsberg HN, Elam MB, Lovato LC, et al. Effects of combination lipid therapy in type 2 diabetes mellitus. N Engl J Med 2010;362: 1563–74.

52. Lee M, Saver JL, Towfighi A, et al. Efficacy of fibrates for cardiovascular risk reduction in persons with atherogenic dyslipidemia: a meta-analysis. Atherosclerosis 2011;217:492–8.

53. Guo J, Meng F, Ma N, et al. Meta-analysis of safety of the coadministration of statin with fenofibrate in patients with combined hyperlipidemia. Am J Cardiol 2012;110:1296–301.

54. Chan DC, Watts GF. Dyslipidaemia in the metabolic syndrome and type 2 diabetes: pathogenesis, priorities, pharmacotherapies. Expert Opin Pharmacother 2011;12:13–30.

55. AIM-HIGH Investigators, Boden WE, Probstfield JL, Anderson T, et al. Niacin in patients with low HDL cholesterol levels receiving intensive statin therapy. N Engl J Med 2011;365:2255–67.

56. Guyton JR, Slee AE, Anderson T, et al. Relationship of lipoproteins to cardiovascular events: the AIM-HIGH Trial (Atherothrombosis intervention in metabolic syndrome with low HDL/high triglycerides and impact on global health outcomes). J Am Coll Cardiol 2013;62:1580–4.

57. HPS2-THRIVE Collaborative Group, Landray MJ, Haynes R, Hopewell JC, et al. Effects of extended-release niacin with laropiprant in high-risk patients. N Engl J Med 2014;371:203–12.

58. Sprecher DL, Abrams J, Allen JW, et al. Low-dose combined therapy with fluvastatin and cholestyramine in hyperlipidemic patients. Ann Intern Med 1994;120: 537–43.

59. Jones MR, Nwose OM. Role of colesevelam in combination lipid-lowering therapy. Am J Cardiovasc Drugs 2013;13:315–23.

60. Ballantyne CM, Bays HE, Kastelein JJ, et al. Efficacy and safety of eicosapentaenoic acid ethyl ester (AMR101) therapy in statin-treated patients with persistent high triglycerides (from the ANCHOR study). Am J Cardiol 2012;110:984–92.

61. Kotwal S, Jun M, Sullivan D, et al. Omega 3 fatty acids and cardiovascular outcomes: systematic review and meta-analysis. Circ Cardiovasc Qual Outcomes 2012;5:808–18.

62. Sattar N, Preiss D, Robinson JG, et al. Lipid-lowering efficacy of the PCSK9 inhibitor evolocumab (AMG 145) in patients with type 2 diabetes: a meta-analysis of individual patient data. Lancet Diabetes Endocrinol 2016;4:403–10.

63. Sabatine MS, Giugliano RP, Keech AC, et al, FOURIER Steering Committee and Investigators. Evolocumab and clinical outcomes in patients with cardiovascular disease. N Engl J Med 2017;376:1713–22.
64. Sabatine MS, Leiter LA, Wiviott SD, et al. Cardiovascular safety and efficacy of the PCSK9 inhibitor evolocumab in patients with and without diabetes and the effect of evolocumab on glycaemia and risk of new-onset diabetes: a prespecified analysis of the FOURIER randomised controlled trial. Lancet Diabetes Endocrinol 2017;5(12):941–50.
65. Heintjes E, Kuiper J, Lucius B, et al. Characterization and cholesterol management in patients with cardiovascular events and/or type 2 diabetes in the Netherlands. Curr Med Res Opin 2017;33:91–100.

Blood Pressure Control and Cardiovascular/Renal Outcomes

Farheen K. Dojki, MD, George L. Bakris, MD*

KEYWORDS

- Diabetes • Hypertension • Cardiovascular outcomes • Diabetic kidney disease
- Blood pressure goals

KEY POINTS

- Type 2 diabetes mellitus is associated with an increased risk of hypertension, kidney disease, and cardiovascular disease.
- Strong evidence from clinical trials and meta-analyses supports targeting blood pressure reduction to at least less than 140/90 mm Hg in all adults with diabetes.
- Lower blood pressure targets that are less than 130/80 mm Hg are beneficial for selected patients with high cardiovascular disease risk if they can be achieved without undue burden.
- Treatment is based on a foundation of lifestyle modifications, especially a reduce sodium diet (<2300 mg/d) and at least 6 hours of uninterrupted sleep nightly, along with medications including renin angiotensin system (RAS) inhibitors, calcium antagonists, and thiazide-like diuretics.
- For patients with albuminuria greater than 300 mg/d, a renin angiotensin system inhibitor must be part of the antihypertensive regimen.

INTRODUCTION

Diabetes mellitus (DM) is a growing epidemic. By 2030, it is projected that there will be at least 400 million individuals with type 2 DM worldwide, with many of those affected being relatively young and living in low- or middle-income countries.[1] Type 2 DM is associated with an increased risk of hypertension. At the age of 45, around 40% of patients with type 2 diabetes are hypertensive, and the proportion increases to 60% by the age of 75.[2] There is also an increased risk of renal disease and a 2-- to 4-fold

Disclosure Statement: F.K. Dojki has nothing to disclose. G.L. Bakris is a consultant for Janssen, AbbVie, Bayer, and Vascular Dynamics and is on the Steering Committee of 3 renal outcome trials (Janssen, AbbVie, Bayer).
Section of Endocrinology, Diabetes, and Metabolism, Department of Medicine, ASH Comprehensive Hypertension Center, University of Chicago Medicine, 5841 South Maryland Avenue, MC 1027, Chicago, IL 60637, USA
* Corresponding author.
E-mail address: gbakris@gmail.com

increased risk for cardiovascular disease (CVD) compared with the general population.[2–4]

CVD is the most common cause of death and disability in patients with type 2 DM.[5,6] Hypertension is an important and modifiable risk factor for CVD associated with DM, and the results of studies suggest that 35% to 75% of the cardiovascular risk in patients with DM can be attributed to the presence of hypertension.[6–8] Hence, management of hypertension contributes significantly to the reduction of burden of CVD in diabetes.[9]

TARGET BLOOD PRESSURE IN PATIENTS WITH DIABETES

The bulk of outcome data about blood pressure (BP) levels in diabetes is based on trials in patients with high cardiovascular risk (generally >7–10 years). Only 2 prospective trials were powered to address the question of BP level and effect on cardiovascular outcome in diabetes, the United Kingdom Prospective Diabetes Study (UKPDS)[9] and the Action to Control Cardiovascular Risk in Diabetes (ACCORD) trial.[10]

In 1998, much enthusiasm was increased by the publication of the post hoc analysis of the Hypertension Optimal Treatment (HOT) trial,[11] and, shortly thereafter, of the UKPDS,[9] both showing that intense BP-lowering treatment significantly reduces cardiovascular morbidity and mortality in hypertensive patients with type 2 DM. These trials are discussed in detail later.

Thereafter, most diabetes and hypertension guidelines published in the first decade of the current century recommended that antihypertensive treatment be initiated at a lower systolic BP (SBP) threshold (130 mm Hg) in individuals with diabetes. They also recommended lower SBP targets (SBP <130 mm Hg in diabetes vs SBP <140 mm Hg in non–diabetic individuals).[12,13] Hence, earlier data from 2000 to 2012 from American Diabetes Association (ADA), Canadian Hypertension Society, Joint National Committee 7 (JNC 7), and Kidney Disease Outcomes Quality Initiative (KDOQI) (National Kindey Foundation [NKF]) all supported a BP goal of less than 130/80 mm Hg in patients with diabetes to reduce cardiovascular risk. After attention was called on the lack of trial evidence for these recommendations,[14] most of the recent guidelines reconsidered their conclusions and now usually recommend that initiation and target of treatment should be similar regardless of diabetes status.[15–19]

The ADA report in 2016, Kidney Disease: Improving Global Outcomes (KDIGO)/ KDOQI (NKF) 2013 and the 2014 Expert Panel Report support a BP goal of less than 140/90 mm Hg for those with diabetes to reduce cardiovascular risk.[18,20,21] The most recent ADA 2017 BP Consensus Report, however, states that although all patients with diabetes must have a BP less than 140/90 mm Hg, a lower BP, that is, less than 130/80 mm Hg, should be achieved for those with high CVD risk. This lower goal should be achieved without undue treatment tolerability issues.[22]

RANDOMIZED CLINICAL TRIALS OF INTENSIVE BLOOD PRESSURE CONTROL

In type 2 diabetes, the UKPDS showed that targeting BP less than 150/85 mm Hg versus less than 180/105 mm Hg reduced composite microvascular and macrovascular diabetes complications by 24%.[9] Events included reduction in deaths related to diabetes, stroke, and heart failure, and in microvascular end points predominantly owing to a reduced risk of retinal photocoagulation. There was a nonsignificant reduction in all-cause mortality. Hence, the SBP goal less than 150 mm Hg improved cardiovascular and cerebrovascular outcomes.

The ACCORD blood pressure (ACCORD BP) trial examined the effects of intensive BP control (goal SBP <120 mm Hg) versus standard BP control (target SBP <140 mm Hg) among people with type 2 diabetes. Although it failed to demonstrate any cardiovascular risk reduction in the intense BP control group less than 120 mm Hg compared with standard 140 mm Hg and did not reduce the rate of a composite outcome of fatal and nonfatal major cardiovascular events (myocardial infarction or cardiovascular death), it did reduce the risk of stroke by 41%.[23] Moreover, a post hoc analysis of this trial demonstrates a major interaction between the intense glycemic control group and the intensive BP group such that even though underpowered a benefit trend was seen in the lower BP group for cardiovascular outcomes. Therefore, the ACCORD BP results suggest that BP targets more intensive than less than 140/90 mm Hg may be reasonable in selected patients who have been educated about added treatment burden, side effects, and costs.[10,24]

Only one trial provides evidence for benefit of a diastolic BP at 80 mm Hg. This benefit was derived from a post hoc analysis of the diabetes subgroup of the HOT trial. This involved the subgroup of those with diabetes randomized to 80 mm Hg who manifested a reduction in composite CVD outcomes[11] (**Tables 1** and **2**). It is notable that in HOT, there were no patients with diabetic kidney disease (DKD).

The Action in Diabetes and Vascular Disease: Preterax and Diamicron MR Controlled Evaluation–Blood Pressure (ADVANCE-BP) trial tested the effects of a fixed-dose combination of antihypertensive interventions versus placebo among people with type 2 diabetes, also informs blood pressure targets.[25] The achieved BP in ADVANCE in the intervention group (136/73 mm Hg) was higher than that achieved in the ACCORD intensive arm (119/64 mm Hg) and would be consistent with a target BP of less than 140/90 mm Hg, although ADVANCE did not explicitly test BP targets[26] (see **Table 1**).

It is noteworthy that ACCORD unlike other diabetes trials measured BP using an ambulatory oscillatory blood pressure device. This approach yields values that are generally lower than typical office BP by approximately 7 to 12 mm Hg.[27] This suggests that implementing the ACCORD protocols in a typical clinic requires a SBP target higher than less than 130 mm Hg. Achieved BPs in Diabetes Outcome Clinical Trials are also summarized in **Table 1**.

Meta-analyses of clinical trials also demonstrate that antihypertensive treatment of cohorts of patients with diabetes and baseline BP ≥140/90 mm Hg reduces risks of atherosclerotic CVD, heart failure, retinopathy, and albuminuria.[28–32] Therefore, patients with type 1 or type 2 diabetes who have hypertension should, at a minimum, be treated to BP targets of less than 140/90 mm Hg.

Notably, there is an absence of high-quality data available to guide BP targets in type 1 diabetes. Associations of BP with macrovascular and microvascular outcomes in type 1 diabetes are generally similar to those in type 2 diabetes and the general population.[33]

Table 1
Summary of clinical outcome trials in patients with diabetes or with the cohort being more than 50% patients with diabetes

Clinical Outcome Trial	Achieved Level of SBP (mm Hg)
ACCORD (primary)	119 (intensive); 133 (conventional)
UKPDS (primary)	144 (intensive); 154 (conventional)
ACCOMPLISH (secondary)	Overall mean 133
INVEST (secondary)	144 (tight control); 149 (conventional)
ONTARGET (secondary)	Averaging around 140
VADT (secondary)	127 (intensive); 125 (conventional)
ADVANCE (secondary)	145 (in both intensive and conventional glucose control)

Table 2
Randomized controlled trials of intensive versus standard hypertension treatment strategies

Clinical Trial	Population	Intensive	Standard	Outcomes
ACCORD BP (18)	4733 participants with type 2 diabetes aged 40–79 y with prior evidence of CVD or multiple cardiovascular risk factors	SBP target: <120 mm Hg Achieved (mean): 119.3/64.4	SBP target: 130–140 mm Hg Achieved (mean) 133.5/70.5	• No benefit in primary end point: composite of nonfatal myocardial infarction (MI), nonfatal stroke, and CVD death • Stroke risk reduced 41% with intensive control, not sustained through follow-up beyond the period of active treatment • Adverse events more common in intensive group, particularly elevated serum creatinine and electrolyte abnormalities
ADVANCE BP (43)	11,140 participants with type 2 diabetes ages 55 y and greater with prior evidence of CVD or multiple cardiovascular risk factors	Intervention: A single-pill, fixed-dose combination of perindopril and indapamide Achieved (mean): 136/73 mm Hg	Control: Placebo Achieved (mean): 141.6/75.2 mm Hg	• Intervention reduced risk of primary composite endpoint of major macrovascular and microvascular events (9%), death from any cause (14%), and death from CVD (18%) • 6-y observational follow-up found reduction in risk of death in intervention group attenuated but still significant (134)
HOT (135)	18,790 participants, including 1501 with diabetes	Diastolic BP target: ≤80 mm Hg	Diastolic BP target: ≤90 mm Hg	• In the overall trial, there was no cardiovascular benefit with more intensive targets • In the subpopulation with diabetes, an intensive diastolic target was associated with a significantly reduced risk (51%) of CVD events
SPRINT (136)	9361 participants without diabetes	SBP target: <120 mm Hg Achieved (mean): 121.4 mm Hg	SBP target <140 mm Hg Achieved (mean): 136.2 mm Hg	• Intensive SBP target lowered risk of the primary composite outcome 25% (MI, ACS, stroke, heart failure, and death, due to CVD) • Intensive target reduced risk of death 27% • Intensive therapy increased risks of electrolyte abnormalities and acute kidney injury

Abbreviation: ACS, acute coronary syndrome.

Adapted from de Boer I, Bangalore S, Benetos A, et al. Diabetes and hypertension: a position statement by the American Diabetes Association. Diabetes Care 2017;40(9):1273–84; with permission.

KIDNEY DISEASE OUTCOMES

Hypertension is highly prevalent in individuals with DKD and is twice that relative to the general population.[9] The prevalence of hypertension increases from ~36% in stage 1 chronic kidney disease (CKD) to ~84% in CKD stage 4 to 5.[29] It is not only the mortality that is of concern, but also the morbidity and high overall costs of care related to DKD. This is due in large part to the strong relationship of DKD with CVD outcomes, such as heart failure, stroke, myocardial infarction, and development of end-stage kidney disease.[30]

In patients with type 1 diabetes, albuminuria or overt nephropathy generally precedes the appearance of hypertension.[34] However, in type 2 diabetes, hypertension in most cases antedates development of albuminuria and reductions in estimated glomerular filtration rate because of shared risk factors, including the presence of obesity, dyslipidemia, and the cardiorenal metabolic syndrome.

The 2014 report from the ADA consensus conference[35] on DKD points out the importance of considering the adverse safety signal in clinical trials when diastolic BP is treated to less than 70 mm Hg. This lower diastolic reading, particularly less than 60 mm Hg in older populations, has recently been reexamined and may not be associated with the same level of CV risk as once thought, however.[36] The 2014 ADA report, however, notes findings from the Kidney Early Evaluation Program that suggest higher incident rates of end-stage renal disease in patients with CKD stage 3 and diastolic BP less than 60 mm Hg.[37]

The 2014 Expert Panel recommends a target BP of less than 140/90 mm Hg in patients of all ages with CKD with or without diabetes.[18] The KDIGO clinical practice guideline for management of BP in CKD also recommends a BP target ≤140/90 mm Hg in patients with diabetes and CKD with urine albumin excretion less than 30 mg/d. The KDIGO and KDOQI guidelines further state that adults with diabetes and CKD with urine albumin excretion greater than 30 mg/d may be treated to a BP that is less than 130/80 mm Hg but with low evidence grade 2C.[38] Hence, although this BP level can be a goal, the evidence supporting benefit on CKD progression is weak.

There are multiple mechanisms in the development of hypertension in patients with DKD, including inappropriate activation of the renin angiotensin aldosterone system and the sympathetic nervous system, volume expansion due to increased sodium (Na^+) reabsorption, peripheral vasoconstriction, increased endothelin-1 levels, inflammation, and generation of reactive oxygen species as well as reduction in nitric oxide release.[22,39] Many of these factors accelerate development of kidney disease and increase risk for CVD among patients with diabetes and hypertension.[34] They, thus, serve as targets for risk reduction by managing hypertension.

APPROACH TO THERAPY

Strategies targeting smoking cessation, reduced sodium intake, exercise, and weight loss have been shown effective in reducing CVD risk as well as progression of DKD as noted in the most recent guidelines.[40,41] A recent Institute of Medicine report, however, indicates insufficient evidence for lowering sodium intake to less than 2.3 g/d with respect to reducing CVD.[42]

The emphasis on treatment of hypertension in patients with DKD should include strategies that address multifactorial risk factor reduction coupled with pharmacotherapy, lifestyle modification, and patient education to improve self-management of these complex medical risk factors. Such strategies require team-based approaches with contribution of primary care physicians, endocrinologists, nephrologists, nutritionists, pharmacists, nurse educators, midlevel providers as well as behavioral health professionals.

Moderation of alcohol intake, weight loss, and increased physical activity as recommended by the ADA position statement Standards of Medical Care in Diabetes and are again reiterated in the ADA BP Consensus Report.[22] The aforementioned lifestyle modifications are all beneficial for management of hypertension in patients with DKD.[35]

Treatment of DM, such as hyperinsulinemia and exogenous insulin, may theoretically lead to hypertension through vasoconstriction, sodium, and fluid retention.[43] However, insulin can also promote vasodilation, and basal insulin compared with standard care was not associated with a change in BP in the Outcome Reduction with an Initial Glargine Intervention trial of people with diabetes or prediabetes.[44]

Sodium glucose cotransport-2 inhibitors are associated with a mild diuretic effect and a reduction in BP of 3 to 6 mm Hg SBP and 1 to 2 mm Hg diastolic BP.[45,46] Glucagon-like peptide-1 receptor agonists are also associated with a reduction in BP of 2 to 3/0 to 1 mm Hg.[47]

Initial treatment of hypertension in diabetes should include drug classes demonstrated to reduce cardiovascular events in patients with diabetes: angiotensin-converting-enzyme (ACE) inhibitors,[48,49] angiotensin receptor blocker (ARBs),[48,49] thiazide-like diuretics, or dihydropyridine calcium channel blockers (CCB).[50] For patients with albuminuria (UACR $\geq$300 mg/g), initial treatment should include an ACE inhibitor or ARB in order to reduce the risk of progressive kidney disease, detailed in later discussion. In the absence of very high albuminuria, where risk of progressive kidney disease is low, ACE inhibitors and ARBs have not been found to afford superior renoprotection when compared with other antihypertensive agents. Beta-blockers may be used for the treatment of coronary disease or heart failure but have not been shown to reduce mortality as BP-lowering agents in the absence of these conditions.[29,51]

Use of ACE inhibitors combined with ARBs are not recommended given the lack of added CVD risk reduction compounded by increased adverse events, namely, hyperkalemia, syncope, and acute kidney injury.[52–54]

Mineralocorticoid receptor antagonists (MRAs) are effective for management of resistant hypertension in patients with type 2 diabetes, when added to existing treatment with an RAS inhibitor, diuretic, and CCB,[55] in part, because they reduce sympathetic nerve activity.[56] MRAs also reduce albuminuria and have additional cardiovascular benefits.[55,57,58] However, adding an MRA to an ACE inhibitor or ARB may increase the risk for hyperkalemic episodes. Hyperkalemia can be managed with dietary potassium restriction, potassium wasting diuretics, or potassium binders,[59,60] but long-term outcome studies are needed to evaluate the role of MRAs (with or without adjunct potassium management) in BP management.

Specific factors to consider are the absolute risk of cardiovascular events[32,61] and the risk of progressive kidney disease as reflected by declines in glomerular filtration rate, adverse effects, age, and overall treatment burden. Patients who have higher risk of cardiovascular events (particularly stroke) who can attain intensive BP control relatively easily and without substantial adverse effects may be best suited to intensive BP control. In contrast, patients with conditions more common in older adults, such as functional limitations, polypharmacy, and multimorbidities, may be best suited to less intensive BP control.

REFERENCES

1. Wild S, Roglic G, Green A, et al. Global prevalence of diabetes: estimates for the year 2000 and projections for 2030. Diabetes Care 2004;27:1047–53.

2. Hypertension in Diabetes Study (HDS): I. Prevalence of hypertension in newly presenting type 2 diabetic patients and the association with risk factors for cardiovascular and diabetic complications. J Hypertens 1993;11: 309–17.

3. Woodward M, Zhang X, Barzi F, et al. The effects of diabetes on the risks of major cardiovascular diseases and death in the Asia-Pacific region. Diabetes Care 2003;26:360–6.

4. Jha V, Garcia-Garcia G, Iseki K, et al. Chronic kidney disease: global dimension and perspectives. Lancet 2013;382:260–72.

5. Go AS, Chertow GM, Fan D, et al. Chronic kidney disease and the risks of death, cardiovascular events, and hospitalization. N Engl J Med 2004;351: 1296–305.

6. Stamler J, Vaccaro O, Neaton JD, et al. Diabetes, other risk factors, and 12-yr cardiovascular mortality for men screened in the multiple risk factor intervention trial. Diabetes Care 1993;16:434–44.

7. Lee WL, Cheung AM, Cape D, et al. Impact of diabetes on coronary artery disease in women and men: a meta-analysis of prospective studies. Diabetes Care 2000;23:962–8.

8. Lloyd-Jones DM, Leip EP, Larson MG, et al. Prediction of lifetime risk for cardiovascular disease by risk factor burden at 50 years of age. Circulation 2006;113:791–8.

9. Tight blood pressure control and risk of macrovascular and microvascular complications in type 2 diabetes: UKPDS 38. UK Prospective Diabetes Study Group. BMJ 1998;317:703–13.

10. ACCORD Study Group, Cushman WC, Evans GW, Byington RP, et al. Effects of intensive blood-pressure control in type 2 diabetes mellitus. N Engl J Med 2010;362:1575–85.

11. Hansson L, Zanchetti A, Carruthers SG, et al. Effects of intensive blood-pressure lowering and low-dose aspirin in patients with hypertension: principal results of the Hypertension Optimal Treatment (HOT) randomised trial. HOT Study Group. Lancet 1998;351:1755–62.

12. Chobanian AV, Bakris GL, Black HR, et al. The seventh report of the Joint National Committee on Prevention, Detection, Evaluation, and Treatment of High Blood Pressure: the JNC 7 report. JAMA 2003;289:2560–72.

13. ESH/ESC Task Force for the Management of Arterial Hypertension. 2013 Practice guidelines for the management of arterial hypertension of the European Society of Hypertension (ESH) and the European Society of Cardiology (ESC): ESH/ESC Task Force for the Management of Arterial Hypertension. J Hypertens 2013;31: 1925–38.

14. Zanchetti A, Grassi G, Mancia G. When should antihypertensive drug treatment be initiated and to what levels should systolic blood pressure be lowered? A critical reappraisal. J Hypertens 2009;27:923–34.

15. Mancia G, Fagard R, Narkiewicz K, et al. 2013 ESH/ESC guidelines for the management of arterial hypertension: the Task Force for the management of arterial hypertension of the European Society of Hypertension (ESH) and of the European Society of Cardiology (ESC). J Hypertens 2013;31:1281–357.

16. Task Force of the SEC for the ESC Guidelines on Diabetes, Prediabetes and Cardiovascular Disease, Expert Reviewers for the ESC Guidelines on Diabetes, Prediabetes And Cardiovascular Disease, Guideliness Committee of the SEC. Comments on the ESC guidelines on diabetes, prediabetes, and cardiovascular diseases developed in collaboration with the European Society for the Study of Diabetes. Rev Esp Cardiol (Engl Ed) 2014;67:87–93.

17. Weber MA, Schiffrin EL, White WB, et al. Clinical practice guidelines for the management of hypertension in the community: a statement by the American Society of Hypertension and the International Society of Hypertension. J Clin Hypertens (Greenwich) 2014;16:14–26.

18. James PA, Oparil S, Carter BL, et al. 2014 evidence-based guideline for the management of high blood pressure in adults: report from the panel members appointed to the Eighth Joint National Committee (JNC 8). JAMA 2014;311:507–20.

19. Standards of medical care in diabetes–2015: summary of revisions. Diabetes Care 2015;38(Suppl):S4.

20. American Diabetes Association. Standards of medical care in diabetes-2016 abridged for primary care providers. Clin Diabetes 2016;34:3–21.

21. Wheeler DC, Becker GJ. Summary of KDIGO guideline. What do we really know about management of blood pressure in patients with chronic kidney disease? Kidney Int 2013;83:377–83.

22. de Boer I, Bangalore S, Benetos A, et al. Diabetes and hypertension: a position statement by the American Diabetes Association. Diabetes Care 2017;40(9):1273–84.

23. Barzilay JI, Howard AG, Evans GW, et al. Intensive blood pressure treatment does not improve cardiovascular outcomes in centrally obese hypertensive individuals with diabetes: the Action to Control Cardiovascular Risk in Diabetes (ACCORD) blood pressure trial. Diabetes Care 2012;35:1401–5.

24. Margolis KL, O'Connor PJ, Morgan TM, et al. Outcomes of combined cardiovascular risk factor management strategies in type 2 diabetes: the ACCORD randomized trial. Diabetes Care 2014;37:1721–8.

25. Zoungas S, de Galan BE, Ninomiya T, et al. Combined effects of routine blood pressure lowering and intensive glucose control on macrovascular and microvascular outcomes in patients with type 2 diabetes: new results from the ADVANCE trial. Diabetes Care 2009;32:2068–74.

26. Patel A, ADVANCE Collaborative Group, MacMahon S, et al. Effects of a fixed combination of perindopril and indapamide on macrovascular and microvascular outcomes in patients with type 2 diabetes mellitus (the ADVANCE trial): a randomised controlled trial. Lancet 2007;370:829–40.

27. Bakris GL. The implications of blood pressure measurement methods on treatment targets for blood pressure. Circulation 2016;134:904–5.

28. Emdin CA, Rahimi K, Neal B, et al. Blood pressure lowering in type 2 diabetes: a systematic review and meta-analysis. JAMA 2015;313:603–15.

29. Ettehad D, Emdin CA, Kiran A, et al. Blood pressure lowering for prevention of cardiovascular disease and death: a systematic review and meta-analysis. Lancet 2016;387:957–67.

30. Bangalore S, Kumar S, Lobach I, et al. Blood pressure targets in subjects with type 2 diabetes mellitus/impaired fasting glucose: observations from traditional and bayesian random-effects meta-analyses of randomized trials. Circulation 2011;123:2799–810, 9 p following 810.

31. Thomopoulos C, Parati G, Zanchetti A. Effects of blood-pressure-lowering treatment on outcome incidence in hypertension: 10-Should blood pressure management differ in hypertensive patients with and without diabetes mellitus? Overview and meta-analyses of randomized trials. J Hypertens 2017;35:922–44.

32. Xie X, Atkins E, Lv J, et al. Effects of intensive blood pressure lowering on cardiovascular and renal outcomes: updated systematic review and meta-analysis. Lancet 2016;387:435–43.

33. de Ferranti SD, de Boer IH, Fonseca V, et al. Type 1 diabetes mellitus and cardiovascular disease: a scientific statement from the American Heart Association and American Diabetes Association. Circulation 2014;130:1110–30.
34. Norgaard K, Feldt-Rasmussen B, Borch-Johnsen K, et al. Prevalence of hypertension in type 1 (insulin-dependent) diabetes mellitus. Diabetologia 1990;33:407–10.
35. Tuttle KR, Bakris GL, Bilous RW, et al. Diabetic kidney disease: a report from an ADA consensus conference. Diabetes Care 2014;37:2864–83.
36. Messerli FH, Mancia G, Conti CR, et al. Dogma disputed: can aggressively lowering blood pressure in hypertensive patients with coronary artery disease be dangerous? Ann Intern Med 2006;144:884–93.
37. Peralta CA, Norris KC, Li S, et al. Blood pressure components and end-stage renal disease in persons with chronic kidney disease: the Kidney Early Evaluation Program (KEEP). Arch Intern Med 2012;172:41–7.
38. Taler SJ, Agarwal R, Bakris GL, et al. KDOQI US commentary on the 2012 KDIGO clinical practice guideline for management of blood pressure in CKD. Am J Kidney Dis 2013;62:201–13.
39. Van Buren PN, Toto R. Hypertension in diabetic nephropathy: epidemiology, mechanisms, and management. Adv Chronic Kidney Dis 2011;18:28–41.
40. American Diabetes Association. Standards of medical care in diabetes-2017 abridged for primary care providers. Clin Diabetes 2017;35:5–26.
41. Whelton PK, Carey RM, Aronow WS, et al. ACC/AHA/AAPA/ABC/ACPM/AGS/APhA/ASH/ASPC/NMA/PCNA guideline for the prevention, detection, evaluation and management of high blood pressure in adults: a report of the American College of Cardiology/American Heart Association Task Force on Clinical Practice Guidelines. Hypertension 2017. [Epub ahead of print].
42. Bibbins-Domingo K. The Institute of Medicine report sodium intake in populations: assessment of evidence: summary of primary findings and implications for clinicians. JAMA Intern Med 2014;174:136–7.
43. Ferrannini E, Cushman WC. Diabetes and hypertension: the bad companions. Lancet 2012;380:601–10.
44. ORIGIN Trial Investigators, Gerstein HC, Bosch J, Dagenais GR, et al. Basal insulin and cardiovascular and other outcomes in dysglycemia. N Engl J Med 2012;367:319–28.
45. Monami M, Nardini C, Mannucci E. Efficacy and safety of sodium glucose cotransport-2 inhibitors in type 2 diabetes: a meta-analysis of randomized clinical trials. Diabetes Obes Metab 2014;16:457–66.
46. Oliva RV, Bakris GL. Sympathetic activation in resistant hypertension: theory and therapy. Semin Nephrol 2014;34:550–9.
47. Sun F, Chai S, Li L, et al. Effects of glucagon-like peptide-1 receptor agonists on weight loss in patients with type 2 diabetes: a systematic review and network meta-analysis. J Diabetes Res 2015;2015:157201.
48. Catala-Lopez F, Macias Saint-Gerons D, Gonzalez-Bermejo D, et al. Cardiovascular and renal outcomes of renin-angiotensin system blockade in adult patients with diabetes mellitus: a systematic review with network meta-analyses. PLoS Med 2016;13:e1001971.
49. Palmer SC, Mavridis D, Navarese E, et al. Comparative efficacy and safety of blood pressure-lowering agents in adults with diabetes and kidney disease: a network meta-analysis. Lancet 2015;385:2047–56.
50. Weber MA, Bakris GL, Jamerson K, et al. Cardiovascular events during differing hypertension therapies in patients with diabetes. J Am Coll Cardiol 2010;56:77–85.

51. Carlberg B, Samuelsson O, Lindholm LH. Atenolol in hypertension: is it a wise choice? Lancet 2004;364:1684–9.

52. Tobe SW, Clase CM, Gao P, et al. Cardiovascular and renal outcomes with telmisartan, ramipril, or both in people at high renal risk: results from the ONTARGET and TRANSCEND studies. Circulation 2011;123:1098–107.

53. Fried LF, Emanuele N, Zhang JH, et al. Combined angiotensin inhibition for the treatment of diabetic nephropathy. N Engl J Med 2013;369:1892–903.

54. Makani H, Bangalore S, Desouza KA, et al. Efficacy and safety of dual blockade of the renin-angiotensin system: meta-analysis of randomised trials. BMJ 2013; 346:f360.

55. Bomback AS, Klemmer PJ. Mineralocorticoid receptor blockade in chronic kidney disease. Blood Purif 2012;33:119–24.

56. Raheja P, Price A, Wang Z, et al. Spironolactone prevents chlorthalidone-induced sympathetic activation and insulin resistance in hypertensive patients. Hypertension 2012;60:319–25.

57. Bakris GL, Agarwal R, Chan JC, et al. Effect of finerenone on albuminuria in patients with diabetic nephropathy: a randomized clinical trial. JAMA 2015;314: 884–94.

58. Williams B, MacDonald TM, Morant S, et al. Spironolactone versus placebo, bisoprolol, and doxazosin to determine the optimal treatment for drug-resistant hypertension (PATHWAY-2): a randomised, double-blind, crossover trial. Lancet 2015; 386:2059–68.

59. Lazich I, Bakris GL. Prediction and management of hyperkalemia across the spectrum of chronic kidney disease. Semin Nephrol 2014;34:333–9.

60. Bakris G. Summary and conclusions. High Blood Press Cardiovasc Prev 2015; 22(Suppl 1):S23.

61. Blood Pressure Lowering Treatment Trialists' Collaboration, Sundstrom J, Arima H, Woodward M, et al. Blood pressure-lowering treatment based on cardiovascular risk: a meta-analysis of individual patient data. Lancet 2014;384:591–8.

Hyperglycemia in Acute Coronary Syndromes

From Mechanisms to Prognostic Implications

Mikhail Kosiborod, MD[a,b,*]

KEYWORDS

- Diabetes • Glucose • Insulin • Myocardial infarction • Review

KEY POINTS

- Hyperglycemia is frequent in the setting of acute coronary syndromes, affects patients with and without established diabetes, and is associated with adverse outcomes.
- Whether interventions to lower glucose in patients with ACS can improve patient outcomes remains unknown, with no definitive randomized controlled trials available to settle this question.
- Until such studies are completed, monitoring glucose levels during ACS is reasonable for prognosis and risk stratification; if targeted glucose control is pursued, conservative treatment initiation thresholds and targets should be used, in line with the recommendations of professional societies.

INTRODUCTION

The observation that elevated blood glucose is common in patients hospitalized with acute coronary syndromes (ACS) was made many decades ago.[1] Since then, numerous studies have documented that hyperglycemia is frequent, affects patients with and without established diabetes, and is associated with adverse outcomes, with incremental increase in the risk of mortality and complications observed across the spectrum of glucose elevations.[2] However, many gaps in knowledge remain. Specifically, it is still unknown whether glucose is a risk marker or mediator of adverse outcomes in patients with ACS (unstable angina, ST-segment elevation myocardial infarction [STEMI], and non-STEMI). Moreover, it remains unclear whether interventions to lower glucose in patients with ACS can improve patient outcomes, and if

Disclosures: Research grants: AstraZeneca, Boehringer Ingelheim. Consultant: AstraZeneca, Boehringer Ingelheim, Amgen, Sanofi, Novo Nordisk, Intarcia, Novartis, Merck (Diabetes), Eisai, Janssen, Glytec, ZS Pharma.
[a] Department of Cardiology, Saint Luke's Mid America Heart Institute, 4401 Wornall Road, Kansas City, MO 64111, USA; [b] Department of Medicine, University of Missouri-Kansas City, 2411 Holmes, Kansas City, MO 64108, USA
* Saint Luke's Mid America Heart Institute, 4401 Wornall Road, Kansas City, MO 64111.
E-mail address: mkosiborod@saint-lukes.org

Endocrinol Metab Clin N Am 47 (2018) 185–202
https://doi.org/10.1016/j.ecl.2017.11.002
0889-8529/18/© 2017 Elsevier Inc. All rights reserved.

so, what the optimal targets, therapeutic strategies, and timing for such interventions should be.

This article reviews what is presently known about the association between glucose levels and outcomes of patients hospitalized with ACS; describes the available data with regards to inpatient glucose management in this patient group, and comparative data across the spectrum of critically ill hospitalized patients; addresses some of the controversies in this field; and offers practical recommendations for patient management based on the existing data.

DEFINITION OF HYPERGLYCEMIA DURING ACUTE CORONARY SYNDROME

There is currently no uniform, accepted definition for hyperglycemia in the setting of ACS. Prior studies used various blood glucose cutpoints, from greater than or equal to 110 mg/dL to greater than or equal to 200 mg/dL.[2] This is compounded by various timing of glucose level assessments in this context. Most prior studies defined hyperglycemia based on the first available (admission or "on-arrival") glucose value,[2–11] whereas others used fasting glucose,[12–17] and glucose values averaged over a period of time, such as the first 24 hours,[18–20] 48 hours, or the entire duration of hospitalization.[21] The American Heart Association (AHA) Scientific Statement on Hyperglycemia and Acute Coronary Syndrome suggests using a random glucose level greater than 140 mg/dL observed at any point over the course of ACS hospitalization as the definition of hyperglycemia.[22] This recommendation is based, in part, on epidemiologic studies demonstrating that admission, mean 24-hour, 48-hour, and hospitalization glucose levels greater than approximately 120 to 140 mg/dL are associated with increased mortality risk[7,18,19,21]; and that decline in glucose levels less than approximately 140 mg/dL during ACS hospitalization is associated with better survival,[23] although no cause-and-effect conclusions can be drawn from these data because of their observational nature.

Importantly, the nature of the relationship between higher glucose levels and greater risk of mortality differs in patients with and without diabetes, with a paradoxically greater magnitude of association in those without versus those with prevalent diabetes.[7,9,10,12,21,23] The risk of mortality gradually rises when glucose levels exceed approximately 110 to 120 mg/dL in patients without diabetes, whereas in patients with established diabetes this risk does not increase significantly until glucose levels exceed approximately 200 mg/dL.[7,21] Thus, different thresholds may be appropriate to define hyperglycemia depending on the presence or absence of known diabetes.

PREVALENCE OF ELEVATED GLUCOSE LEVELS IN ACUTE CORONARY SYNDROME

Multiple studies have documented that elevated glucose occurs commonly in patients with ACS.[2] Prior investigations show that the prevalence of hyperglycemia (>140 mg/dL) at the time of hospitalization varies between 51% and 58%.[7,21] Furthermore, more than 50% of patients with ACS that are hyperglycemic on hospital arrival do not have known diabetes.[6]

Although glucose levels normalize in some ACS patients following admission (either spontaneously or because of targeted pharmacologic interventions),[24] the prevalence of persistent hyperglycemia remains greater than 40% throughout the course of hospitalization; and the prevalence of severe, sustained hyperglycemia (average hospitalization glucose >200 mg/dL) is around 14%.[21,25] Although persistent hyperglycemia occurs more commonly in patients with versus without established diabetes (78% vs 26%, respectively),[26] more than 40% of patients with persistent hyperglycemia do not have known diabetes.[20]

GLUCOSE LEVELS AND MORTALITY IN ACUTE CORONARY SYNDROME

Many studies have demonstrated an independent relationship between higher glucose and increased mortality and other adverse outcomes in patients with ACS.[2] Plausible pathophysiologic mechanisms potentially contributing to these observed associations derive from numerous *ex vivo*, animal and human studies, which show that hyperglycemia may mediate adverse effects on inflammation, cell injury, apoptosis, ischemic myocardial metabolism, endothelial function, the coagulation cascade, and enhanced platelet aggregation in the setting of acute ischemia.[22,27] The association between higher glucose and greater mortality risk has been established across various glucose metrics,[28] across the spectrum of ACS,[3] and applies to short- and longer-term outcomes.[7,21]

The relationship between hyperglycemia and adverse outcomes in ACS has been quantitatively summarized based on data from a large series of small human studies collected over a period of three decades by Capes and colleagues.[2] This systematic overview demonstrated that among ACS patients without known diabetes, the relative risk of in-hospital mortality was 3.9-times higher in those with initial glucose of greater than or equal to 110 mg/dL compared with patients with normoglycemia. Among ACS patients with established diabetes, those with initial glucose greater than or equal to 180 mg/dL had a 70% increase in the relative risk of in-hospital mortality, as compared with patients with normoglycemia. More recent studies confirmed these findings and extended them across the broader range of ACS to include STEMI, non-STEMI, and unstable angina, demonstrating a significant increase in the risk of short- and long-term mortality, and incident heart failure in ACS patients with hyperglycemia with and without diabetes.[3,9,10] In the largest observational study to date, using data from the Cooperative Cardiovascular Project, there was a near-linear relationship between higher admission glucose and greater risk of mortality at 30 days and at 1 year in more than 140,000 patients hospitalized with acute MI (AMI).[7] A similar relationship between elevated glucose and increased risk of death was also shown with other glucose metrics, such as postadmission fasting glucose,[12,15–17] and with outcomes other than mortality, including a "no-reflow phenomenon" following percutaneous coronary intervention (PCI),[29] greater infract size,[7,21] worse left ventricular systolic function,[5] and contrast-mediated acute kidney injury.[28,30]

The association between hyperglycemia and increased risk of death is not limited to the initial stages of ACS hospitalization. In a study of approximately 17,000 patients hospitalized with AMI in the United States, persistently elevated glucose was a better discriminator of adverse events than hyperglycemia on admission.[21] There was a significant, gradual increase in the risk of in-hospital mortality with rising mean hospitalization glucose levels. Observational analyses from randomized clinical trials of glucose-insulin-potassium (GIK) therapy and of targeted glucose control in ACS also confirm the relationship between persistent hyperglycemia and increased mortality risk.[18,20]

Importantly, the nature of the relationship between higher glucose levels and increased mortality differs in patients with and without established diabetes.[7,21] Regardless of the glucose metrics used, the mortality risk starts rising at lower glucose levels, and increases at steeper slope in patients without known diabetes. This phenomenon has been recently observed in other critically ill patient populations,[31] and is not well understood. Several possible explanations have been proposed. Many patients presenting with hyperglycemia in the absence of known diabetes actually have diabetes that simply has not been recognized or treated before hospitalization,[32] representing a higher-risk cohort because other undiagnosed and untreated cardiovascular risk factors may be more prevalent in this group. Moreover, although the effect of targeted glucose control and insulin therapy in this clinical setting remains uncertain, ACS patients without diabetes with hyperglycemia are less likely to be treated with insulin than those with established diabetes, even when glucose levels are markedly elevated.[7,33] Finally, it is possible that higher degrees of illness severity are required to produce similar degrees of hyperglycemia in patients without known diabetes compared with those that have established diabetes.

DYNAMIC CHANGES IN GLUCOSE LEVELS DURING ACUTE CORONARY SYNDROME AND MORTALITY

Adding to the growing body of data on the relationship between hyperglycemia and adverse events in hospitalized ACS patients, several studies have shown that dynamic changes in glucose values are also strongly associated with patient survival. In post hoc analyses of data from the Complement And ReDuction of INfarct size after Angioplasty or Lytics (CARDINAL) trial, a decline in glucose of greater than or equal to 30 mg/dL during the first 24 hours of hospitalization was associated with lower risk of 30-day mortality compared with the groups who had either no change or an increase in glucose values.[23] Similarly, in a study of approximately 8000 patients hospitalized with ACS in the United States who had hyperglycemia (glucose >140 mg/dL) on arrival, glucose normalization following admission was associated with better patient survival.[24] Interestingly, improved survival was observed regardless of whether glucose normalization occurred as the result of insulin therapy, or happened spontaneously. In fact, it was glucose normalization, and not insulin therapy *per se*, that was associated with better outcomes. These observational analyses highlight the uncertainty in regards to whether normalization of glucose levels during hospitalization simply identifies a lower-risk group of patients, reflects differences in patient care, or has a direct beneficial impact on survival.

CLINICAL TRIALS OF GLUCOSE CONTROL IN PATIENTS WITH ACUTE CORONARY SYNDROME

Although the strong relationship between elevated glucose levels and greater risk of death in ACS is clear, the critical question in regards to whether hyperglycemia is a direct mediator of increased mortality and complications in patients with ACS, or is simply a marker of greater disease severity remains unanswered. To address this question, large randomized clinical trials of target-driven intensive glucose control in hospitalized ACS patients are required. Because no such clinical outcomes trial has been performed to date, this issue continues to be highly controversial, and cannot be presently addressed with certainty. However, some insights may be gained from critical review of small clinical trials of targeted glucose control in the ACS setting, trials of GIK therapy, and data from studies of targeted glucose control conducted in non-ACS settings.

Because of marked variability in the insulin-infusion strategies used and the hypotheses tested across the clinical trials to date, several key parameters need to be established to appropriately identify those randomized studies that provide useful information with regard to the effect of targeted glucose control in the ACS setting. These parameters include the following:

1. The presence of hyperglycemia at the time of patient randomization, because targeted glucose management is unlikely to yield benefit in the absence of hyperglycemia.

2. Target-driven glucose control as the primary tested intervention, with significantly lower glucose targets in the intervention and control arms.
3. The achievement of a clinically and statistically significant difference in glucose values between intervention and control groups after randomization.
4. The assessment of treatment effects on meaningful patient outcomes.

To date, no ACS trial has fulfilled all of these criteria. A few studies fulfilling some but not all of these criteria are summarized in **Table 1**. One study most closely satisfying the listed parameters is the Diabetes Mellitus, Insulin Glucose Infusion in Acute Myocardial Infarction (DIGAMI) trial.[34] In DIGAMI, patients presenting within 24 hours of ACS symptoms with diabetes or initial glucose greater than 198 mg/dL were randomized to an acute and chronic insulin treatment regime versus usual care. Those randomized to the insulin arm received greater than or equal to 24 hours of intravenous (IV) dextrose-insulin infusion titrated to maintain glucose levels of 126 to 180 mg/dL, followed by subcutaneous insulin injections three times daily for the subsequent 3 months. The trial enrolled 620 patients, 80% of whom had previously diagnosed diabetes. By 24 hours, those randomized to insulin achieved significantly lower glucose levels compared with the control arm (173 vs 211 mg/dL; $P<.0001$), although average glucose values remained significantly elevated in both groups; the differences between the groups were smaller by hospital discharge but remained significant (148 vs 162 mg/dL; $P<.01$). Hemoglobin (Hb) A_{1C} levels were also significantly lower in the intervention versus control group at 3 months (7.0% vs 7.5%; $P<.01$). Hypoglycemia was observed in 15% of the insulin infusion patients compared with none in the usual care group. For the primary end point of all-cause mortality at 3 months, there was no significant difference between the treatment groups (38 vs 49 deaths).[34] However, subsequent analyses of mortality at 1-year and 3.5-year follow-up showed significant reductions in mortality in the insulin-treated group versus control (at 1 year: 18.6% vs 26.1%, $P = .027$; at 3.5 years: 33% vs 44%, $P = .011$, respectively).[34,35] If one accepts the validity of the mortality reduction observed in the longer-term analyses, the relative contributions of the various aspects of the trial remain uncertain, including the effects of the acute dextrose-insulin infusion; or the effects of multidose insulin injection in the outpatient setting. Therefore, although the DIGAMI data are compelling, the relative attribution of improved survival to acute, in-hospital glucose lowering remains uncertain.

Beyond DIGAMI, a few other studies satisfy some (but not all) of the proposed parameters of validity and generalizability with regard to targeted glycemic control in ACS. The Hyperglycemia: Intensive Insulin Infusion in Infarction (HI-5) trial was designed to assess the effect of dextrose-insulin infusion versus usual care in patients with MI and hyperglycemia. Similar to DIGAMI, the therapeutic target for the insulin arm was 72 to 180 mg/dL and IV dextrose was infused with the insulin (either D_5W or $D_{10}W$); however, the insulin dose was much lower in HI-5 at 2 U/h (contrasted with 5 U/h used in DIGAMI).[36] The HI-5 trial was terminated early because of slow enrollment, and failed to achieve a statistically significant difference in glucose values between the intensive and conventional glucose groups (149 vs 162 mg/dL; 24 hours postrandomization; $P = $ NS).[18] Mortality assessments at hospital discharge, 30-days, and 6-month all numerically favored usual care over targeted glucose control with insulin treatment, although none of these comparisons were statistically significant because of low numbers of events (6 month: 10 vs 7 deaths; $P = .62$).

The DIGAMI-2 multicenter study attempted to determine whether potential survival benefit seen with glucose control in the original DIGAMI study was attributable to acute or chronic glucose lowering.[37] In DIGAMI-2, a total of 1253 patients with acute

Table 1
Clinical trials of glucose control in ACS

Trial	Targeted Glucose Control	Elevated BG on Entry	Glucose Targets Specified	BG Contrast Achieved	Clinical End Points	Results
DIGAMI (1995)	+/–	+ ≈280 mg/dL	+ 126–180 mg/dL vs usual care acutely 90–126 mg/dL fasting BG vs usual care afterward	+/– 173 vs 211 mg/dL during first 24 h; difference in hemoglobin A_{1c} but not fasting BG afterward	+	+/– Mortality neutral at 3 mo (primary end point), improved survival in glucose control arm by 1 y
DIGAMI2 (2005)	+/–	+ 229 mg/dL	+ 126–180 mg/dL in-hospital vs usual care acutely 90–126 mg/dL fasting BG (Group 1 only) vs usual care afterward	+/– 164 vs 180 mg/dL at 24 h, no difference afterward	+	– Mortality neutral among three groups
HI-5 (2006)	+/–	+ ≈198 mg/dL	+ 72–180 mg/dL vs usual care	– 149 vs 162 mg/dL (P = NS) during first 24 h	+	– Mortality neutral in-hospital, at 3 and 6 mo
Marfella (2009)	+	+ ≥140 mg/dL	+ 80–140 vs 180–200 mg/dL	+ 163 vs 192 mg/dL	–	+/– Higher ejection fraction, less oxidative stress, less inflammation and apoptosis in the intensive vs standard group
Marfella (2012)	+	+ ≥140 mg/dL	+ 80–140 vs 180–200 mg/dL or GIK	+ 161 vs 194 vs 182 mg/dL	–	+/– More regenerative potential in the peri-infarcted areas in the intensive vs conventional and GIK groups

Study								
Marfella (2013, myocardial salvage)	+	≥140 mg/dL	+	80–140 vs 180–200 mg/dL	+	144 vs 201 mg/dL	−	+/− Greater myocardial salvage in the intensive vs standard group
Marfella (2013, ISR)	+	≥140 mg/dL	+	80–140 vs 180–200 mg/dL	+	145 vs 191 mg/dL	−	+/− Lower ISR in the intensive vs standard group
RECREATE pilot (2012)	+	≥144 mg/dL	+	90–117 mg/dL vs usual care	+	117 vs 143 mg/dL	−	+/− Significant difference in glucose between intensive and standard groups (primary end point) No difference in mortality (small number of events)
BIOMArKS2 (2013)	+	≥140 mg/dL	+	85–110 mg/dL during day, 85–139 mg/dL at night vs <288 mg/dL	+	112 mg/dL vs ~130 mg/dL	+	− No difference in infract size by high-sensitive troponin; composite of in-hospital and reinfraction higher in the intensive vs standard group (very small number of events)

Abbreviations: BG, blood glucose; BIOMArKS2, Biomarker Study to Identify the Acute Risk of a Coronary Syndrome-2; DIGAMI, Diabetes Mellitus, Insulin Glucose Infusion in Acute Myocardial Infarction; HI-5, The Hyperglycemia: Intensive Insulin Infusion in Infarction; ISR, in-stent restenosis; RECREATE, Researching Coronary Reduction by Appropriately Targeting Euglycemia.

MI and diabetes or admission glucose greater than 198 mg/dL were randomized to one of three subgroups: (1) 24-hour insulin-glucose infusion targeting glucose of 126 to 180 mg/dL, followed by a subcutaneous insulin-based long-term glucose control (Group 1, identical to the original DIGAMI intervention group); (2) same 24-hour insulin-glucose infusion, but followed by standard glucose control (Group 2); and (3) routine glucose management (Group 3). Of note, the trial was stopped prematurely because of slow recruitment. Glucose levels on arrival were similar among the three arms (approximately 229 mg/dL). At 24 hours postrandomization glucose levels were modestly lower in the two groups assigned to acute glucose lowering versus control (164 vs 180 mg/dL; $P<.01$). This difference, although statistically significant, was clinically small and considerably less than expected. There was no difference in either glucose or HbA_{1C} levels among the three groups at any other time point, with up to 3 years of follow-up. Importantly, patients in Group 1 failed to achieve the targeted fasting glucose range of 90 to 126 mg/dL during the outpatient management phase. Mortality over 2 years was not statistically different among the three groups. Because of its limitations (primarily lack of substantial contrast in glucose levels among the three groups), the DIGAMI-2 study did not provide a definitive answer on whether targeted glucose lowering (whether acute or chronic) has any clinical value in patients with ACS.

Several additional, smaller clinical trials of intensive versus conventional glucose control in ACS have tested mechanistic hypotheses, and the effectiveness of streamlined insulin infusion protocol in lowering glucose compared with usual care, and feasibility of its implementation internationally (including resource-limited areas).[27,38–41] Marfella and colleagues randomized 50 patients with AMI and hyperglycemia (admission blood glucose $\geq$140 mg/dL) who had coronary angiography and were referred for coronary bypass surgery to either intensive or conventional glucose control for 3 days preoperatively; 38 AMI patients requiring coronary artery bypass graft (CABG) who had normal admission glucose levels served as control subjects.[27] Two-dimensional echocardiography was performed on admission and after achieving glucose treatment goals. All patients underwent myocardial biopsies from peri-infracted areas that were subjected to a variety of immunohistochemical and biochemical analyses. Patients in the intensive treatment group achieved greater reduction in glucose values (78 vs 10 mg/dL), but also had higher hypoglycemia rates. Compared with conventional treatment group, patients in the intensive group had higher ejection fraction, less oxidative stress, and less inflammation and apoptosis in peri-infarcted specimens. However, the study was too small to evaluate clinically meaningful outcomes.

The same group subsequently embarked on an additional small randomized trial with almost identical design, except that patients could be randomized to three different arms: (1) intensive glucose control, (2) conventional control, or (3) GIK.[39] Patients in the intensive control group exhibited more regenerative potential (as analyzed by myocyte precursor cells) in the peri-infarcted areas than those in the conventional and GIK groups. Two subsequent randomized trials by the same investigators evaluated the effect of intensive glucose control (vs conventional management) on myocardial salvage index among 106 patients with hyperglycemia with STEMI undergoing PCI[38]; and on in-stent restenosis in 165 patients with hyperglycemia with STEMI undergoing PCI.[40] Despite small sample size, both studies showed clinically and statistically significant benefits of intensive versus conventional periprocedural glucose control in terms of greater myocardial salvage (15% vs 7%; $P<.05$) and lower rates of in-stent restenosis at 6 months (24% vs 46%; $P<.05$). These clinical trials, although elegant, and intriguing, require confirmation in larger studies before their results are extrapolated to routine clinical care.

The International Multicentre Randomized Controlled Trial of Intensive Insulin Therapy Targeting Normoglycemia In Acute Myocardial Infarction: RECREATE (REsearching Coronary REduction by Appropriately Targeting Euglycemia) was a randomized open-label pilot study of targeted glucose control in patients with STEMI, with the main objective of testing the feasibility and safety of implementing a streamlined glucose control protocol across international sites, many in resource-limited environments.[41] A total of 287 patients presenting with STEMI and initial glucose value greater than or equal to 144 mg/dL were randomly assigned to either intensive glucose control with a streamlined IV insulin infusion protocol or usual care. Patients in the intensive arm were treated with IV infusion of insulin glulisine for at least 24 hours and for as long as cardiac care unit–level care was required, with a target glucose range of 90 to 117 mg/dL. Once transferred to the ward, patients in the intensive arm were switched to insulin glargine and continued this treatment for a total duration of 30 days postrandomization. Patients in the control arm receive usual care for ACS, according to local practice of each participating center. Because RECREATE was a pilot study designed to demonstrate the feasibility of targeted glucose control in STEMI with a simplified insulin infusion protocol, the primary end point was 24-hour difference in mean glucose between the two study groups. At 24 hours, mean glucose was significantly lower in the intervention arm versus standard care (117 vs 143 mg/dL); however, at 30 days HbA_{1c} was similar between the groups. Although the overall rates of hypoglycemia (<70 mg/dL) were significantly higher in the intensive versus standard groups (22.7% vs 4.4%; $P<.05$), there was only one episode of severe hypoglycemia (<50 mg/dL). The rates of mortality at 90 days were not different in the intensive versus standard groups (12 vs 13 events); however, the study lacked statistical power to provide answers in regards to clinical outcomes.

The most recent study of glucose control in AMI was the Randomized BIOMarker Study to Identify the Acute Risk of a Coronary Syndrome-2 (BIOMArCS-2) study,[42] a prospective, single-center, open-label clinical trial that randomized 294 patients with ACS (280 patients in the final analytical dataset; 82% with STEMI) and admission glucose between 140 and 288 mg/dL to either intensive glucose control for 48 hours (target glucose of 85–110 mg/dL during the day; 85–139 mg/dL at night) or conventional management (target glucose <288 mg/dL). Primary outcome was high-sensitivity troponin T value 72 hours postadmission (hsTropT72, as a marker of infarct size). The extent of myocardial injury was also measured at 6 weeks using myocardial perfusion scintigraphy (myocardial perfusion imaging single-photon emission computed tomography). Glucose values were significantly lower in the intensive versus the conventional group at 6, 12, 24, and 36 hours, and equalized by 72 hours. Severe hypoglycemia (<50 mg/dL) occurred in 13 patients (9%) randomized to the intensive glucose control. There was no significant difference in hsTropT72 between the groups (1197 vs 1354 ng/L; $P = .41$). The median extent of myocardial injury by myocardial perfusion imaging single-photon emission computed tomography was numerically lower in the intensive versus conventional group, but this difference did not reach significance (2% vs 4% respectively; $P = .07$). The number of in-hospital deaths and recurrent MI was small (nine events in total), but occurred more frequently in the intensive versus conventional groups (eight vs one event, respectively; $P = .04$). The results of the BIOMArCS-2 study suggest that intensive glucose control after AMI does not reduce infarct size as measured by high-sensitivity troponin essay, while increasing the risk of hypoglycemia and, possibly, composite of in-hospital death and recurrent MI. However, given that the number of events in the study was small, its single-center and open-label design, and that the findings conflict with other small clinical trials that showed reduction in infarct size with intensive versus conventional glucose control,[38] and no difference in mortality between the groups (despite the higher number of events),[41] the results of BIOMArCS-2 are difficult to interpret.

The remaining trials evaluating the effects of insulin infusion on clinical outcomes in the ACS setting have predominantly tested the GIK hypothesis (ie, hyperinsulinemic, hyperglycemic therapy), as summarized in published quantitative analyses,[43] and have little to do with target-driven glucose control (**Table 2**). Studies like the Glucose-Insulin-Potassium (GIPS) trial,[44] or the much larger Clinical Trial of Reviparin and Metabolic Modulation in Acute Myocardial Infarction Treatment and Evaluation - Estudios Cardiológicos Latinoamérica (CREATE-ECLA) and the Organization for the Assessment of Strategies for Ischemic Syndromes (OASIS)-6 trials (which in total randomized nearly 23,000 participants),[19] assigned patients to fixed-dose GIK infusion regardless of their initial glucose values or diabetes status, and did not prespecify targets for glucose control. In these studies, as dictated by the infusion protocols, high-dose delivery of insulin was supported by IV glucose administration to affect modest hyperglycemia, defined by protocol as a range of 126 to 198 mg/dL. For example, in the (CREATE-ECLA) trial that enrolled more than 20,000 patients with ACS and demonstrated no discernible treatment benefit with GIK therapy,[19] 6-hour postrandomization glucose values were significantly higher in the GIK group than in the control group (187 vs 148 mg/dL). Thus, the GIK studies were not designed to

Table 2
Clinical trials of GIK in ACS

Trial	Targeted Glucose Control	Elevated BG on Entry	Glucose Targets Specified	BG Contrast Achieved	Clinical End Points	Results
Pol-GIK (1999)	−	− 124 mg/dL	−	N/A 106 vs 112 mg/dL in intervention vs control arms	+	Significantly higher mortality in intervention vs control arm at 35 d
CREATE-ECLA (2005)	−	+ 162 mg/dL	−	N/A Glucose higher in intervention arm vs control (187 vs 148 mg/dL)	+	Mortality neutral
IMMEDIATE (2012)	−	Not specified	−	N/A	+	No difference in progression to AMI, 30-d mortality or HF Composite of in-hospital mortality or cardiac arrest lower in the GIK vs placebo groups

Abbreviations: BG, blood glucose; CREATE-ECLA, Clinical Trial of Reviparin and Metabolic Modulation in Acute Myocardial Infarction Treatment and Evaluation - Estudios Clinicos Latino America; IMMEDIATE, Immediate Myocardial Metabolic Enhancement During Initial Assessment and Treatment in Emergency Care; N/A, not applicable; Pol-GIK, Poland Glucose-Insulin-Potassium trial.

evaluate targeted glucose control with insulin, and their findings should not be used in guiding the decisions about glucose management in ACS.

The Poland Glucose-Insulin-Potassium (Pol-GIK) trial randomized 954 patients with acute MI to either to fixed low-dose GIK, which included a much lower rate of insulin infusion (0.8–1.3 U/h) than typical GIK regimens, versus normal saline infusion.[45] Pol-GIK also cannot be considered a study of targeted glucose control, because it randomized patients with normoglycemia (initial glucose ≈ 124 mg/dL in both groups). It is, therefore, not surprising that excess hypoglycemia was observed in the intervention arm. Similar to other GIK studies, no glucose goals were prespecified or aimed for and the dose of GIK infusion was fixed, and not adjusted to maintain a certain range of glucose values. As the result, there was no significant difference in glucose levels 24 hours postrandomization (106 mg/dL in GIK vs 112 mg/dL in the control arm). The study was stopped prematurely because of excess mortality in the GIK arm at 35 days (8.9% vs 4.8% in the control arm; $P = .01$). However, because of the serious limitations of interpretation stemming from the intent of the trial to evaluate the effect of fixed-dose administration of insulin rather than targeted glucose control hypothesis, no valuable lessons are learned about glucose-lowering and patient outcomes in AMI based on its results.

The Immediate Myocardial Metabolic Enhancement During Initial Assessment and Treatment in Emergency Care Trial (IMMEDIATE) was a randomized, placebo-controlled, multicenter clinical trial of GIK infusion (1.5 mL/kg/h, continuous infusion for total of 12 hours) versus matching placebo administered in the setting of suspected ACS in the prehospital emergency medical service setting.[46] The IMMEDIATE trial was designed to test the GIK hypothesis, and was not a study of targeted glucose control in ACS. Similar to previous GIK trials, the presence of hyperglycemia was not required, and there were no prespecified goals for glucose control. The primary hypothesis was that early GIK administration would prevent progression of suspected ACS to AMI within 24 hours, as determined by biomarker and electrocardiogram evidence of myocardial damage. A small biologic cohort substudy also evaluated the impact of GIK infusion on infract size.

A total of 871 patients (411 in the GIK group, 460 in the placebo group) were evaluated. There was no significant difference between the GIK and placebo groups in progression to AMI (48.7% vs 52.6%; $P = .28$), 30-day mortality (4.4% vs 6.1%; $P = .27$), or 30-day heart failure (1.5% vs 2.2%; $P = .43$).[46] The rates of prespecified composite of cardiac arrest or in-hospital mortality were significantly lower in the GIK group (4.4% vs 8.7%; $P = .01$). In a small biologic mechanism cohort (110 patient total), GIK significantly reduced infract size compared with placebo (2% vs 10% of left ventricular mass, respectively; $P = .01$). Although the results from this small substudy of IMMEDIATE are intriguing, overall, the results of IMMEDIATE showed no significant clinical benefit of early GIK administration among patients with suspected ACS.

In summary, no definitive clinical trial of targeted glucose control in ACS has been performed, and the data from the existing small studies are conflicting and inconclusive. In this context, one might be tempted to look for more definitive answers in the broader critical care field of patients in other clinical settings. In 2001, van den Berghe and colleagues[47] reported marked beneficial effects associated with normalization of blood glucose using an insulin infusion compared with usual care among patients hospitalized in a surgical intensive care unit (ICU). These observations fueled enthusiasm to endorse a strategy of targeted glucose control in critically ill hospitalized populations.[48] However, in the 8 years that followed, several additional randomized trials in various ICU patient populations have failed to reproduce these results.[49–53] Key among these include the same investigators testing intensive glucose lowering in the medical ICU patients, and showing lower morbidity, but no difference in the trial primary end point of mortality with intensive glucose lowering versus usual care.[53] In addition, the Normoglycemia in Intensive Care Evaluation–Survival Using Glucose Algorithm Regulation (NICE-SUGAR) trial, which was the largest trial of targeted glucose control in critically ill patients across ICU settings, demonstrated significantly higher mortality with intensive versus more conservative glucose control.[50] These results have substantially tempered enthusiasm for aggressive glucose lowering in the ICU setting. However, the results of NICE-SUGAR need to be interpreted in the context of the study design; NICE-SUGAR compared "very intensive" glucose control with "good" glucose control, not with "usual care." Specifically, an IV insulin protocol was used in more than two-thirds of patients in the control arm, producing an average glucose of 142 mg/dL. This degree of glucose control is more intensive than what was achieved in control groups of other critical care studies, and lower than what was achieved in the intensive arm of many ACS studies. Thus, the most appropriate conclusion from NICE-SUGAR study is that "moderate" glucose control (with values somewhere between 140 and 180 mg/dL) is sufficient, and more aggressive glucose lowering provides no additive benefit, and may be harmful.

Finally, the most recent clinical trial to evaluate the potential effects of intensive versus conventional glucose control in critically ill patients was Randomized Controlled Trial of Intensive versus Conservative Glucose Control in Patients Undergoing Coronary Artery Bypass Graft Surgery (GLUCO-CABG Trial).[54] In this study, the investigators randomized patients with hyperglycemia with and without diabetes (n = 152 and n = 150, respectively) undergoing CABG to more intensive glucose control (target, 100–140 mg/dL) or more conservative control (target, 141–180 mg/dL), using software-directed IV insulin infusion for both treatment groups. Primary outcome was a composite of mortality and multiple postoperative complications, including wound infection, pneumonia, bacteremia, respiratory failure, acute kidney injury, and major cardiovascular events. The investigators achieved significantly lower mean glucose levels in the intensive versus conservative arms (132 vs 154 mg/dL; $P < .001$). The primary end point occurred less frequently in the intensive versus conservative groups (42% vs 52%; $P = .08$), but this difference did not reach statistical significance, likely because of the trial being underpowered. There was no difference in complications among patients with diabetes treated with intensive or conservative regimens (49% vs 48%; $P = .87$), but a significantly lower rate of complications in patients without diabetes (34% vs 55%; $P = .008$). These results, although suggestive of possible benefit from lower target glucose targets in patients with hyperglycemia without diabetes undergoing CABG, should be considered as hypothesis generating, and in need for confirmation in larger trials.

Regardless, extrapolation of observations from trials outside of the ACS setting is problematic. Specifically, the findings from patients hospitalized with surgical illness, trauma, and sepsis cannot be simply extended to those with ACS. The pathophysiology of these conditions is different, and the treatment thresholds and targets may be distinct. Prior studies have shown that the relationship between glucose values and mortality may vary significantly across various cardiovascular conditions[7,55]; thus, it can also vary substantially between cardiac and noncardiac disease states.

THE PROGNOSTIC IMPORTANCE OF HYPOGLYCEMIA IN PATIENTS WITH ACUTE CORONARY SYNDROME

Because therapy for hyperglycemia in the hospital necessitates the use of insulin, it is expected that glucose lowering in the in-patient setting will produce excess hypoglycemia. Several studies suggested that glucose values in the hypoglycemic range may adversely affect mortality in ACS (93% increase in the adjusted odds of 2-year mortality in one study),[25,56] and demonstrated a J-shaped relationship between average glucose values during hospitalization and in-hospital mortality.[21] Whether hypoglycemia is directly harmful in patients with ACS, or whether it is simply a marker for the most critically ill patients was evaluated in a large observational study.[57] The risk associated with low blood glucose was confined to those who developed hypoglycemia spontaneously, most likely as the result of severe underlying illness. In contrast, hypoglycemia that occurred after insulin initiation was not associated with worse survival. Two subsequent analyses of data from the DIGAMI-2 and CREATE-ECLA trials also found no significant association between hypoglycemia and mortality, after adjustment for confounders.[58,59] These findings suggest that hypoglycemia is a marker of severe illness, rather than a direct cause of adverse outcomes. Although continuous efforts to avoid hypoglycemia are certainly warranted, these studies cast some doubt on the assumption that the lack of clinical benefit from intensive glycemic control in clinical trials is simply a consequence of excess hypoglycemia.

CURRENT PATTERNS OF GLUCOSE CONTROL IN ACUTE CORONARY SYNDROME

The current practice of glucose management in the United States is highly variable.[33] Large proportions of ACS patients with hyperglycemia do not receive glucose-lowering therapy, even in the setting of marked hyperglycemia; this is particularly evident among those without known diabetes.[7,26] A study from the United Kingdom showed that 64% of patients without diabetes with admission glucose greater than or equal to 11 mmol/L (~200 mg/dL) received no glucose-lowering treatments during hospitalization.[60] Similar findings were observed in the recent analysis of 4297 admissions with ACS and mean hospitalization glucose of greater than or equal to 200 mg/dL; insulin was used 63% of the time, and IV insulin infusion was used only in 13% of these admissions, with substantial variation between hospitals that did not change over 10 years of observation.[61] Many factors contribute to this inconsistency of clinical practice, such as the lack of convincing clinical outcomes data, concerns about hypoglycemia, institutional barriers, and clinical inertia, underscoring the critical importance of continued investigation with regard to the efficacy and safety of glucose management in the setting of ACS.

SUMMARY AND RECOMMENDATIONS

There is a clear need for well-designed, large clinical trials of target-driven glucose control in ACS with sufficient statistical power to detect a clinically important difference in mortality and other adverse clinical outcomes. Until such trials are completed, any specific recommendations in regards to glucose management in ACS are based on epidemiologic observations, mechanistic hypotheses, and expert consensus, and not grounded in solid clinical evidence.

Reflecting this uncertainty, in 2008 the AHA published an update on its position regarding glucose targets for ACS/MI patients, which substantially liberalized previous recommendations.[22] This AHA position advocates for a glucose treatment threshold of greater than 180 mg/dL. A similar position was adopted by the 2009 focused update of STEMI guidelines,[62] the 2012 focused update of non-STEMI guidelines,[63] and endorsed by the revised American Association of Clinical Endocrinologists/American Diabetes Association guidelines.[64] These guidelines now recommend the same glucose threshold for therapeutic intervention in critically ill patients of greater than 180 mg/dL, with suggested therapeutic target of glucose control specified at 140 to

180 mg/dL, a substantially more liberal approach than prior documents.[48] Although even these targets represent an expert consensus, it is likely the most prudent approach in the presence of the accumulated data.

Until more information becomes available, several practical suggestions are reasonable in regards to glucose management during ACS hospitalization:

1. Assessment of glucose values at the time of admission, and glucose monitoring during hospitalization, provide useful information in regards to risk stratification and prognosis.
2. If targeted glucose control is being considered, several precautions should be observed:
   a. Conservative treatment initiation thresholds and glucose targets (as outlined previously) should be used, in line with the recommendations of professional societies. Aggressive glucose lowering, including "normalization of blood glucose" as previously recommended, does not clearly offer additional benefit, and may be harmful.
   b. Evidence-based protocols should be used when and if glucose control strategies are implemented. Such protocols should
      i. have demonstrated effectiveness and safety with regard to targeted glucose control in the variety of clinical settings;
      ii. incorporate the rate of change in glucose values and insulin sensitivity in determination of insulin infusion rates and adjustments;
      iii. provide specific directions on the frequency of glucose testing and hypoglycemia management.
3. Lastly, and importantly, continued efforts are necessary for the design and execution of definitive clinical trials assessing glucose control targets, therapies, and timing, so that more evidence-based recommendations may be provided to clinicians in regards to glucose management during ACS.

REFERENCES

1. Datey K, Nanda N. Hyperglycemia after acute myocardial infarction: its relation to diabetes mellitus. N Engl J Med 1967;276(5):262–5.
2. Capes SE, Hunt D, Malmberg K, et al. Stress hyperglycaemia and increased risk of death after myocardial infarction in patients with and without diabetes: a systematic overview. Lancet 2000;355(9206):773–8.
3. Foo K, Cooper J, Deaner A, et al. A single serum glucose measurement predicts adverse outcomes across the whole range of acute coronary syndromes. Heart 2003;89:512–6.
4. Hadjadj S, Coisne D, Mauco G, et al. Prognostic value of admission plasma glucose and HbA in acute myocardial infarction. Diabet Med 2004;21:305–10.
5. Ishihara M, Inoue I, Kawagoe T, et al. Impact of acute hyperglycemia on left ventricular function after reperfusion therapy in patients with a first anterior wall acute myocardial infarction. Am Heart J 2003;146:674–8.
6. Kadri Z, Danchin N, Vaur L, et al. Major impact of admission glycaemia on 30 day and one year mortality in non-diabetic patients admitted for myocardial infarction: results from the nationwide French USIC 2000 study. Heart 2006;92:910–5.
7. Kosiborod M, Rathore SS, Inzucchi SE, et al. Admission glucose and mortality in elderly patients hospitalized with acute myocardial infarction: implications for patients with and without recognized diabetes. Circulation 2005;111:3078–86.
8. Meier JJ, Deifuss S, Klamann A, et al. Plasma glucose at hospital admission and previous metabolic control determine myocardial infarct size and survival in

patients with and without type 2 diabetes: the Langendreer Myocardial Infarction and Blood Glucose in Diabetic Patients Assessment (LAMBDA). Diabetes Care 2005;28:2551–3.

9. Stranders I, Diamant M, van Gelder RE, et al. Admission blood glucose level as risk indicator of death after myocardial infarction in patients with and without diabetes mellitus. Arch Intern Med 2004;164:982–8.

10. Wahab NN, Cowden EA, Pearce NJ, et al. Is blood glucose an independent predictor of mortality in acute myocardial infarction in the thrombolytic era? J Am Coll Cardiol 2002;40:1748–54.

11. Yudkin JS, Oswald GA. Stress hyperglycemia and cause of death in non-diabetic patients with myocardial infarction. Br Med J (Clin Res Ed) 1987;294:773.

12. Aronson D, Hammerman H, Kapeliovich MR, et al. Fasting glucose in acute myocardial infarction: incremental value for long-term mortality and relationship with left ventricular systolic function. Diabetes Care 2007;30:960–6.

13. Mak KH, Mah PK, Tey BH, et al. Fasting blood sugar level: a determinant for in-hospital outcome in patients with first myocardial infarction and without glucose intolerance. Ann Acad Med Singapore 1993;22:291–5.

14. O'Sullivan JJ, Conroy RM, Robinson K, et al. In-hospital prognosis of patients with fasting hyperglycemia after first myocardial infarction. Diabetes Care 1991;14:758–60.

15. Porter A, Assali AR, Zahalka A, et al. Impaired fasting glucose and outcomes of ST-elevation acute coronary syndrome treated with primary percutaneous intervention among patients without previously known diabetes mellitus. Am Heart J 2008;155:284–9.

16. Suleiman M, Hammerman H, Boulos M, et al. Fasting glucose is an important independent risk factor for 30-day mortality in patients with acute myocardial infarction: a prospective study. Circulation 2005;111:754–60.

17. Verges B, Zeller M, Dentan G, et al. Impact of fasting glycemia on short-term prognosis after acute myocardial infarction. J Clin Endocrinol Metab 2007;92:2136–40.

18. Cheung NW, Wong VW, McLean M. The Hyperglycemia: Intensive Insulin Infusion in Infarction (HI-5) study: a randomized controlled trial of insulin infusion therapy for myocardial infarction. Diabetes Care 2006;29:765–70.

19. Diaz R, Goyal A, Mehta SR, et al. Glucose-insulin-potassium therapy in patients with ST-segment elevation myocardial infarction. JAMA 2007;298:2399–405.

20. Goyal A, Mehta SR, Gerstein HC, et al. Glucose levels compared with diabetes history in the risk assessment of patients with acute myocardial infarction. Am Heart J 2009;157:763–70.

21. Kosiborod M, Inzucchi SE, Krumholz HM, et al. Glucometrics in patients hospitalized with acute myocardial infarction: defining the optimal outcomes-based measure of risk. Circulation 2008;117:1018–27.

22. Deedwania P, Kosiborod M, Barrett E, et al. Hyperglycemia and acute coronary syndrome: a scientific statement from the American Heart Association Diabetes Committee of the Council on Nutrition, Physical Activity, and Metabolism. Circulation 2008;117:1610–9.

23. Goyal A, Mahaffey KW, Garg J, et al. Prognostic significance of the change in glucose level in the first 24 h after acute myocardial infarction: results from the CARDINAL study. Eur Heart J 2006;27:1289–97.

24. Kosiborod M, Inzucchi SE, Krumholz HM, et al. Glucose normalization and outcomes in patients with acute myocardial infarction. Arch Intern Med 2009;169:438–46.

25. Svensson AM, McGuire DK, Abrahamsson P, et al. Association between hyper- and hypoglycaemia and 2 year all-cause mortality risk in diabetic patients with acute coronary events. Eur Heart J 2005;26:1255–61.

26. Kosiborod M, Inzucchi S, Clark B, et al. National patterns of glucose control among patients hospitalized with acute myocardial infarction. J Am Coll Cardiol 2007;49:1018–183, 283A.

27. Marfella R, Di Filippo C, Portoghese M, et al. Tight glycemic control reduces heart inflammation and remodeling during acute myocardial infarction in hyperglycemic patients. J Am Coll Cardiol 2009;53:1425–36.

28. Kosiborod MMP, Rao S, Inzucchi SE, et al. Hyperglycemia and risk of acute kidney injury after coronary angiography in patients hospitalized with acute myocardial infarction. J Am Coll Cardiol 2009;53:1028. A382.

29. Iwakura K, Ito H, Ikushima M, et al. Association between hyperglycemia and the no-reflow phenomenon in patients with acute myocardial infarction. J Am Coll Cardiol 2003;41:1–7.

30. Naruse H, Ishii J, Hashimoto T, et al. Pre-procedural glucose levels and the risk for contrast-induced acute kidney injury in patients undergoing emergency coronary intervention. Circ J 2012;76:1848–55.

31. Krinsley JS, Egi M, Kiss A, et al. Diabetic status and the relation of the three domains of glycemic control to mortality in critically ill patients: an international multi-center cohort study. Crit Care 2013;17:R37.

32. Conaway DG, O'Keefe JH, Reid KJ, et al. Frequency of undiagnosed diabetes mellitus in patients with acute coronary syndrome. Am J Cardiol 2005;96:363–5.

33. Kosiborod M, Inzucchi S, Clark B, et al. Variability in the hospital use of insulin to control sustained hyperglycemia among acute myocardial infarction patients. J Am Coll Cardiol 2007;49:1018–186, 284A.

34. Malmberg K, Ryden L, Efendic S, et al. Randomized trial of insulin-glucose infusion followed by subcutaneous insulin treatment in diabetic patients with acute myocardial infarction (DIGAMI study): effects on mortality at 1 year. J Am Coll Cardiol 1995;26:57–65.

35. Malmberg K. Prospective randomised study of intensive insulin treatment on long term survival after acute myocardial infarction in patients with diabetes mellitus. DIGAMI (Diabetes Mellitus, Insulin Glucose Infusion in Acute Myocardial Infarction) Study Group. BMJ 1997;314:1512–5.

36. Gnaim CI, McGuire DK. Glucose-insulin-potassium therapy for acute myocardial infarction: what goes around comes around. Am Heart J 2004;148:924–30.

37. Malmberg K, Ryden L, Wedel H, et al. Intense metabolic control by means of insulin in patients with diabetes mellitus and acute myocardial infarction (DIGAMI 2): effects on mortality and morbidity. Eur Heart J 2005;26:650–61.

38. Marfella R, Rizzo MR, Siniscalchi M, et al. Peri-procedural tight glycemic control during early percutaneous coronary intervention up-regulates endothelial progenitor cell level and differentiation during acute ST-elevation myocardial infarction: effects on myocardial salvage. Int J Cardiol 2013;168(4):3954–62.

39. Marfella R, Sasso FC, Cacciapuoti F, et al. Tight glycemic control may increase regenerative potential of myocardium during acute infarction. J Clin Endocrinol Metab 2012;97:933–42.

40. Marfella R, Sasso FC, Siniscalchi M, et al. Peri-procedural tight glycemic control during early percutaneous coronary intervention is associated with a lower rate of in-stent restenosis in patients with acute ST-elevation myocardial infarction. J Clin Endocrinol Metab 2012;97:2862–71.

41. Nerenberg KA, Goyal A, Xavier D, et al. Piloting a novel algorithm for glucose control in the coronary care unit: the RECREATE (REsearching Coronary REduction by Appropriately Targeting Euglycemia) trial. Diabetes Care 2012;35:19–24.

42. de Mulder M, Umans V, Cornel JH, et al. Intensive glucose regulation in hyperglycemic acute coronary syndrome: results of the randomized BIOMarker study to identify the acute risk of a coronary syndrome-2 (BIOMArCS-2) glucose trial. JAMA Intern Med 2013;173(20):1896–904.

43. Fath-Ordoubadi F, Beatt KJ. Glucose-insulin-potassium in acute myocardial infarction. Lancet 1999;353:1968.

44. van der Horst IC, Zijlstra F, van't Hof AW, et al. Glucose-insulin-potassium infusion inpatients treated with primary angioplasty for acute myocardial infarction: the glucose-insulin-potassium study: a randomized trial. J Am Coll Cardiol 2003;42:784–91.

45. Ceremuzynski L, Budaj A, Czepiel A, et al. Low-dose glucose-insulin-potassium is ineffective in acute myocardial infarction: results of a randomized multicenter Pol-GIK trial. Cardiovasc Drugs Ther 1999;13:191–200.

46. Selker HP, Beshansky JR, Sheehan PR, et al. Out-of-hospital administration of intravenous glucose-insulin-potassium in patients with suspected acute coronary syndromes: the IMMEDIATE randomized controlled trial. JAMA 2012;307(18):1925–33.

47. van den Berghe G, Wouters P, Weekers F, et al. Intensive insulin therapy in the critically ill patients. N Engl J Med 2001;345:1359–67.

48. Garber AJ, Moghissi E, Bransome ED, et al. American College of Endocrinology position statement on inpatient diabetes and metabolic control. Endocr Pract 2004;10:77–82.

49. Brunkhorst FM, Engel C, Bloos F, et al. Intensive insulin therapy and pentastarch resuscitation in severe sepsis. N Engl J Med 2008;358:125–39.

50. Finfer S, Chittock DR, Su SY, et al. Intensive versus conventional glucose control in critically ill patients. N Engl J Med 2009;360:1283–97.

51. Gandhi GY, Nuttall GA, Abel MD, et al. Intensive intraoperative insulin therapy versus conventional glucose management during cardiac surgery: a randomized trial. Ann Intern Med 2007;146:233–43.

52. Gray CS, Hildreth AJ, Sandercock PA, et al. Glucose-potassium-insulin infusions in the management of post-stroke hyperglycaemia: the UK Glucose Insulin in Stroke Trial (GIST-UK). Lancet Neurol 2007;6:397–406.

53. Van den Berghe G, Wilmer A, Hermans G, et al. Intensive insulin therapy in the medical ICU. N Engl J Med 2006;354:449–61.

54. Umpierrez G, Cardona S, Pasquel F, et al. Randomized controlled trial of intensive versus conservative glucose control in patients undergoing coronary artery bypass graft surgery: GLUCO-CABG trial. Diabetes Care 2015;38:1665–72.

55. Kosiborod M, Inzucchi SE, Spertus JA, et al. Elevated admission glucose and mortality in elderly patients hospitalized with heart failure. Circulation 2009;119:1899–907.

56. Pinto DS, Skolnick AH, Kirtane AJ, et al. U-shaped relationship of blood glucose with adverse outcomes among patients with ST-segment elevation myocardial infarction. J Am Coll Cardiol 2005;46:178–80.

57. Kosiborod M, Inzucchi SE, Goyal A, et al. Relationship between spontaneous and iatrogenic hypoglycemia and mortality in patients hospitalized with acute myocardial infarction. JAMA 2009;301:1556–64.

58. Goyal A, Mehta SR, Diaz R, et al. Differential clinical outcomes associated with hypoglycemia and hyperglycemia in acute myocardial infarction. Circulation 2009;120:2429–37.
59. Mellbin LG, Malmberg K, Waldenstrom A, et al. Prognostic implications of hypoglycaemic episodes during hospitalisation for myocardial infarction in patients with type 2 diabetes: a report from the DIGAMI 2 trial. Heart 2009;95:721–7.
60. Weston C, Walker L, Birkhead J. Early impact of insulin treatment on mortality for hyperglycaemic patients without known diabetes who present with an acute coronary syndrome. Heart 2007;93:1542–6.
61. Venkitachalam L, McGuire DK, Gosch K, et al. Temporal trends and hospital variation in the management of severe hyperglycemia among patients with acute myocardial infarction in the United States. Am Heart J 2013;166:315–24.e1.
62. Kushner FG, Hand M, Smith SC Jr, et al. 2009 focused updates: ACC/AHA guidelines for the management of patients with ST-elevation myocardial infarction (updating the 2004 guideline and 2007 focused update) and ACC/AHA/SCAI guidelines on percutaneous coronary intervention (updating the 2005 Guideline and 2007 Focused Update): a report of the American College of Cardiology Foundation/American Heart Association Task Force on Practice Guidelines. Circulation 2009;120:2271–306.
63. Jneid H, Anderson JL, Wright RS, et al. 2012 ACCF/AHA focused update of the guideline for the management of patients with unstable angina/Non-ST-elevation myocardial infarction (updating the 2007 guideline and replacing the 2011 focused update): a report of the American College of Cardiology Foundation/American Heart Association Task Force on practice guidelines. Circulation 2012;126:875–910.
64. Moghissi ES, Korytkowski MT, Dinardo M, et al. American Association of Clinical Endocrinologists and American Diabetes Association consensus statement on inpatient glycemic control. Endocr Pract 2009;15:1–17.

Perioperative Management of Hyperglycemia and Diabetes in Cardiac Surgery Patients

 CrossMark

Rodolfo J. Galindo, MD, Maya Fayfman, MD,
Guillermo E. Umpierrez, MD, CDE*

KEYWORDS

- Perioperative hyperglycemia • Diabetes • Cardiac surgery • Stress hyperglycemia
- Hospital diabetes • CABG

KEY POINTS

- Perioperative hyperglycemia is common after cardiac surgery and is associated with higher health care resource utilization, longer length of stay, and greater perioperative mortality.
- Improvement in glycemic control, in patients with stress hyperglycemia and diabetes, has a positive impact on morbidity and mortality.
- A target blood glucose level between 140 mg/dL and 180 mg/dL is recommended for most patients during the perioperative period.
- Insulin given by continuous insulin infusion is the preferred regimen for treating hyperglycemia in critically ill patients.
- Subcutaneous administration of basal bolus or basal plus correctional bolus is the preferred treatment of non–critically ill patients.

INTRODUCTION

The prevalence of diabetes mellitus is rising at an alarming rate, affecting 415 million people worldwide and approximately 30 million people in the United States in 2015.[1] Approximately half a million patients undergo coronary artery bypass graft surgery (CABG) each year in the United States.[2] Nearly 30% to 40% of patients undergoing

Disclosure: G.E.U. is partly supported by research grants NIH/NATS UL1 TR002378 from Clinical and Translational Science Award program, and 1P30DK111024-01 from the National Institutes of Health and National Center for Research Resources. The other authors have nothing to disclose.
Division of Endocrinology, Metabolism and Lipids, Emory University School of Medicine, 69 Jesse Hill Jr Drive, Glenn Building, Suite 202, Atlanta, GA 30303, USA
* Corresponding author. Emory University School of Medicine, 69 Jesse Hill Jr Drive, Atlanta, GA 30303.
E-mail address: geumpie@emory.edu

cardiac surgery have a history of diabetes[3,4] and approximately 60% of patients without diabetes develop stress hyperglycemia, defined as a blood glucose greater than 140 mg/dL.[5–7]

Numerous studies have reported that, in critically ill and cardiac surgery patients, those who develop hyperglycemia are at increased risk for morbidity and mortality.[7–16] Perioperative hyperglycemia, in patients with and without diabetes, is associated with higher rates of wound infections, acute renal failure, longer hospital stay, and higher perioperative mortality compared with those without hyperglycemia.[8–13] Patients without diabetes who develop stress hyperglycemia during CABG surgery[14] or during intensive care unit (ICU) stay[15] have worse outcomes compared with those with previous history of diabetes. Stress hyperglycemia in patients without diabetes undergoing surgery has been associated with up to a 4-fold increase in complications and a 2-fold increase in death compared with patients with normoglycemia[16–18] and to subjects with diabetes.[16,19–24]

Stress mediators, namely stress hormones and cytokines, and the central nervous system interfere with insulin secretion and action leading to increased hepatic glucose production and reduced glucose uptake in peripheral tissues.[25,26] The adverse outcomes associated with hyperglycemia may be attributed to hyperglycemia-induced inflammatory and oxidative stress as well as its prothrombotic and vascular abnormalities. This article discusses the pathophysiology of stress-induced hyperglycemia, the impact of hyperglycemia on clinical outcomes, and strategies for the management of hyperglycemia and diabetes in cardiac surgery patients with and without a history of diabetes.

EPIDEMIOLOGY OF STRESS HYPERGLYCEMIA

Hyperglycemia, defined as a blood glucose level greater than 140 mg/dL, is common in critically ill and cardiac surgery patients, reported in 60% to 80% of cardiac surgery patients[5–7] and in and 40% to 60% of general ICU patients.[24,27–29] Most critically ill and cardiac surgery patients with hyperglycemia have a previous diagnosis of diabetes.[12,24] Most patients with diabetes experience worsening glycemic control due to the stress of surgery and anesthesia or the use of corticosteroids and nutritional support.[30] 40% to 60% of patients without a history of diabetes experience transient hyperglycemia due to the stress of surgery,[31–33] which resolves in many patients at the time of discharge. A third group of patients with inpatient hyperglycemia includes those who are newly diagnosed during hospitalization.[33–36] Thus, all patients admitted to the hospital should undergo laboratory glucose testing. Subjects without a history of diabetes with blood glucose greater than 140 mg/dL should have bedside point-of-care glucose testing.[37–39] In patients with hyperglycemia, measurement of hemoglobin A_{1c} (HbA_{1c}) differentiates stress hyperglycemia from diabetes in those who were previously undiagnosed.[32,33] The American Diabetes Association and Endocrine Society guidelines indicate that patients with hyperglycemia and an HbA_{1c} of 6.5% or higher can be classified as having diabetes.[37] It is important to emphasize, however, that despite a high specificity (100%), the HbA_{1c} cutoff of greater than 6.5% has a poor sensitivity (57%)[32] and its use is limited in patients with hemoglobinopathies, recent blood transfusion, severe kidney or liver disease, high-dose of salicylates, pregnancy, and iron deficiency anemia.[40] It is important to identify and track patients with stress hyperglycemia, because up to 60% of patients may have confirmed diabetes after 1 year of follow-up.[32]

REGULATION OF BLOOD GLUCOSE IN HEALTHY INDIVIDUALS AND DURING STRESS

Maintenance of normoglycemia is essential for normal physiology in the body and is maintained by dynamic, minute-to-minute regulation of endogenous glucose production from the liver and kidneys and of glucose utilization by peripheral tissues.[25,30,31,41] Glucose production is accomplished by gluconeogenesis and glycogenolysis. Insulin as the main regulatory hormone inhibits hepatic glucose production and stimulates glucose uptake by peripheral tissues (**Fig. 1**). During prolonged fasting, a reduction in insulin concentration leads to increased lipolysis (fat breakdown) releasing glycerol and to proteolysis (protein breakdown) releasing lactate and amino acids (alanine) that serve as the most important gluconeogenesis precursors.[41] Excess glucose is polymerized to glycogen, which is mainly stored in the liver and muscle. Glycogenolysis, mediated primarily by glucagon, breaks down glycogen to the individual glucose units for mobilization during times of metabolic need. These steps are dependent on the interaction between insulin and counter-regulatory hormones.[25]

During stress, the release of counter-regulatory hormones (glucagon, catecholamines, cortisol, and growth hormone) antagonizes the action of insulin, leading to increased gluconeogenesis in the liver and impaired insulin action in peripheral tissues resulting in hyperglycemia. Glucagon excess counteracts the action of insulin on glucose metabolism by stimulating glycogenolysis and gluconeogenesis.[42] Furthermore, catecholamines stimulate glucagon secretion and inhibit insulin release by pancreatic ß-cells as well as suppression of glucose uptake in peripheral tissues.[43] High levels of circulating corticosteroids have been shown to increase gluconeogenesis and lipolysis and to inhibit insulin release.[44] Growth hormone increases hepatic glucose production and is known to cause insulin resistance in humans; however, its role during stress is less understood.[44]

The normal response to stress is associated with activation of central nervous system and neuroendocrine axes with subsequent release of counter-regulatory

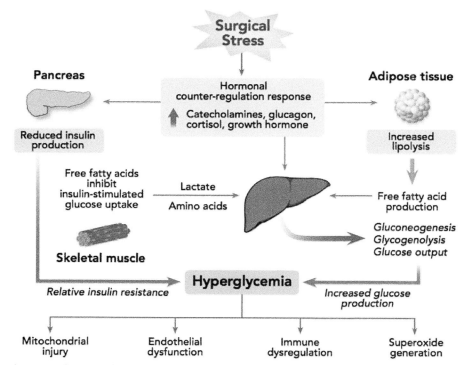

Fig. 1. Mechanism of stress hyperglycemia and its complications in surgical patients.

hormones. These hormones modify the inflammatory response, especially cytokine release that results in several alterations in carbohydrate metabolism, including insulin resistance, increased hepatic glucose production, impaired peripheral glucose utilization, and relative insulin deficiency. Acute stress increases proinflammatory cytokines, such as tumor necrosis factor α (TNF-α), interleukin (IL)-6, and IL-1, resulting in increased insulin resistance by interfering with insulin signaling.[45] Thus, stress adversely affects multiple biological processes, resulting in diminished insulin action, and if the pancreas is unable to compensate by increasing insulin production, the result is the development of hyperglycemia. Furthermore, in the presence of hyperglycemia, the pancreatic ß-cells develop desensitization (glucose toxicity) that results in further blunting of insulin secretion and increasing serum glucose levels.[46]

Increasing evidence indicates that development of hyperglycemia leads to the generation of reactive oxygen species (ROS), which affect different biological signaling pathways.[47] ROS are formed from the reduction of molecular oxygen or by oxidation of water to yield products, such as superoxide anion, hydrogen peroxide, and hydroxyl radical. The mitochondria and NADPH oxidase system are the major sources of ROS production.[48] In moderate amounts, ROS are involved in several physiologic processes that produce desired cellular responses. Large quantities of ROS, however, can lead to cellular damage of lipids, membranes, proteins, and DNA. In addition, oxidative stress has also been implicated as a contributor to ß-cell dysfunction and mitochondrial dysfunction, which can lead to the development and worsening of hyperglycemia.[49]

CONSEQUENCES OF HYPERGLYCEMIA IN HOSPITALIZED PATIENTS

Although the underlying causes have not been completed elucidated, several mechanisms have been proposed to explain the higher risk of complications and mortality of hyperglycemia in critically ill patients (see **Fig. 1**). Severe hyperglycemia causes osmotic diuresis that leads to hypovolemia, decreased glomerular filtration rate, and prerenal azotemia. Hyperglycemia has been shown to increase rates of hospital infections and to impair collagen synthesis and wound healing among patients with poorly controlled diabetes.[25,40,50] It is also associated with impaired leukocyte function, including decreased phagocytosis, impaired bacterial killing, and chemotaxis. In addition, acute hyperglycemia results in nuclear factor kB (NF-κB) activation and production of inflammatory cytokines, such as TNF-α, IL-6, and plasminogen activator inhibitor-1, which cause increased vascular permeability and leukocyte and platelet activation.[51] Furthermore, high glucose concentrations have deleterious effects on endothelial function by suppressing formation of nitric oxide and impairing endothelium-dependent flow-mediated dilation as well as abnormalities in hemostasis, including: increased platelet activation, adhesion, and aggregation and; reduced plasma fibrinolytic activity.[52] Adding to the effects of hyperglycemia in acute coronary syndrome, high free fatty acid levels seen in diabetes and stress can also aggravate ischemia/reperfusion damage by limiting the ability of cardiac muscle to uptake glucose for anaerobic metabolism.[25,53]

Several studies have shown that the hormonal and proinflammatory aberrations associated with stress hyperglycemia return to normal after treatment with insulin and resolution of hyperglycemia.[45] The anti-inflammatory and antihyperglycemic effects of insulin are well established.[54,55] Insulin acts to suppress counter-regulatory hormones and proinflammatory transcription factors and may even suppress the formation of reactive oxidation species.[56] Insulin suppresses major proinflammatory transcription factors: NF-κB, , activator protein 1, and early growth response 1.

Correction of hyperglycemia has been shown to improve the inflammatory response and to reduce generation of ROS (including superoxide radical) generation.[56,57] In addition, insulin induces vasodilation and inhibits lipolysis and platelet aggregation. The vasodilation that accompanies insulin administration may be attributed to its ability to stimulate nitric oxide release and induce the expression of endothelial nitric oxide synthase.[58] The impaired lipolysis and reduction in free fatty acids that accompany insulin administration may be associated with decreases in thrombosis and inflammation.[53]

EVIDENCE FOR CONTROLLING PERIOPERATIVE HYPERGLYCEMIA IN CARDIAC SURGERY PATIENTS

The negative impact of hyperglycemia in patients admitted for cardiac surgery merits a comprehensive and multidisciplinary approach. This plan should include dietary modifications, glucose monitoring, personalized glycemic targets to improve hyperglycemia while preventing hypoglycemia, a safe transitioning plan from the ICU to the regular floors and/or home, and proper outpatient follow-up.[39,59,60]

Intraoperative Period

In a retrospective study of 409 patients undergoing cardiac surgery, Gandhi and colleagues[61] reported that for each incremental increase in intraoperative glucose by 20 mg/dL above 100 mg/dL, there was a 30% increase in occurrence of adverse events, including pulmonary and renal complications and death. In contrast to this retrospective study, a randomized controlled trial of 400 diabetic and nondiabetic surgery patients assigned to receive continuous insulin infusion (CII) to maintain intraoperative glucose level between 80 mg/dL and 100 mg/dL versus a glucose target less than 200 mg/dL reported no improvement in clinical outcome or complications.[62] A meta-analysis of 5 randomized controlled trials in 706 cardiac surgery patients reported that rigorous intraoperative glycemic control decreased the infection rate compared with the conventional therapy but did not decrease mortality.[63]

Postoperative Period

Several randomized controlled trials in cardiac surgery patients have evaluated the impact of hyperglycemia and ideal blood glucose target during the postoperative period to optimize outcomes.[14,64–68] Desai and colleagues[64] randomized 189 patients to an intensive target of 90 mg/dL to 120 mg/dL and to a conventional target between 121 mg/dL and 180 mg/dL in first-time CABG surgery patients. They reported no differences in deep sternal wound infection, pneumonia, perioperative renal failure, or mortality. Similarly, Pezzella and colleagues[67] and Lazar and colleagues[65] reported no differences in perioperative complications, hospital length of stay, and mortality between intensive insulin targeting glucose of 90 mg/dL to 120 mg/dL versus 120 mg/dL to 180 mg/dL. In a recent study, Umpierrez and colleagues[14] aimed to determine if the lower end of the recommended glucose target can reduce hospital complications in patients undergoing CABG surgery randomized patients with hyperglycemia to an intensive insulin therapy aimed to maintain a blood glucose between 100 mg/dL and 140 mg/dL or to a conservative therapy aimed to maintain a glucose value between 141 mg/dL and 180 mg/dL in an ICU.[14] The primary outcome of this trial was to determine differences between a composite of complications, including wound infection, pneumonia, bacteremia, acute kidney injury, major adverse cardiovascular events, and mortality. The authors found no differences in a composite of complications (42% vs 52%, $P = .08$).The authors observed, however, heterogeneity in treatment effect according to diabetes status, with no differences in complications among patients with prior history of diabetes treated with intensive or conservative regimens (49% vs 48%, $P = .87$) but a significantly lower rate of complications in patients without diabetes treated with an intensive treatment regimen compared with the conservative treatment regimen (34% vs 55%, $P = .008$). In agreement with these findings, a recent study by Blaha and colleagues[68] in 2383 cardiac surgery patients treated to a target glucose range between 80 mg/dL and 110 mg/dL reported a reduction in postoperative complications only in nondiabetic patients (21% vs 33%; relative risk, 0.63; 95% CI, 0.54–0.74), whereas no significant benefit of intensive therapy was seen in patients with diabetes. Moreover, a subgroup analysis by Van den Berghe and colleagues[69] of surgical and medical ICU patients reported that whereas glucose lowering effectively reduced mortality in those without a previous history of diabetes, no significant benefit from treatment was observed in patients with diabetes.

Clinical guidelines on inpatient management of hyperglycemia recommend the use of IV CII in critically ill and in cardiac surgery patients with and without a history of diabetes.[37,39,60,70,71] Several cohort and randomized controlled trials in cardiac surgery patients have reported that improvement in glycemic control can reduce short-term and long-term complications and hospital mortality.[14,68,72,73] A target glucose level between 140 mg/dL and 180 mg/dL is recommended for most ICU and cardiac surgery patients with hyperglycemia and diabetes, but lower targets between 110 mg/dL and 140 mg/dL could be appropriate in a select group of ICU patients (ie, centers with extensive experience and cardiac surgical patients).[39] Recent studies in mixed ICU populations and in cardiac surgery patients have shown that intensive insulin therapy (glucose target <110 mg/dL) does not reduce complications compared with conventional control but increases the risk of hypoglycemia.[65,74]

Table 1 presents a comprehensive review of observational and prospective randomized trials addressing intensive glycemic control in patients undergoing cardiac surgery.[14,62,64–68,72,73,75–78] Although the readers should use caution with extrapolating data from the medical or surgical ICUs and combined trials into the cardiothoracic ICU practice, the overall consensus is that hyperglycemia management, targeting less stringent goals (140–180 mg/dL), represents the standard of care in hospitalized patients.[38,39,59,60,79]

MANAGEMENT OF PERIOPERATIVE HYPERGLYCEMIA DURING CARDIAC SURGERY
Management of Hyperglycemia in Intensive Care Unit Settings

Insulin therapy is effective in achieving and maintaining glycemic control in patients with diabetes and with stress hyperglycemia in an ICU.[25,38,39,60] Several protocols have been published, both nursing-driven and computer-generated algorithms, which have been validated for their safety and efficacy.[80–82]

There is no ideal protocol for the management of hyperglycemia in the critical patient. In addition, there is no clear evidence demonstrating the benefit of one protocol/algorithm versus another. Most institutions have standard nursing-driven protocols to facilitate insulin titration and to avoid errors in insulin dosing. Essential elements that increase protocol success are (1) rate adjustment that considers the current and previous glucose values and the current rate of insulin infusion, (2) rate adjustment that considers the rate of change (or lack of change) from the previous reading, and (3) frequent glucose monitoring (hourly until stable glycemia is established and then every 2–3 hours). Several computer-based algorithms aiming at directing the nursing staff adjusting insulin infusion rate have become commercially available (Glucommander [Glytec, Greenville, South Carolina], EndoTool System

[MD Scientific, Charlotte, North Carolina], GlucoStabilizer [Medical Decision Network, Charlottesville, Virginia], and GlucoTab [Joanneum Research, Graz, Austria, and Medical University of Graz, Graz, Austria]).[83] These devices may be especially useful in hospitals with no diabetes management teams or diabetes experts on staff; however, some come at a considerable financial cost to institutions. **Table 2** shows an example of the authors' paper-based IV insulin infusion and hypoglycemia protocol. This protocol was specifically developed to be used in cardiac surgery ICU patients in the authors' hospitals.

It has been shown that glucose targets are usually achieved with most protocols within approximately 4 hours.[84] The onset of regular insulin after IV administration is within 15 minutes to 30 minutes, with a half-life of approximately 9 minutes and duration of action between 30 minutes and 60 minutes. These features allow a rapid up-titration or down-titration of insulin rate in anticipated (ie, rapid decline of blood glucose and use of vasopressors) or unanticipated (ie, acute clinical status deteriorations and hypoglycemia) situations.[60,81,82] Insulin infusion requirements are usually higher during the first few hours of infusion in patients with severe hyperglycemia. Postoperative stress, pain, presence of infection or administration of pressors are factors that have an impact on on insulin requirements.[82] Thus, it is recommended to monitor glucose values every 1 hours to 2 hours and to adjust insulin infusion rates accordingly.[85] Insulin infusion should be continued until clinical and hemodynamic stability has been achieved, until patients are tolerating oral intake or receiving nutritional support, and after several hours of stable glycemic control.

Management of Hyperglycemia in Non-intensive Care Unit Settings

Subcutaneous insulin is the preferred therapeutic agent for glucose control in cardiac surgery patients after stopping CII or after transition to non-ICU areas. Transition to subcutaneous insulin should be considered in hemodynamically stable patients who are off pressors and are tolerating oral intake.[82] Use of protocols for insulin transition leads to better glucose control than nonprotocol therapy, with lower rates of complications and hypoglycemia. A protocol-based transition to a subcutaneous regimen, using basal insulin early after initiation of CII, has also been shown to decrease rebound hyperglycemia after infusion discontinuation.[86]

The basal-bolus (or basal-prandial) insulin regimen is considered the physiologic approach because it addresses the 3 components of insulin requirement: basal (required in the fasting state), nutritional (required for peripheral glucose disposal following a meal), and supplemental (required for unexpected glucose elevations or for disposal of glucose in hyperglycemia).[37,39,60] In insulin-naïve patients, the calculation of basal and bolus insulin dosing requirements should be based on a patient's previous rate of IV insulin infusion and carbohydrate intake.[82,85] Due to the short IV insulin half-life, administration of the initial subcutaneous basal dose is recommended at least 2 hours to 4 hours before stopping the insulin infusion to prevent rebound hyperglycemia.

Most nondiabetic patients with stress hyperglycemia requiring less than 1 U/h to 2 U/h frequently do not require transition to scheduled subcutaneous basal-bolus therapy but rather just correctional insulin scale. Those requiring insulin infusion at a rate of greater than 2 U/h can be started to at 50% of the calculated 24-hour insulin requirements. Most patients with a history of diabetes, however, require transition to subcutaneous insulin therapy. Patients with type 2 diabetes mellitus can be started at 80% of the calculated daily IV insulin requirements.[87-89] The total insulin dose is given 50% as basal and 50% as bolus (prandial) insulin.[82,85,90-92]

Several randomized controlled trials using subcutaneous basal or basal-bolus insulin regimens have been shown successful and are preferred over the use of

Table 1
Studies of intensive glycemic control in cardiac surgery populations

Study	Patients	Population	Target Blood Glucose (mg/dL)	Clinical Outcomes
Furnary et al,[76] 1999	N = 2467 I: 1499 (CII) C: 968 (subcutaneous)	DM Cardiac surgery 85% CABG	I: 150–200 C: >200	65% reduction in risk of deep sternal wound infections
Van den Berghe et al,[72] 2001	N = 1548 I: 544 C: 557	DM and no-DM 62% cardiac surgery 57% CABG 13% DM	I: 80–110 C: 180–200	32% reduction in adjusted mortality risk
Furnary et al,[73] 2003	N = 3554 I: 2612 C: 942	DM CABG	Variable: <200 before 1991, 150–200 between 1991–1998, 125–175 between 1999 and 2001 and between 100 and 150 after 2001	50% reduction in adjusted mortality risk
Lazar et al,[66] 2004	N = 141 I: 72 C: 69	DM CABG	I: 125–200 C: <250	60% reduction in postoperative atrial fibrillation
Ingels et al,[77] 2006	N = 970 C: 477 I: 493	DM and no-DM Cardiac surgery <20% DM	I: <110 C: <220	41% reduction in unadjusted mortality risk at 2 y and 22% at 3 y No significant (12.7%) reduction at 4 y
Li et al,[78] 2006	N = 93 C: 42 I: 51	DM CABG	I: 150–200 C: 150–200	No differences in mortality, wound infections, or ICU LOS
Gandhi et al,[62] 2007	N = 371 C: 185 I: 186	DM and no-DM, Cardiac surgery Approximately 20% DM	I: 80–100 C: <200	No significant differences in mortality or morbidity

Study	N	Population	BG	Findings
Chan et al,[75] 2009	N = 99 C: 55 I: 54	DM and no-DM, Cardiac surgery Approximately 30% DM Approximately 34% CABG	I: 80–130 C: 160–200	No differences in 30-d mortality
Lazar et al,[65] 2011	N = 82 C: 42 I: 40	DM CABG	I: 90–120 C: 120–180	No differences in 30-d mortality, myocardial infarction, stroke, infection, atrial fibrillation, ventilator time, ICU LOS
Desai et al,[64] 2012	N = 189 C: 82 I: 107	DM and no-DM CABG Approximately 41%–45% DM	I: 90–120 C: 121–180	No differences in deep sternal wound infections, pneumonia, renal failure, or mortality
Pezzella et al,[67] 2014	N = 189 C: 98 I: 91	DM and no-DM CABG Approximately 41%–45% DM	I: 90–120 C: 121–180	No differences in perioperative complications No differences in mortality at 40 mo of follow-up
Blaha et al,[68] 2015	N = 2383 C: 1134 I: 1249	DM and no-DM, Cardiac surgery Approximately 70% CABG Approximately 23%–27% DM	I: 80–110 C: 80–150	37% reduction in risk of postoperative complications in no-DM No differences in complications in DM
Umpierrez et al,[14] 2015	N = 338 C: 151 I: 151	DM and no-DM CABG 50% DM	I: 100–140 C: 141–180	62% reduction in risk of postoperative complications in no-DM No difference in complications in DM

Abbreviations: BG, blood glucose; C, control/conventional treatment group; DM, diabetes mellitus; I, intervention/intensive treatment group; LOS, length of stay; N, number of patients; no-DM, no history of DM.

Table 2
Emory healthcare protocol for intravenous insulin infusion in critically ill patients undergoing cardiothoracic surgery with hyperglycemia

Initiating the insulin drip

History of diabetes or HbA$_{1c}$ >6.5%: begin insulin drip with first BG >180 mg/dL

No history of diabetes and HbA$_{1c}$ <6.5%: begin if BG >180 mg/dL × 2 consecutive occasions

Calculating initial IV insulin infusion rate

BG/100 = U/h (round to the nearest 0.1; U/h = mL/h)

Target range: 110–140 mg/dL

Adjusting the insulin drip

Blood glucose (mg/dL)	Any increase in blood glucose from prior blood glucose	Blood glucose decrease less than 30 mg/dL from prior blood glucose	Blood glucose decrease greater than 30 mg/dL from prior blood glucose
>241	Increase rate by 3 U/h	Increase rate by 3 U/h	No change
211–240	Increase rate by 2 U/h	Increase rate by 2 U/h	No change
181–210	Increase rate by 1 U/h	Increase rate by 1 U/h	No change
141–180	Increase rate by 0.5 U/h	Increase rate by 0.5 U/h	No change
110–140	No change	No change	No change
91–109	Decrease rate by 50%	No change	Decrease rate by 50%
71–90	1. HOLD insulin drip 2. Check BG every 30 min, when BG >90 mg/dL, check BG every hour 3. Restart infusion rate at 50% of prior insulin rate when BG >140 mg/dL		
70 or less	1. HOLD insulin drip and ADMINISTER IV dextrose 50% as follows: 2. If BG 41–70 mg/dL: give half ampule of dextrose 50% IV or 235 mL of juice PO 3. If BG ≤40 mg/dL: give 1 ampule of dextrose 50% IV 4. Repeat BG every 15 min until BG >70 mg/dL, then every 30 min until BG >90. When BG >90 mg/dL, check BG every 1 h 5. Restart infusion at half of prior infusion rate when BG >140 mg/dL		

sliding-scale insulin alone in hospitalized patients with type 2 diabetes mellitus.[93–95] Basal insulin analogs, such as glargine and detemir, are generally preferred over NPH insulin or premixed insulin, because the latter has been associated with lower glycemic variability and less severe hypoglycemia.[96,97] Recently, a study comparing the 2 most commonly used basal insulins, glargine and detemir, in the management of inpatient hyperglycemia and diabetes reported similar efficacy in glycemic control and hypoglycemia rates between these 2 insulin formulations.[98] Renal dysfunction, a common complication in hospitalized patients, increases the risk of insulin and non–insulin-related hypoglycemia.[99] Baldwin and colleagues[100] studied 2 basal-bolus (glargine-glulisine) insulin-dosing regimens in hospitalized patients with diabetes and chronic kidney disease (estimated glomerular filtration rate <45 mL/min). The investigators found that a weight-based insulin regimen of 0.25 U/kg/d was associated with 50% less hypoglycemia (15.8% vs 30%, $P = .08$) compared with a traditional approach of a total daily dose of 0.5 U/kg. In patients with reduced oral intake, the administration of a single dose of basal once-daily dose plus correctional premeal doses of rapid-acting insulin per sliding scale (basal-plus approach) may be an alternative to basal-bolus regimen.[101]

GLUCOSE MONITORING DURING THE PERIOPERATIVE PERIOD

All patients with a diagnosis of diabetes and those with newly discovered hyperglycemia should be monitor closely during the perioperative period. The frequency of monitoring and the schedule of the blood glucose checks are dependent on the nutritional intake, patient treatment, and schedule of insulin. Current guidelines recommend glucose monitoring every 1 hour to 2 hours in critically ill patients receiving IV insulin administration.[60] There is some controversy regarding the best method to monitor blood glucose. A recent international consensus meeting recommended against relying solely on the use of capillary blood glucose, given the poor reliability of meters in critically ill patients.[102] In patients with permanent vascular access (arterial and/or venous), samples for glucose monitoring could be easily drawn after standard safety precautions. Arterial catheters may be preferred in patients with shock, severe peripheral edema, and/or on vasopressor therapy.[102] Considering the convenience and wide availability, however, capillary point-of-care testing is the most widely used approach in the hospital setting. When using point-of-care testing, clinicians should account for conditions that might alter the meter accuracy of glucose measurement, such as hemoglobin level, perfusion, and medications. In addition, safety standards should be established for blood glucose monitoring that prohibits the sharing of finger-stick lancing devices, lancets, and needles.[30]

The use of continuous glucose monitoring (CGM) has been proposed as an alternative to capillary glucose testing in the hospital setting.[103–107] CGM provides frequent measurements of glucose levels as well as direction and magnitude of glucose trends facilitating short and long-term therapy adjustments and limiting glycemic excursions. CGM devices can sample glucose intravascularly (venous or arterial blood) or subcutaneously by way of interstitial fluid.[104] CGM devices can be highly invasive (intravascular devices), minimally invasive (subcutaneous), or even noninvasive (transdermal). Sampling and measurement frequencies typically range from 1 minute to 15 minutes, but most commonly are done every 5 minutes. There are currently 5 CGMs approved for use in Europe and 1 CGM system approved by the Food and Drug Administration for use in US hospitals.[104] Although the use of CGM in the ICU population has the potential for improving glucose control from an accuracy standpoint, there are several concerns. Technological limitations that impede accuracy of CGMs include buildup of tissue deposits (biofilm), the need for regular calibration due to sensor drift, measurement lag, and substance interference (acetaminophen, maltose, ascorbic acid, dopamine, mannitol, heparin, uric acid, and salicylic acid). In addition, the intravascular CGM devices carry the risk of thrombus formation, catheter occlusion, and catheter-related infections.[108]

HYPOGLYCEMIA AND OUTCOMES IN PATIENTS HOSPITALIZED WITH CARDIAC CONDITIONS

Hypoglycemia (<70 mg/dL) is the most common adverse event associated with insulin administration[99,109–111] and has been associated with poor clinical outcomes and higher mortality.[74,112] Hypoglycemia is associated with increased risk of arrhythmias, ranging from bradycardia to ventricular ectopic beats and QT prolongation, mostly because of sympathetic and adrenal activation.[113] The relationship between mortality and glycemic control in hospitalized patients with acute cardiovascular disease follows a U-shape curve,[114–116] with a 2-fold increase in mortality in patients with hypoglycemia.[74] In the NICE-SUGAR (The Normoglycemia in Intensive Care Evaluation–Survival Using Glucose Algorithm Regulation) trial, the adjusted hazard ratios for death among patients with moderate (<70 mg/dL) or severe (<40 mg/dL) hypoglycemia, compared with those without hypoglycemia, were 1.41 (95% CI, 1.21–1.62; $P<.001$) and 2.10 (95% CI, 1.59–2.77; $P<.001$), respectively. Several studies have reported that spontaneous hypoglycemia is associated with worse outcomes and higher mortality than iatrogenic hypoglycemia in hospitalized patients,[110,111,114] suggesting that spontaneous hypoglycemia may be a marker of disease severity. Because hypoglycemia may go unrecognized in patients under anesthesia or those who are critically ill,[30] frequent glucose monitoring, conservative glucose targets, excellent perioperative provider communication, and treatment algorithms are needed to reduce the risk of intraoperative and postoperative hypoglycemia.

MANAGEMENT OF DIABETES AFTER HOSPITAL DISCHARGE

The transition of care from inpatient to the outpatient settings has been determined as a national priority in patients with diabetes.[117] The Joint Commission National Patient Safety Goals document includes goals and requirements for hospital discharge planning and transitional care. Hospital discharge represents an opportune time to address glycemic control and to adjust home diabetes therapy if necessary. Few studies, however, have focused on the optimal management of hyperglycemia and diabetes after hospital discharge. Clinical guidelines have recommended that patients with diabetes and hyperglycemia have an HbA_{1c} measured to assess preadmission glycemic control and to tailor treatment regimen at discharge. In a recent randomized control trial, the authors' group validated a discharged patient algorithm based on admission HbA_{1c}, as shown in **Fig. 2**. Patients with acceptable diabetes control ($HbA_{1c} <8\%$) may be discharged on their prehospitalization treatment regimen (oral agents and/or insulin therapy). Patients with suboptimal glucose control and HbA_{1c} between 8% and 10% should have intensification of therapy, either by adding or increasing the dose of oral agents or by adjusting the dose of basal insulin (approximately 50%). Those with HbA_{1c} greater than 10% should be considered candidates for insulin therapy alone (basal-bolus) or in combination to oral agents.[118] When a patient is discharged from the hospital with poorly controlled diabetes or with insulin therapy, a clear strategy for the management of hyperglycemia and hypoglycemia, and a titration of therapy should be communicated to the community diabetes team and/or primary care team.

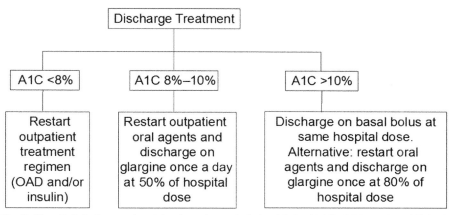

Fig. 2. Hospital discharge algorithm based on admission HbA$_{1c}$ (A1C). OAD, oral antidiabetic drugs. (*Adapted from* Umpierrez GE, Reyes D, Smiley D, et al. Hospital discharge algorithm based on admission HbA1c for the management of patients with type 2 diabetes. Diabetes Care 2014;37(11):2934–9; with permission.)

REFERENCES

1. Federation ID 2015. Available at: http://www.diabetesatlas.org/. Accessed May, 2017.
2. Centers for disease control and prevention. National diabetes statistics report, 2015. Atlanta (GA): Centers for Disease Control and Prevention, US Department of Health and Human Services; 2015.
3. Whang W, Bigger JT Jr. Diabetes and outcomes of coronary artery bypass graft surgery in patients with severe left ventricular dysfunction: results from The CABG Patch Trial database. The CABG Patch Trial Investigators and Coordinators. J Am Coll Cardiol 2000;36(4):1166–72.
4. Szabo Z, Hakanson E, Svedjeholm R. Early postoperative outcome and medium-term survival in 540 diabetic and 2239 nondiabetic patients undergoing coronary artery bypass grafting. Ann Thorac Surg 2002;74(3):712–9.
5. McAlister FA, Man J, Bistritz L, et al. Diabetes and coronary artery bypass surgery: an examination of perioperative glycemic control and outcomes. Diabetes Care 2003;26(5):1518–24.
6. Carvalho G, Moore A, Qizilbash B, et al. Maintenance of normoglycemia during cardiac surgery. Anesth Analg 2004;99(2):319–24.
7. Schmeltz LR, DeSantis AJ, Thiyagarajan V, et al. Reduction of surgical mortality and morbidity in diabetic patients undergoing cardiac surgery with a combined intravenous and subcutaneous insulin glucose management strategy. Diabetes Care 2007;30(4):823–8.
8. Morricone L, Ranucci M, Denti S, et al. Diabetes and complications after cardiac surgery: comparison with a non-diabetic population. Acta Diabetol 1999; 36(1–2):77–84.
9. Thourani VH, Weintraub WS, Stein B, et al. Influence of diabetes mellitus on early and late outcome after coronary artery bypass grafting. Ann Thorac Surg 1999; 67(4):1045–52.
10. Herlitz J, Wognsen GB, Karlson BW, et al. Mortality, mode of death and risk indicators for death during 5 years after coronary artery bypass grafting among

patients with and without a history of diabetes mellitus. Coron Artery Dis 2000; 11(4):339–46.

11. Carson JL, Scholz PM, Chen AY, et al. Diabetes mellitus increases short-term mortality and morbidity in patients undergoing coronary artery bypass graft surgery. J Am Coll Cardiol 2002;40(3):418–23.

12. Bucerius J, Gummert JF, Walther T, et al. Impact of diabetes mellitus on cardiac surgery outcome. Thorac Cardiovasc Surg 2003;51(1):11–6.

13. Weintraub WS, Stein B, Kosinski A, et al. Outcome of coronary bypass surgery versus coronary angioplasty in diabetic patients with multivessel coronary artery disease. J Am Coll Cardiol 1998;31(1):10–9.

14. Umpierrez G, Cardona S, Pasquel F, et al. Randomized controlled trial of intensive versus conservative glucose control in patients undergoing coronary artery bypass graft surgery: GLUCO-CABG trial. Diabetes Care 2015;38(9):1665–72.

15. Krinsley JS, Maurer P, Holewinski S, et al. Glucose control, diabetes status, and mortality in critically ill patients: the continuum from intensive care unit admission to hospital discharge. Mayo Clin Proc 2017;92(7):1019–29.

16. Kotagal M, Symons RG, Hirsch IB, et al. Perioperative hyperglycemia and risk of adverse events among patients with and without diabetes. Ann Surg 2015; 261(1):97–103.

17. Buehler L, Fayfman M, Alexopoulos AS, et al. The impact of hyperglycemia and obesity on hospitalization costs and clinical outcome in general surgery patients. J Diabetes Complications 2015;29(8):1177–82.

18. Kwon S, Thompson R, Dellinger P, et al. Importance of perioperative glycemic control in general surgery: a report from the Surgical Care and Outcomes Assessment Program. Ann Surg 2013;257(1):8–14.

19. Szekely A, Levin J, Miao Y, et al. Impact of hyperglycemia on perioperative mortality after coronary artery bypass graft surgery. J Thorac Cardiovasc Surg 2011; 142(2):430–7.e1.

20. Ascione R, Rogers CA, Rajakaruna C, et al. Inadequate blood glucose control is associated with in-hospital mortality and morbidity in diabetic and nondiabetic patients undergoing cardiac surgery. Circulation 2008;118(2):113–23.

21. Falciglia M, Freyberg RW, Almenoff PL, et al. Hyperglycemia-related mortality in critically ill patients varies with admission diagnosis. Crit Care Med 2009;37(12): 3001–9.

22. Mendez CE, Mok KT, Ata A, et al. Increased glycemic variability is independently associated with length of stay and mortality in noncritically ill hospitalized patients. Diabetes Care 2013;36(12):4091–7.

23. Frisch A, Chandra P, Smiley D, et al. Prevalence and clinical outcome of hyperglycemia in the perioperative period in noncardiac surgery. Diabetes Care 2010; 33(8):1783–8.

24. Umpierrez GE, Isaacs SD, Bazargan N, et al. Hyperglycemia: an independent marker of in-hospital mortality in patients with undiagnosed diabetes. J Clin Endocrinol Metab 2002;87(3):978–82.

25. McDonnell ME, Umpierrez GE. Insulin therapy for the management of hyperglycemia in hospitalized patients. Endocrinol Metab Clin North Am 2012;41(1): 175–201.

26. McCowen KC, Malhotra A, Bistrian BR. Stress-induced hyperglycemia. Crit Care Clin 2001;17(1):107–24.

27. Cook CB, Kongable GL, Potter DJ, et al. Inpatient glucose control: a glycemic survey of 126 U.S. hospitals. J Hosp Med 2009;4(9):E7–14.

28. Swanson CM, Potter DJ, Kongable GL, et al. Update on inpatient glycemic control in hospitals in the United States. Endocr Pract 2011;17(6):853–61.
29. Wexler DJ, Meigs JB, Cagliero E, et al. Prevalence of hyper- and hypoglycemia among inpatients with diabetes: a national survey of 44 U.S. hospitals. Diabetes Care 2007;30(2):367–9.
30. Duggan EW, Carlson K, Umpierrez GE. Perioperative hyperglycemia management: an update. Anesthesiology 2017;126(3):547–60.
31. Dungan KM, Braithwaite SS, Preiser JC. Stress hyperglycaemia. Lancet 2009; 373(9677):1798–807.
32. Greci LS, Kailasam M, Malkani S, et al. Utility of HbA(1c) levels for diabetes case finding in hospitalized patients with hyperglycemia. Diabetes Care 2003;26(4): 1064–8.
33. Wexler DJ, Nathan DM, Grant RW, et al. Prevalence of elevated hemoglobin A1c among patients admitted to the hospital without a diagnosis of diabetes. J Clin Endocrinol Metab 2008;93(11):4238–44.
34. Clement S, Braithwaite SS, Magee MF, et al. Management of diabetes and hyperglycemia in hospitals. Diabetes Care 2004;27(2):553–91.
35. Farrokhi F, Smiley D, Umpierrez GE. Glycemic control in non-diabetic critically ill patients. Best Pract Res Clin Endocrinol Metab 2011;25(5):813–24.
36. Mazurek JA, Hailpern SM, Goring T, et al. Prevalence of hemoglobin A1c greater than 6.5% and 7.0% among hospitalized patients without known diagnosis of diabetes at an urban inner city hospital. J Clin Endocrinol Metab 2010;95(3): 1344–8.
37. Umpierrez GE, Hellman R, Korytkowski MT, et al. Management of hyperglycemia in hospitalized patients in non-critical care setting: an endocrine society clinical practice guideline. J Clin Endocrinol Metab 2012;97(1):16–38.
38. American Diabetes Association. 14. Diabetes care in the hospital. Diabetes Care 2017;40(Suppl 1):S120–7.
39. Moghissi ES, Korytkowski MT, DiNardo M, et al. American Association of Clinical Endocrinologists and American Diabetes Association consensus statement on inpatient glycemic control. Diabetes Care 2009;32(6):1119–31.
40. Lansang MC, Umpierrez GE. Inpatient hyperglycemia management: A practical review for primary medical and surgical teams. Cleve Clin J Med 2016;83(5 Suppl 1):S34–43.
41. Edgerton DS, Ramnanan CJ, Grueter CA, et al. Effects of insulin on the metabolic control of hepatic gluconeogenesis in vivo. Diabetes 2009;58(12): 2766–75.
42. Boden G. Gluconeogenesis and glycogenolysis in health and diabetes. J Investig Med 2004;52(6):375–8.
43. Barth E, Albuszies G, Baumgart K, et al. Glucose metabolism and catecholamines. Crit Care Med 2007;35(9 Suppl):S508–18.
44. Riad M, Mogos M, Thangathurai D, et al. Steroids. Curr Opin Crit Care 2002; 8(4):281–4.
45. Stentz FB, Umpierrez GE, Cuervo R, et al. Proinflammatory cytokines, markers of cardiovascular risks, oxidative stress, and lipid peroxidation in patients with hyperglycemic crises. Diabetes 2004;53(8):2079–86.
46. Ferrannini E. The stunned beta cell: a brief history. Cell Metab 2010;11(5): 349–52.
47. Esposito K, Nappo F, Marfella R, et al. Inflammatory cytokine concentrations are acutely increased by hyperglycemia in humans: role of oxidative stress. Circulation 2002;106(16):2067–72.

48. Valko M, Leibfritz D, Moncol J, et al. Free radicals and antioxidants in normal physiological functions and human disease. Int J Biochem Cell Biol 2007; 39(1):44–84.

49. Duchen MR. Roles of mitochondria in health and disease. Diabetes 2004; 53(Suppl 1):S96–102.

50. Montori VM, Bistrian BR, McMahon MM. Hyperglycemia in acutely ill patients. JAMA 2002;288(17):2167–9.

51. Pandolfi A, Giaccari A, Cilli C, et al. Acute hyperglycemia and acute hyperinsulinemia decrease plasma fibrinolytic activity and increase plasminogen activator inhibitor type 1 in the rat. Acta Diabetol 2001;38(2):71–6.

52. Gresele P, Guglielmini G, De Angelis M, et al. Acute, short-term hyperglycemia enhances shear stress-induced platelet activation in patients with type II diabetes mellitus. J Am Coll Cardiol 2003;41(6):1013–20.

53. Tripathy D, Mohanty P, Dhindsa S, et al. Elevation of free fatty acids induces inflammation and impairs vascular reactivity in healthy subjects. Diabetes 2003;52(12):2882–7.

54. Dandona P. Endothelium, inflammation, and diabetes. Curr Diab Rep 2002;2(4): 311–5.

55. Chaudhuri A, Umpierrez GE. Oxidative stress and inflammation in hyperglycemic crises and resolution with insulin: implications for the acute and chronic complications of hyperglycemia. J Diabetes Complications 2012;26(4):257–8.

56. Dandona P, Mohanty P, Chaudhuri A, et al. Insulin infusion in acute illness. J Clin Invest 2005;115(8):2069–72.

57. Mohanty P, Hamouda W, Garg R, et al. Glucose challenge stimulates reactive oxygen species (ROS) generation by leucocytes. J Clin Endocrinol Metab 2000;85(8):2970–3.

58. Aljada A, Ghanim H, Mohanty P, et al. Insulin inhibits the pro-inflammatory transcription factor early growth response gene-1 (Egr)-1 expression in mononuclear cells (MNC) and reduces plasma tissue factor (TF) and plasminogen activator inhibitor-1 (PAI-1) concentrations. J Clin Endocrinol Metab 2002; 87(3):1419–22.

59. Deedwania P, Kosiborod M, Barrett E, et al. Hyperglycemia and acute coronary syndrome: a scientific statement from the American Heart Association Diabetes Committee of the Council on nutrition, physical activity, and metabolism. Anesthesiology 2008;109(1):14–24.

60. Jacobi J, Bircher N, Krinsley J, et al. Guidelines for the use of an insulin infusion for the management of hyperglycemia in critically ill patients. Crit Care Med 2012;40(12):3251–76.

61. Gandhi GY, Nuttall GA, Abel MD, et al. Intraoperative hyperglycemia and perioperative outcomes in cardiac surgery patients. Mayo Clin Proc 2005;80(7): 862–6.

62. Gandhi GY, Nuttall GA, Abel MD, et al. Intensive intraoperative insulin therapy versus conventional glucose management during cardiac surgery: a randomized trial. Ann Intern Med 2007;146(4):233–43.

63. Hua J, Chen G, Li H, et al. Intensive intraoperative insulin therapy versus conventional insulin therapy during cardiac surgery: a meta-analysis. J Cardiothorac Vasc Anesth 2012;26(5):829–34.

64. Desai SP, Henry LL, Holmes SD, et al. Strict versus liberal target range for perioperative glucose in patients undergoing coronary artery bypass grafting: a prospective randomized controlled trial. J Thorac Cardiovasc Surg 2012; 143(2):318–25.

65. Lazar HL, McDonnell MM, Chipkin S, et al. Effects of aggressive versus moderate glycemic control on clinical outcomes in diabetic coronary artery bypass graft patients. Ann Surg 2011;254(3):458–63 [discussion: 63–4].
66. Lazar HL, Chipkin SR, Fitzgerald CA, et al. Tight glycemic control in diabetic coronary artery bypass graft patients improves perioperative outcomes and decreases recurrent ischemic events. Circulation 2004;109(12):1497–502.
67. Pezzella AT, Holmes SD, Pritchard G, et al. Impact of perioperative glycemic control strategy on patient survival after coronary bypass surgery. Ann Thorac Surg 2014;98(4):1281–5.
68. Blaha J, Mraz M, Kopecky P, et al. Perioperative tight glucose control reduces postoperative adverse events in nondiabetic cardiac surgery patients. J Clin Endocrinol Metab 2015;100(8):3081–9.
69. Van den Berghe G, Wouters PJ, Bouillon R, et al. Outcome benefit of intensive insulin therapy in the critically ill: Insulin dose versus glycemic control. Crit Care Med 2003;31(2):359–66.
70. Schnipper JL, Magee M, Larsen K, et al. Society of Hospital Medicine Glycemic Control Task Force summary: practical recommendations for assessing the impact of glycemic control efforts. J Hosp Med 2008;3(5 Suppl):66–75.
71. Seley JJ, D'Hondt N, Longo R, et al. Position statement: inpatient glycemic control. Diabetes Educ 2009;35(Suppl 3):65–9.
72. Van den Berghe G, Wouters P, Weekers F, et al. Intensive insulin therapy in critically ill patients. N Engl J Med 2001;345(19):1359–67.
73. Furnary AP, Gao G, Grunkemeier GL, et al. Continuous insulin infusion reduces mortality in patients with diabetes undergoing coronary artery bypass grafting. J Thorac Cardiovasc Surg 2003;125(5):1007–21.
74. Finfer S, Liu B, Chittock DR, et al. Hypoglycemia and risk of death in critically ill patients. N Engl J Med 2012;367(12):1108–18.
75. Chan RP, Galas FR, Hajjar LA, et al. Intensive perioperative glucose control does not improve outcomes of patients submitted to open-heart surgery: a randomized controlled trial. Clinics (Sao Paulo) 2009;64(1):51–60.
76. Furnary AP, Zerr KJ, Grunkemeier GL, et al. Continuous intravenous insulin infusion reduces the incidence of deep sternal wound infection in diabetic patients after cardiac surgical procedures. Ann Thorac Surg 1999;67(2):352–60 [discussion: 60–2].
77. Ingels C, Debaveye Y, Milants I, et al. Strict blood glucose control with insulin during intensive care after cardiac surgery: impact on 4-years survival, dependency on medical care, and quality-of-life. Eur Heart J 2006;27(22):2716–24.
78. Li JY, Sun S, Wu SJ. Continuous insulin infusion improves postoperative glucose control in patients with diabetes mellitus undergoing coronary artery bypass surgery. Tex Heart Inst J 2006;33(4):445–51.
79. Task Force on the management of ST-segment elevation acute myocardial infarction of the European Society of Cardiology (ESC), Steg PG, James SK, Atar D, et al. ESC Guidelines for the management of acute myocardial infarction in patients presenting with ST-segment elevation. Eur Heart J 2012;33(20):2569–619.
80. Davidson PC, Steed RD, Bode BW. Glucommander: a computer-directed intravenous insulin system shown to be safe, simple, and effective in 120,618 h of operation. Diabetes Care 2005;28(10):2418–23.
81. Goldberg PA, Siegel MD, Sherwin RS, et al. Implementation of a safe and effective insulin infusion protocol in a medical intensive care unit. Diabetes Care 2004;27(2):461–7.

82. Kreider KE, Lien LF. Transitioning safely from intravenous to subcutaneous insulin. Curr Diab Rep 2015;15(5):23.

83. Gianchandani R, Umpierrez GE. Inpatient use of computer-guided insulin devices moving into the non-intensive care unit setting. Diabetes Technol Ther 2015;17(10):673–5.

84. Newton CA, Smiley D, Bode BW, et al. A comparison study of continuous insulin infusion protocols in the medical intensive care unit: computer-guided vs. standard column-based algorithms. J Hosp Med 2010;5(8):432–7.

85. Dungan K, Hall C, Schuster D, et al. Comparison of 3 algorithms for Basal insulin in transitioning from intravenous to subcutaneous insulin in stable patients after cardiothoracic surgery. Endocr Pract 2011;17(5):753–8.

86. Hsia E, Seggelke S, Gibbs J, et al. Subcutaneous administration of glargine to diabetic patients receiving insulin infusion prevents rebound hyperglycemia. J Clin Endocrinol Metab 2012;97(9):3132–7.

87. Ramos P, Childers D, Maynard G, et al. Maintaining glycemic control when transitioning from infusion insulin: a protocol-driven, multidisciplinary approach. J Hosp Med 2010;5(8):446–51.

88. Schmeltz LR, DeSantis AJ, Schmidt K, et al. Conversion of intravenous insulin infusions to subcutaneously administered insulin glargine in patients with hyperglycemia. Endocr Pract 2006;12(6):641–50.

89. O'Malley CW, Emanuele M, Halasyamani L, et al. Bridge over troubled waters: safe and effective transitions of the inpatient with hyperglycemia. J Hosp Med 2008;3(5 Suppl):55–65.

90. Dungan K, Hall C, Schuster D, et al. Differential response between diabetes and stress-induced hyperglycaemia to algorithmic use of detemir and flexible mealtime aspart among stable postcardiac surgery patients requiring intravenous insulin. Diabetes Obes Metab 2011;13(12):1130–5.

91. Olansky L, Sam S, Lober C, et al. Cleveland Clinic cardiovascular intensive care unit insulin conversion protocol. J Diabetes Sci Technol 2009;3(3):478–86.

92. DeSantis AJ, Schmeltz LR, Schmidt K, et al. Inpatient management of hyperglycemia: the Northwestern experience. Endocr Pract 2006;12(5):491–505.

93. Umpierrez GE, Smiley D, Zisman A, et al. Randomized study of basal-bolus insulin therapy in the inpatient management of patients with type 2 diabetes (RABBIT 2 trial). Diabetes Care 2007;30(9):2181–6.

94. Umpierrez GE, Smiley D, Jacobs S, et al. Randomized study of basal-bolus insulin therapy in the inpatient management of patients with type 2 diabetes undergoing general surgery (RABBIT 2 surgery). Diabetes Care 2011;34(2):256–61.

95. Umpierrez GE, Hor T, Smiley D, et al. Comparison of inpatient insulin regimens with detemir plus aspart versus neutral protamine hagedorn plus regular in medical patients with type 2 diabetes. J Clin Endocrinol Metab 2009;94(2):564–9.

96. Bueno E, Benitez A, Rufinelli JV, et al. Basal-bolus regimen with insulin analogues versus human insulin in medical patients with type 2 diabetes: a randomized controlled trial in Latin America. Endocr Pract 2015;21(7):807–13.

97. Bellido V, Suarez L, Rodriguez MG, et al. Comparison of basal-bolus and premixed insulin regimens in hospitalized patients with type 2 diabetes. Diabetes Care 2015;38(12):2211–6.

98. Galindo RJ, Davis GM, Fayfman M, et al. Comparison of efficacy and safety of glargine and detemir insulin in the management of inpatient hyperglycemia and diabetes. Endocr Pract 2017;23(9):1059–66.

99. Farrokhi F, Klindukhova O, Chandra P, et al. Risk factors for inpatient hypoglycemia during subcutaneous insulin therapy in non-critically ill patients with type 2 diabetes. J Diabetes Sci Technol 2012;6(5):1022–9.

100. Baldwin D, Zander J, Munoz C, et al. A randomized trial of two weight-based doses of insulin glargine and glulisine in hospitalized subjects with type 2 diabetes and renal insufficiency. Diabetes Care 2012;35(10):1970–4.

101. Umpierrez GE, Smiley D, Hermayer K, et al. Randomized study comparing a Basal-bolus with a basal plus correction insulin regimen for the hospital management of medical and surgical patients with type 2 diabetes: basal plus trial. Diabetes Care 2013;36(8):2169–74.

102. Finfer S, Wernerman J, Preiser JC, et al. Clinical review: consensus recommendations on measurement of blood glucose and reporting glycemic control in critically ill adults. Crit Care 2013;17(3):229.

103. Kosiborod M, Gottlieb RK, Sekella JA, et al. Performance of the Medtronic Sentrino continuous glucose management (CGM) system in the cardiac intensive care unit. BMJ Open Diabetes Res Care 2014;2(1):e000037.

104. Wallia A, Umpierrez GE, Nasraway SA, et al. Round table discussion on inpatient use of continuous glucose monitoring at the International Hospital Diabetes Meeting. J Diabetes Sci Technol 2016;10(5):1174–81.

105. Brunner R, Kitzberger R, Miehsler W, et al. Accuracy and reliability of a subcutaneous continuous glucose-monitoring system in critically ill patients. Crit Care Med 2011;39(4):659–64.

106. Thabit H, Hovorka R. Glucose control in non-critically ill inpatients with diabetes: towards closed-loop. Diabetes Obes Metab 2014;16(6):500–9.

107. Gomez AM, Umpierrez GE, Munoz OM, et al. Continuous glucose monitoring versus capillary point-of-care testing for inpatient glycemic control in type 2 diabetes patients hospitalized in the general ward and treated with a basal bolus insulin regimen. J Diabetes Sci Technol 2015;10(2):325–9.

108. Klonoff DC, Buckingham B, Christiansen JS, et al. Continuous glucose monitoring: an Endocrine Society Clinical Practice Guideline. J Clin Endocrinol Metab 2011;96(10):2968–79.

109. Akirov A, Grossman A, Shochat T, et al. Mortality among hospitalized patients with hypoglycemia: insulin-related and non-insulin related. J Clin Endocrinol Metab 2017;102(2):416–24.

110. Boucai L, Southern WN, Zonszein J. Hypoglycemia-associated mortality is not drug-associated but linked to comorbidities. Am J Med 2011;124(11):1028–35.

111. Garg R, Hurwitz S, Turchin A, et al. Hypoglycemia, with or without insulin therapy, is associated with increased mortality among hospitalized patients. Diabetes Care 2013;36(5):1107–10.

112. Investigators N-SS, Finfer S, Chittock DR, et al. Intensive versus conventional glucose control in critically ill patients. N Engl J Med 2009;360(13):1283–97.

113. Chow E, Bernjak A, Williams S, et al. Risk of cardiac arrhythmias during hypoglycemia in patients with type 2 diabetes and cardiovascular risk. Diabetes 2014;63(5):1738–47.

114. Kosiborod M, Inzucchi SE, Goyal A, et al. Relationship between spontaneous and iatrogenic hypoglycemia and mortality in patients hospitalized with acute myocardial infarction. JAMA 2009;301(15):1556–64.

115. Pinto DS, Skolnick AH, Kirtane AJ, et al. U-shaped relationship of blood glucose with adverse outcomes among patients with ST-segment elevation myocardial infarction. J Am Coll Cardiol 2005;46(1):178–80.

116. Svensson AM, McGuire DK, Abrahamsson P, et al. Association between hyper- and hypoglycaemia and 2 year all-cause mortality risk in diabetic patients with acute coronary events. Eur Heart J 2005;26(13):1255–61.
117. JCAHO. Available at: http://www.jointcommission.org/standards_information/npsgs.aspx. Accessed May, 2017.
118. Umpierrez GE, Reyes D, Smiley D, et al. Hospital discharge algorithm based on admission HbA1c for the management of patients with type 2 diabetes. Diabetes Care 2014;37(11):2934–9.

Antiplatelet Therapy in Diabetes

Arjun Majithia, MD[a], Deepak L. Bhatt, MD, MPH[b],*

KEYWORDS

- Cardiovascular disease • Diabetes • Antiplatelet therapy • Thrombosis
- Antithrombotic therapy

KEY POINTS

- Patients with diabetes mellitus (DM) are higher risk for atherothrombotic events than patients without DM, in part due to increased platelet reactivity.
- Aspirin is effective for secondary prevention of cardiovascular events in DM.
- The role of aspirin for primary prevention in DM is uncertain.
- There is no role for dual antiplatelet therapy in DM patients without a history of cardiovascular disease.
- Using more potent antiplatelet therapy in DM patients with a history of myocardial infarction or acute coronary syndrome provides similar or greater risk reduction for ischemic events than in non-DM patients.

INTRODUCTION

Cardiovascular disease (CVD) is a significant cause of morbidity and mortality among patients with diabetes mellitus (DM). Common cardiovascular comorbidities include coronary artery disease (CAD), stroke, and peripheral artery disease (PAD). The presence of DM alone is predictive of the risk of future cardiovascular events. Some older studies have suggested that patients with DM without a history of CAD have a future risk similar to non-DM patients with a history of myocardial infarction (MI).[1] In 2010, among those aged 20 years or older with DM, hospitalization for MI and stroke were 1.8 and 1.5 times higher, respectively, compared with those without DM. Among

Disclosures: D.L. Bhatt has received research funding from Amarin, Amgen, AstraZeneca, Bristol-Myers Squibb, Chiesi, Eisai, Ethicon, Forest Laboratories, Ironwood, Ischemix, Lilly, Medtronic, Pfizer, Roche, Sanofi Aventis, and The Medicines Company. A. Majithia has nothing to disclose.
[a] Division of Cardiovascular Medicine, Lahey Hospital and Medical Center, 41 Burlington Mall Road, Burlington, MA 01805, USA; [b] Division of Cardiovascular Medicine, Brigham and Women's Hospital Heart and Vascular Center and Harvard Medical School, 75 Francis Street, Boston, MA 02115, USA
* Corresponding author.
E-mail address: dlbhattmd@post.harvard.edu

Endocrinol Metab Clin N Am 47 (2018) 223–235
https://doi.org/10.1016/j.ecl.2017.10.009
0889-8529/18/© 2017 Elsevier Inc. All rights reserved.

those with clinical CVD, DM status is also predictive of worse clinical outcomes. In 2003 to 2006, cardiovascular death rates were 1.7 times higher in patients diagnosed with DM that in those without DM.[2] An analysis of the Reduction of Atherothrombosis for Continued Health (REACH) registry of 45,227 patients at high risk of atherothrombosis or with established atherothrombosis suggested that DM was associated with an increased hazard for cardiovascular death, MI, or stroke, as well as an increase in both cardiovascular death and overall mortality.[3,4]

Although the mechanisms for predisposition to atherosclerosis in DM have not been entirely elucidated, the process is thought to be multifactorial and involve metabolic stress from hyperglycemia, increased oxidative stress, endothelial dysfunction, inflammation, and a hypercoagulable state with heightened platelet reactivity.[5] For these reasons, there has been tremendous interest in exploring the role of antiplatelet therapies in DM to reduce the frequency of cardiovascular events.[6]

PLATELET ACTIVATION AND AGGREGATION

Platelet activation and aggregation are integral to both normal hemostasis and pathologic atherothrombosis. Circulating platelets flow in the blood as smooth disks and are normally separated from the subendothelial connective tissue matrix by vascular endothelial cells. Healthy endothelium secretes nitric oxide and prostacyclin, which help keep platelets in an inactive state.[7] On the endothelial cell surface, adenosine diphosphate (ADP), a potent platelet activator, is normally converted to adenosine monophosphate (AMP) through the action of CD39, and AMP is further converted to adenosine through the action of CD79, additionally promoting platelet inactivity.[7]

If there is disruption in the integrity of the vascular endothelium, platelets are exposed to subendothelial collagen and von Willebrand factor. These subendothelial ligands interact with platelet membrane receptors glycoprotein (Gp)VI and GpIb/IX/V to promote platelet adhesion and subsequent activation.[8,9] These interactions induce conformational changes, allowing platelets to spread along collagen fibrils and promote the release of potent stimulants of platelet activation and aggregation, including thromboxane A2 (TXA2) and ADP, into the circulation. Activated platelets cross-link through the interaction of fibrinogen and the GpIIb/IIIa receptor. Platelet activation is further influenced by initiation of the coagulation cascade, which occurs when exposed tissue factor binds circulating factor VIIa, leading to the downstream production of thrombin, a highly potent platelet agonist, and fibrinogen.[8,9]

Antiplatelet therapies prevent thrombosis by disrupting platelet activation and aggregation at various steps along this pathway. Antiplatelet agents may interfere with activation of platelet membrane surface receptors, including the ADP (P2Y12) receptor, the GpIIb/IIIa receptor, and the thrombin (protease activated receptor [PAR]-1) receptor. Depending on the specific agent, this may occur through competitive or noncompetitive inhibition, reversibly or irreversibly, and with variable potency, influenced by drug metabolism pathways. Additional mechanisms for antiplatelet agents include disruption of prostaglandin synthesis and interference with cyclic AMP generation. The ultimate goal is to try to prevent the development of ischemic events (primary prevention of CAD, cerebrovascular disease, and PAD), or to prevent recurrent ischemic events (secondary prevention).

ASPIRIN

During the process of platelet activation, phospholipase A2 is stimulated by an increase in cytosolic calcium and releases arachidonic acid through enzymatic cleavage within the platelet. Through the action of cycloxygenase-1 (COX-1), arachidonic acid is metabolized into TXA2, a potent stimulator of platelet activation. Aspirin irreversibly acetylates and inactivates COX-1, effectively blocking synthesis of TXA2 for the lifetime of the platelet.

The clinical utility of aspirin in primary and secondary prevention of cardiovascular events has been widely explored. The Antithrombotic Trialists' Collaboration (ATT) meta-analysis of randomized trials of antiplatelet therapy in high-risk patients included 287 studies with 212,000 subjects.[10] The study evaluated the efficacy of antiplatelet therapy in reducing serious vascular events (nonfatal MI, nonfatal stroke, or vascular death), among patients with acute or previous MI, stroke, or clinical features that increased their risk for vascular events (including DM). Aspirin was the most widely studied antiplatelet agent, with doses of 75 to 100 mg shown to be at least as effective as higher doses, with doses less than 75 mg of uncertain benefit. Overall, there was a significant reduction in cardiovascular events among subjects treated with antiplatelet therapy (13.2% vs 10.7%; 22% odds reduction, $P<.0001$), with greatest odds reduction among subjects with acute MI. The absolute risk reduction for serious vascular events was 36 per 1000 subjects treated for 2 years. Among subjects with other conditions, including CAD, high embolic risk, and PAD, and high-risk clinical features, including hemodialysis status, carotid disease, and DM, there was a significant reduction in the rate of vascular events with antiplatelet therapy compared with controls (10.2% vs 8.1%; $P<.0001$). Among 9 clinical trials with 4961 subjects with DM, both with and without preexisting cardiac disease, antiplatelet therapy was associated with a 7% odds reduction for serious vascular events, though this finding individually did not meet statistical significance. Overall, the study findings strongly supported aspirin for prevention of cardiovascular events among patients with a previous history of CVD (secondary prevention), and among those with other high-risk clinical conditions, with a nonstatistically significant signal for benefit among patients with DM.

Additional studies have explored the role of aspirin in primary prevention of CVD in DM. A meta-analysis evaluating the efficacy of low-dose aspirin among DM patients without CVD included 6 randomized studies with a total 10,117 subjects and found that aspirin use was not associated with a reduction in major cardiovascular events, cardiovascular mortality, or all-cause mortality.[11] However, when stratified by sex, aspirin reduced the risk of MI in men but not in women. Overall, the study did not demonstrate a clear benefit with aspirin for primary prevention in patients with DM, though sex may have been an important effect modifier. An updated meta-analysis that included 90,000 subjects was similarly unable to demonstrate a statistically significant benefit in total cardiovascular events, nonfatal MI, stroke, and cardiovascular or all-cause mortality with aspirin.[12]

Despite clear evidence supporting the use of aspirin for secondary prevention, the role of aspirin for primary prevention, particularly among patients with DM, remains uncertain. Recent studies have suggested the possibility of aspirin nonresponsiveness in DM may be mediated by reduced bioavailability.[13] Ongoing studies may provide additional insight into the role of aspirin for primary prevention in DM. These studies include the ASCEND (A Study of Cardiovascular Events in Diabetes) trial (NCT00135226), which is evaluating the efficacy of aspirin with or without the addition of omega-3 fatty acid supplementation for prevention of vascular events among DM patients without known occlusive arterial disease. Separately, the ACCEPT-D (Aspirin and Simvastatin Combination for Cardiovascular Events Prevention Trial in Diabetes) trial (CCT ISRCTN48110081) is assessing whether the addition of aspirin to simvastatin reduces cardiovascular events among DM patients without clinically manifest vascular disease.

GLYCOPROTEIN IIb/IIIa INHIBITORS

GpIIb/IIIa inhibitors receptor antagonists (abciximab, tirofiban, eptifibatide) inhibit fibrinogen-mediated platelet cross-linking. Though the clinical role of GpIIb/IIIa inhibitors is more limited in the current era, the rationale for use of GpIIb/IIIa inhibitors, particularly in DM, is to complement percutaneous coronary intervention (PCI) by counteracting the heightened thrombotic state.[14]

Multiple studies evaluated the efficacy of GpIIb/IIIa inhibitors for reduction of ischemic outcomes in DM subjects undergoing PCI. A pooled analysis that included 3 placebo-controlled trials and 1462 subjects sought to determine whether abciximab at the time of PCI would favorably affect 1-year mortality in patients with diabetes.[15] Abciximab use was associated with reduction in mortality from 4.5% to 2.5% ($P = .031$). Among subjects with clinical insulin resistance (DM, hypertension, and obesity), mortality reduction was from 5.1% to 2.3% ($P = .044$). Among non-DM subjects, it was observed that those who received placebo had a 2.6% mortality rate compared with a 1.9% rate with abciximab treatment. Thus, the event rate for DM subjects treated with abciximab was comparable to that of placebo-treated non-DM subjects.

Additional studies have evaluated the interaction of GpIIb/IIIa inhibitors and DM in subjects undergoing PCI for acute coronary syndrome (ACS). In a meta-analysis of 6 large trials including 6458 DM subjects treated with GpIIb/IIIa inhibition for non-ST-segment elevation ACS, treatment was associated with a significant 30-day mortality reduction (6.2% to 4.6%, $P = .007$), not evident in non-DM subjects.[16] The impact on mortality reduction was even greater among DM subjects undergoing PCI.

ADENOSINE DIPHOSPHATE RECEPTOR ANTAGONISTS

The platelet P2Y1 and P2Y12 G-protein coupled receptors bind ADP, which is stored in platelet-dense granules and released at the time of platelet activation.[8,9] The normal interaction of ADP with the G-protein coupled receptors inhibits downstream formation of cyclic AMP, which promotes sustained platelet aggregation.[8,9] In DM, insulin resistance promotes platelet dysfunction. Insulin normally inhibits platelet aggregation by suppressing the P2Y12 pathway.[17] However, loss of responsiveness to insulin leads to upregulation of the P2Y12 pathway and increased platelet reactivity, leading to a prothrombotic state in DM.[17] This is further exaggerated in insulin-dependent DM, and is thought to confer additional risk for atherothrombosis.[17,18] A variety of P2Y12 receptor antagonists are now commonly used in conjunction with aspirin to prevent atherothrombotic events in patients presenting with ACS, as well as among patients who undergo PCI (for stable CAD and ACS). A summary of commonly used ADP receptor antagonists is provided in **Table 1**.

CLOPIDOGREL

Clopidogrel is a thienopyridine, competitive, irreversible, P2Y12 receptor antagonist. Several large clinical studies of subjects across a wide spectrum of atherothrombotic risk inform the understanding of the role of clopidogrel for reduction of cardiovascular events. A summary of pivotal trials of antiplatelet therapies is provided in **Table 2**.

The safety and efficacy of clopidogrel was compared with aspirin for the treatment of patients with ischemic stroke, MI, or established PAD in the Clopidogrel versus Aspirin in Patients at Risk of Ischemic Events (CAPRIE) trial.[19] A total of 19,185 subjects were randomized to treatment with clopidogrel or aspirin, and treatment with clopidogrel resulted in greater reduction in the composite of MI, ischemic stroke, or vascular death (5.32% vs 5.83% annual risk, relative risk [RR] reduction 8.7%, $P = .043$). A substudy of

Table 1
Summary of commonly used adenosine diphosphate receptor blocking agents

	Clopidogrel	Prasugrel	Ticagrelor	Cangrelor
Drug Class	Thienopyridine	Thienopyridine	Triazolopyrimidine	Nonthienopyridine, adenosine triphosphate analogue
Mechanism	Competitive, irreversible, P2Y12 receptor blockade	Competitive, irreversible, P2Y12 receptor blockade	Noncompetitive, reversible, P2Y12 receptor blockade	Noncompetitive, reversible, P2Y12 receptor blockade
Duration of action	5–7 d	7–10 d	3–5 d	60 min
Administration and frequency	Oral, once daily	Oral, once daily	Oral, twice daily	Intravenous
Indications	ACS ± PCI; PCI (elective); Ischemic stroke, MI, or symptomatic PAD	ACS + PCI	ACS ± PCI	PCI (adjunctive)

subjects with coexisting DM suggested that baseline ischemic risk may influence risk reduction with antiplatelet therapy. Subjects without DM treated with clopidogrel experienced a reduction of 9 events per 1000 subjects per year compared with aspirin.[20] Among higher risk, insulin-dependent subjects, a 38 events per 1000 subjects per year reduction was observed versus aspirin. Additionally, subjects with DM treated with clopidogrel experienced a lower rate of bleeding compared with aspirin-treated subjects. These early studies suggested that that clopidogrel is superior to aspirin in reducing ischemic events, with an amplified benefit among patients with DM.

The efficacy of clopidogrel in addition to aspirin for treatment of patients with non-ST-segment elevation ACS was evaluated in the Clopidogrel in Unstable Angina to Prevent Recurrent Events (CURE) trial.[21] The addition of clopidogrel to aspirin decreased ischemic events by approximately 20% during the first 30 days of treatment, with a similar reduction from 30 days to the end of the follow-up period of 12 months, suggesting both an early and late clinical benefit in reduction of ischemic events. Among CURE trial participants with DM, the incremental reduction with addition of clopidogrel to standard therapy was maintained, while the absolute benefit was amplified.

The Clopidogrel for High Atherothrombotic Risk and Ischemic Stabilization, Management, and Avoidance (CHARISMA) study evaluated whether the combination of aspirin and clopidogrel versus aspirin alone would reduce atherothrombotic events in subjects at high risk for atherothrombosis.[22] The study included 15,603 subjects with clinically evident atherosclerotic disease or multiple risk factors (including DM) for development for vascular disease. The composite endpoint of cardiovascular death, MI, or stroke was not significantly different between the 2 arms of the study, though the secondary endpoint was significantly reduced with clopidogrel added to aspirin. A total of 42% of the overall study population had DM, including 83% of asymptomatic subjects. Overall, these findings suggested that among patients with DM, without clinical atherosclerotic CVD, the addition of clopidogrel to aspirin for primary prevention does not confer clinical benefit. In contrast, among all symptomatic

Table 2
Summary of pivotal trials of antiplatelet therapies

Trial, Year	Study Design	Subject Population	Treatment Groups	Endpoints
CAPRIE, 1996	Randomized, double-blind; n = 19,185	Subjects with ischemic stroke, MI, or symptomatic PAD	Clopidogrel vs ASA	CV death, MI, or CVA: 5.3% with clopidogrel vs 5.83% with ASA (RR 0.91, 95% CI 0.3–16.5) Severe bleeding: 1.38% with clopidogrel vs 1.55% with aspirin
CURE, 2003	Randomized, double-blind, placebo-controlled; n = 12,562	Patients with non-ST-segment elevation ACS	ASA + clopidogrel vs ASA + placebo	CV death, MI, or CVA: 9.3% with DAPT vs 11.4% with ASA alone (RR 0.80, 95% CI 0.72–0.90) Major bleeding: 3.7% with DAPT vs 2.7% with ASA alone (RR 1.38, 95% CI 1.13–1.67)
CHARISMA, 2006	Randomized, double-blind, placebo-controlled; n = 15,603	Subjects age 45 y or greater, atherothrombotic risk factors, or documented CAD, CVD, or PAD	ASA + clopidogrel vs ASA + placebo	CV death, MI, or CVA: 6.8% with clopidogrel vs 7.3% with placebo (RR 0.93, 95% CI 0.83–1.05) GUSTO severe bleeding: 1.7% with clopidogrel vs 1.3% with placebo (RR 1.25, 95% CI 0.97–1.61)
TRITON-TIMI 38, 2007	Randomized, double-blind, placebo-controlled; n = 13,608	Subjects with ACS undergoing PCI	ASA + prasugrel vs ASA + clopidogrel	CV death, MI, CVA: 9.9% with prasugrel vs 12.1% with clopidogrel (RR 0.81, 95% CI 0.73–0.90) Major bleeding: 2.4% with prasugrel vs 1.8% with clopidogrel (RR 1.32; CI 1.03–1.68)
PLATO, 2009	Randomized, double-blind, placebo-controlled; n = 18,624	Subjects with ACS and symptoms within 24 h	ASA + ticagrelor vs ASA + clopidogrel	CV death, MI, or CVA: 9.8% with ticagrelor vs 11.7% with clopidogrel (RR 0.84, 95% CI 0.77–0.92) Major bleeding: 11.6% with ticagrelor vs 11.2% with clopidogrel (RR 1.04, 95% CI 0.95–1.13)

Trial	Design	Population	Comparison	Outcomes
TRA-2P TIMI-50, 2012	Randomized, double-blind, placebo-controlled; n = 26,449	Subjects with a history of MI, ischemic stroke, or PAD	Vorapaxar vs placebo	CV death, MI, or stroke: 9.3% with vorapaxar vs 10.5% with placebo (RR 0.87, 95% CI 0.80–0.94); Moderate to severe bleeding: 4.2% with vorapaxar vs 2.5% with placebo (RR 1.66, 95% CI 1.43–1.93)
CHAMPION PHOENIX, 2013	Randomized, double-blind, placebo-controlled; n = 11,145	Patients with atherosclerosis who required PCI for stable angina, non-ST-segment elevation ACS, or ST-segment elevation MI	Cangrelor vs clopidogrel	Death, MI, revascularization, or stent thrombosis: 4.7% with cangrelor vs 5.9% with clopidogrel (OR 0.78, 95% CI 0.66–0.93); GUSTO severe bleeding: 0.16% with cangrelor vs 0.11% with clopidogrel (OR 1.50, 95% CI 0.53–4.22)
PEGASUS-TIMI 54, 2015	Randomized, double-blind, placebo-controlled; n = 21,162	Patients with a history of MI1-3 y before enrollment, age >50 y, and additional CV risk factor	ASA + ticagrelor 90 mg or ASA + ticagrelor 60 mg vs ASA + placebo	CV death, MI, CVA: 7.85% with ticagrelor 90 mg (RR 0.85, 95% CI 0.75–0.96), 7.77% with ticagrelor 60 mg (RR 0.84, 95% CI 0.74–0.95), and 9.04% with placebo; Major bleeding: 2.60% with ticagrelor 90 mg (RR 2.69, 95% CI 1.96–3.70), 2.30% with ticagrelor 60 mg (RR 2.32, 95% CI 1.68–3.21), and 1.06% with placebo

Abbreviations: ASA, aspirin; CAPRIE, Clopidogrel versus Aspirin in Patients at Risk of Ischemic Events; CHAMPION PHOENIX, Cangrelor versus Standard Therapy to Achieve Optimal Management of Platelet Inhibition PHOENIX; CHARISMA, Clopidogrel for High Atherothrombotic Risk and Ischemic Stabilization, Management, and Avoidance; CURE, Clopidogrel in Unstable Angina to Prevent Recurrent Events; CV, cardiovascular; CVA, cerebrovascular accident; DAPT, dual antiplatelet therapy; OR, odds ratio; PEGASUS-TIMI 54, Prevention of Cardiovascular Events in Patients with Prior Heart Attack Using Ticagrelor Compared to Placebo on a Background of Aspirin–Thrombolysis in Myocardial Infarction 54; PLATO, Study of Platelet Inhibition and Patient Outcome; RR, relative risk; TRA-2P TIMI-50, Thrombin Receptor Antagonist in Secondary Prevention of Atherothrombotic Ischemic Events-Thrombolysis in Myocardial Infraction 50; TRITON-TIMI 38, Trial to Assess Improvement in Therapeutic Outcomes by Optimizing Platelet Inhibition with Prasugrel-Thrombolysis in Myocardial Infarction 38.

subjects with clinically evident atherothrombosis, the composite event rate was 6.9% with clopidogrel and 7.9% with placebo (RR 0.88, 95% CI 0.77–0.998, $P = .046$). In a post hoc analysis of 9478 trial participants with a history of MI, stroke, or symptomatic PAD, dual antiplatelet therapy was associated with a reduction in cardiovascular death, MI, or stroke (7.3% vs 8.8%; hazard ratio [HR] 0.83, 95% CI 0.72–0.96, $P = .01$).[23]

Additional studies have assessed the efficacy of clopidogrel in preventing cardiovascular events following MI specifically among subjects with DM. A large observational Danish study examined 58,851 subjects with MI, 7247 of whom had DM, and found that 25% of the subjects with DM versus 15% without DM experienced the composite endpoint of recurrent MI or all-cause mortality at 1 year.[24] Interestingly, among subjects with DM, clopidogrel provided less effective reduction in all-cause mortality (HR 0.89, 95% CI 0.79–1.00 vs HR 0.75, 95% CI 0.70–0.80, $P_{interaction}$ 0.001) and cardiovascular mortality (HR 0.93, 95% CI 0.81–1.06 vs HR 0.77, 95% CI 0.72–0.83, $P_{interaction}$ 0.01). The study particularly highlights the elevated risk of recurrent MI and cardiovascular mortality among patients with DM following MI. At least some portion of this excess risk is likely due to increased platelet reactivity in DM.[24,25]

PRASUGREL

Prasugrel is a competitive, irreversible, thienopyridine ADP (P2Y12) receptor antagonist, approved for treatment of patients with ACS who undergo PCI. Compared with clopidogrel, prasugrel is metabolized more efficiently and provides more reliable, potent antiplatelet activity.[26]

The Trial to Assess Improvement in Therapeutic Outcomes by Optimizing Platelet Inhibition with Prasugrel-Thrombolysis in Myocardial Infarction (TRITON-TIMI 38) study assessed the efficacy of prasugrel versus clopidogrel among 13,608 subjects with unstable angina or MI who were undergoing planned PCI.[27] Prasugrel reduced the composite endpoint of cardiovascular death, MI, or stroke (9.9% vs 12.1%; HR 0.81, 95% CI 0.73–0.90, $P<.001$), driven primarily by reduction in MI. However, this occurred at the expense of increased bleeding, including major and life-threatening bleeding (1.4% vs 0.9%; $P = .01$). Additional subgroup analyses revealed increased rates of the primary outcome and more frequent bleeding (including intracranial bleeding) among those with a history of stroke or transient ischemic attack, and lack of net clinical benefit among subjects with low body weight (less than 60 kg), and age greater than or equal to 75 years. However, the clinical benefit of prasugrel was most apparent among subjects with ST-segment elevation MI and subjects with DM.[28]

In a TRITON-TIMI 38 substudy of subjects with DM, among those treated with prasugrel, the composite endpoint occurred less frequently both in subjects with DM (12.2% vs 17.0%; HR 0.70, $P = .001$, $P_{interaction} = 0.09$) and without DM (9.2% vs 10.6%; HR 0.86, $P = .02$). Among prasugrel-treated subjects, MI was reduced by 18% among subjects without DM (7.2% vs 8.7%; HR 0.82, $P = .006$) and by 40% among subjects with DM (8.2% vs 13.2%; HR 0.60, $P = .001$, $P_{interaction} = 0.02$). Notably, although TIMI major hemorrhage was increased among prasugrel-treated subjects without DM (2.4% vs 1.6%; HR 1.43, $P = .02$), the bleeding rates were similar among subjects with DM for clopidogrel and prasugrel (2.6% vs 2.5%; HR 1.06, $P = .81$, $P_{interaction} = 0.29$). Overall, the net clinical benefit with prasugrel, accounting for both ischemic events and bleeding, was greater among subjects with DM (14.6% vs 19.2%; HR 0.74, $P = .001$) than for subjects without DM (11.5% vs 12.3%; HR 0.92, $P = .16$, $P_{interaction} = 0.05$).

Overall, these studies suggest that patients with DM tend to have a greater reduction in ischemic events with prasugrel compared with clopidogrel, suggesting that the more intensive antiplatelet therapy provided with prasugrel may be of particular benefit in this patient population.

TICAGRELOR

Ticagrelor is a direct, rapidly acting, noncompetitive, reversible triazolopyrimidine ADP receptor (P2Y12) antagonist.[29] Ticagrelor was evaluated against clopidogrel for the treatment of patients with ACS in the Study of Platelet Inhibition and Patient Outcomes (PLATO).[30] A total of 18,624 subjects with ACS were randomly assigned to receive ticagrelor or clopidogrel in addition to aspirin. During the 12-month follow-up period, there was a significant reduction in the composite endpoint of cardiovascular mortality, MI, or stroke with ticagrelor (9.8% vs 11.7%; HR 0.84, 95% CI 0.77–0.92, $P<.001$). Notably, there was a significant reduction in cardiovascular mortality, as well as all-cause mortality with ticagrelor. However, major bleeding unrelated to coronary artery bypass grafting was increased, and there was a trend toward increased intracranial bleeding with ticagrelor. In a substudy of the PLATO trial examining 4662 subjects with preexisting DM, the reduction in the primary composite endpoint, all-cause mortality, and stent thrombosis with ticagrelor was consistent in subjects with DM.[31] Additionally, there was no heterogeneity among subjects with or without ongoing insulin treatment.

The Prevention of Cardiovascular Events in Patients with Prior Heart Attack Using Ticagrelor Compared to Placebo on a Background of Aspirin–Thrombolysis in Myocardial Infarction 54 (PEGASUS-TIMI 54) trial provided an additional opportunity to study the efficacy of long-term dual antiplatelet therapy with aspirin and ticagrelor in patients with a history of MI.[32] A total of 21,162 subjects with a history of MI 1 to 3 years before enrollment were randomized to receive ticagrelor 90 mg twice daily, ticagrelor 60 mg twice daily, or placebo in addition to low-dose aspirin. After 33 months, the composite endpoint of cardiovascular death, MI, or stroke was significantly reduced with ticagrelor. Rates of major bleeding were higher with ticagrelor than placebo in the overall cohort.

In a substudy of the PEGASUS-TIMI 54 study examining 6806 subjects with DM, the relative risk reduction in major adverse cardiovascular events with ticagrelor was consistent in subjects with and without DM.[33] However, the absolute risk reduction tended to be greater in subjects with DM (1.5% vs 1.1%, with a corresponding 3-year number needed to treat of 67 vs 91, respectively), with even greater absolute benefit in subjects with DM requiring pharmacologic therapy (absolute risk reduction 1.9%, number needed to treat of 53 for 3 years). A PEGASUS-TIMI 54 platelet function substudy demonstrated a consistent inhibitory effect with ticagrelor, regardless of DM status.[34] Additionally, patients with DM did not demonstrate an increased incidence of high platelet reactivity, and the pharmacokinetics of ticagrelor was not affected by DM status.

Overall, these studies suggest that patients with DM experience a preserved relative but greater absolute benefit with ticagrelor for treatment of ACS and for, in patients with a history of MI, long-term prevention of ischemic events.

CANGRELOR

Cangrelor is a nonthienopyridine, intravenous, adenosine triphosphate analogue, P2Y12 receptor blocker. Cangrelor provides rapid, potent, and reversible platelet inhibition. Two early trials of cangrelor administered before or after PCI did not demonstrate statistically significant reductions in the composite primary outcome of death, MI, or ischemia-driven revascularization, though there were positive signals when the analysis used more specific definitions of periprocedural MI, with 1 trial showing significant reductions in stent thrombosis and in mortality as well.[35,36] The pivotal Cangrelor versus Standard Therapy to Achieve Optimal Management of Platelet Inhibition (CHAMPION) PHOENIX trial, which randomized 11,145 subjects undergoing urgent or elective PCI to cangrelor or a loading dose of clopidogrel, demonstrated a significant reduction in the composite primary efficacy endpoint of death, MI, ischemia-driven revascularization, or stent thrombosis at 48 hours with cangrelor (4.7% vs 5.9%; odds ratio 0.78, 95% CI 0.66–0.93, $P = .005$).[37] The reduction in ischemic endpoints was consistent across several subgroups, including among subjects with DM. A pooled analysis of subjects-level data from the 3 trials of cangrelor additionally supported this finding and demonstrated that cangrelor was associated with a 19% reduction in the odds for the composite primary outcome of death, MI, ischemia-driven revascularization, or stent thrombosis at 48 hours.[38] The efficacy of cangrelor was again demonstrated to be consistent across several subject subsets, including subjects with DM.

THROMBIN RECEPTOR ANTAGONIST

Vorapaxar is a potent antiplatelet agent that inhibits thrombin-induced platelet activation through competitive inhibition of the PAR-1 receptor. The safety and efficacy of vorapaxar was evaluated in the Thrombin Receptor Antagonist in Secondary Prevention of Atherothrombotic Ischemic Events (TRA 2P)–Thrombolysis in Myocardial Infraction (TIMI) 50 trial, which randomly assigned 26,449 subjects with a history of atherothrombotic events to vorapaxar or placebo.[39] The study was stopped early in the subset of subjects with stroke due to an increased risk of intracranial hemorrhage. At 3 years, there was a reduction in the composite endpoint of cardiovascular death, MI, or stroke with vorapaxar (HR for the vorapaxar group 0.87, 95% CI 0.80–0.94, $P<.001$), primarily driven by reduction in MI. However, this came at the expense of increased moderate or severe bleeding (HR 1.66, 95% CI 1.43–1.93, $P<.001$), and an increase in the rate of intracranial hemorrhage in the vorapaxar group (1.0% vs 0.5% in the placebo group; $P<.001$).

A substudy of the TRA 2P-TIMI 50 trial examined the effect of vorapaxar for secondary prevention of cardiovascular events in DM subjects with previous MI.[40] The composite endpoint of cardiovascular death, MI, or stroke occurred more frequently in subjects with DM than in subjects without DM (14.3% vs 7.6%; adjusted HR 1.47, $P<.001$). However, among DM subjects randomized to vorapaxar, the frequency of the composite endpoint was significantly reduced (11.4% vs 14.3%; HR 0.73, 95% CI 0.60–0.89, $P = .002$) with a number needed to treat of 29, compared with 74 in subjects without DM, with an overall improvement in net clinical outcomes when integrating reduction in ischemic endpoints and bleeding risk.

SUMMARY

Patients with DM are at higher risk for atherothrombotic events than patients without DM. The mechanism for this is in part increased platelet reactivity, which is exacerbated by insulin resistance. For patients with a history of atherothrombosis (secondary prevention), aspirin is beneficial for prevention of cardiovascular events. For patients with diabetes without a history of atherothrombotic events, the benefit of aspirin for primary prevention is unclear. Additional studies may elucidate the role of aspirin in primary prevention among patients with diabetes. The use of more potent single antiplatelet agents, namely clopidogrel, confers greater benefit to patients with DM in the setting of high-risk secondary prevention, and can also be considered in patients who have contraindications or intolerance to aspirin. In patients with DM without a history of atherothrombotic events, there is no role for treatment with dual antiplatelet therapy. In patients with DM presenting with ACS, more potent antiplatelet inhibition with the addition of prasugrel (in those who were treated with PCI), or ticagrelor (instead of clopidogrel), in addition to low-dose aspirin, provides similar or greater risk reduction for future cardiovascular events than in non-DM patients. For patients with DM and a history of MI who remain at high ischemic risk but who are at low bleeding risk, longer term treatment with aspirin plus either clopidogrel or reduced-dose ticagrelor reduces the risk of ischemic events.

REFERENCES

1. Haffner SM, Lehto S, Ronnemaa T, et al. Mortality from coronary heart disease in subjects with type 2 diabetes and in nondiabetic subjects with and without prior myocardial infarction. N Engl J Med 1998;339(4):229–34.

2. Gregg EW, Cheng YJ, Saydah S, et al. Trends in death rates among U.S. adults with and without diabetes between 1997 and 2006: findings from the National Health Interview Survey. Diabetes Care 2012;35(6):1252–7.

3. Bhatt DL, Eagle KA, Ohman EM, et al. Comparative determinants of 4-year cardiovascular event rates in stable outpatients at risk of or with atherothrombosis. JAMA 2010;304(12):1350–7.

4. Cavender MA, Steg PG, Smith SC Jr, et al. Impact of diabetes mellitus on hospitalization for heart failure, cardiovascular events, and death: outcomes at 4 years from the Reduction of Atherothrombosis for Continued Health (REACH) Registry. Circulation 2015;132(10):923–31.

5. Eckel RH. Prevention conference VI: diabetes and cardiovascular disease: writing group II: pathogenesis of atherosclerosis in diabetes. Circulation 2002; 105(18):e138–43.

6. Majithia A, Bhatt DL. Optimal duration of dual antiplatelet therapy after percutaneous coronary intervention. Interv Cardiol Clin 2017;6(1):25–37.

7. Bhatt DL. Intensifying platelet inhibition–navigating between Scylla and Charybdis. N Engl J Med 2007;357(20):2078–81.

8. Gremmel T, Frelinger AL 3rd, Michelson AD. Platelet physiology. Semin Thromb Hemost 2016;42(3):191–204.

9. Jackson SP. The growing complexity of platelet aggregation. Blood 2007;109(12): 5087–95.

10. Antithrombotic Trialists C. Collaborative meta-analysis of randomised trials of antiplatelet therapy for prevention of death, myocardial infarction, and stroke in high risk patients. BMJ 2002;324(7329):71–86.

11. De Berardis G, Sacco M, Strippoli GF, et al. Aspirin for primary prevention of cardiovascular events in people with diabetes: meta-analysis of randomised controlled trials. BMJ 2009;339:b4531.

12. Bartolucci AA, Tendera M, Howard G. Meta-analysis of multiple primary prevention trials of cardiovascular events using aspirin. Am J Cardiol 2011;107(12): 1796–801.

13. Bhatt DL, Grosser T, Dong JF, et al. Enteric coating and aspirin nonresponsiveness in patients with type 2 diabetes mellitus. J Am Coll Cardiol 2017;69(6): 603–12.

14. Lincoff AM. Important triad in cardiovascular medicine: diabetes, coronary intervention, and platelet glycoprotein IIb/IIIa receptor blockade. Circulation 2003; 107(11):1556–9.

15. Bhatt DL, Marso SP, Lincoff AM, et al. Abciximab reduces mortality in diabetics following percutaneous coronary intervention. J Am Coll Cardiol 2000;35(4): 922–8.

16. Roffi M, Chew DP, Mukherjee D, et al. Platelet glycoprotein IIb/IIIa inhibitors reduce mortality in diabetic patients with non-ST-segment-elevation acute coronary syndromes. Circulation 2001;104(23):2767–71.

17. Angiolillo DJ, Bernardo E, Ramirez C, et al. Insulin therapy is associated with platelet dysfunction in patients with type 2 diabetes mellitus on dual oral antiplatelet treatment. J Am Coll Cardiol 2006;48(2):298–304.

18. Angiolillo DJ, Fernandez-Ortiz A, Bernardo E, et al. Influence of aspirin resistance on platelet function profiles in patients on long-term aspirin and clopidogrel after percutaneous coronary intervention. Am J Cardiol 2006;97(1):38–43.

19. CAPRIE Steering Committee. A randomised, blinded, trial of clopidogrel versus aspirin in patients at risk of ischaemic events (CAPRIE). Lancet 1996; 348(9038):1329–39.

20. Bhatt DL, Marso SP, Hirsch AT, et al. Amplified benefit of clopidogrel versus aspirin in patients with diabetes mellitus. Am J Cardiol 2002;90(6):625–8.

21. Yusuf S, Zhao F, Mehta SR, et al. Effects of clopidogrel in addition to aspirin in patients with acute coronary syndromes without ST-segment elevation. N Engl J Med 2001;345(7):494–502.

22. Bhatt DL, Fox KA, Hacke W, et al. Clopidogrel and aspirin versus aspirin alone for the prevention of atherothrombotic events. N Engl J Med 2006;354(16):1706–17.

23. Bhatt DL, Flather MD, Hacke W, et al. Patients with prior myocardial infarction, stroke, or symptomatic peripheral arterial disease in the CHARISMA trial. J Am Coll Cardiol 2007;49(19):1982–8.

24. Andersson C, Lyngbaek S, Nguyen CD, et al. Association of clopidogrel treatment with risk of mortality and cardiovascular events following myocardial infarction in patients with and without diabetes. JAMA 2012;308(9):882–9.

25. Bhatt DL. Antiplatelet therapy following myocardial infarction in patients with diabetes. JAMA 2012;308(9):921–2.

26. Bhatt DL. Prasugrel in clinical practice. N Engl J Med 2009;361(10):940–2.

27. Wiviott SD, Braunwald E, McCabe CH, et al. Prasugrel versus clopidogrel in patients with acute coronary syndromes. N Engl J Med 2007;357(20):2001–15.

28. Wiviott SD, Braunwald E, Angiolillo DJ, et al. Greater clinical benefit of more intensive oral antiplatelet therapy with prasugrel in patients with diabetes mellitus in the trial to assess improvement in therapeutic outcomes by optimizing platelet inhibition with prasugrel-thrombolysis in myocardial infarction 38. Circulation 2008; 118(16):1626–36.

29. Bhatt DL. Antiplatelet therapy: ticagrelor in ACS-what does PLATO teach us? Nat Rev Cardiol 2009;6(12):737–8.

30. Wallentin L, Becker RC, Budaj A, et al. Ticagrelor versus clopidogrel in patients with acute coronary syndromes. N Engl J Med 2009;361(11):1045–57.

31. James S, Angiolillo DJ, Cornel JH, et al. Ticagrelor vs. clopidogrel in patients with acute coronary syndromes and diabetes: a substudy from the PLATelet inhibition and patient Outcomes (PLATO) trial. Eur Heart J 2010;31(24):3006–16.

32. Bonaca MP, Bhatt DL, Cohen M, et al. Long-term use of ticagrelor in patients with prior myocardial infarction. N Engl J Med 2015;372(19):1791–800.

33. Bhatt DL, Bonaca MP, Bansilal S, et al. Reduction in ischemic events with ticagrelor in diabetic patients with prior myocardial infarction in PEGASUS-TIMI 54. J Am Coll Cardiol 2016;67(23):2732–40.
34. Thomas MR, Angiolillo DJ, Bonaca MP, et al. Consistent platelet inhibition with ticagrelor 60 mg twice-daily following myocardial infarction regardless of diabetes status. Thromb Haemost 2017;117(5):940–7.
35. Bhatt DL, Lincoff AM, Gibson CM, et al. Intravenous platelet blockade with cangrelor during PCI. N Engl J Med 2009;361(24):2330–41.
36. Harrington RA, Stone GW, McNulty S, et al. Platelet inhibition with cangrelor in patients undergoing PCI. N Engl J Med 2009;361(24):2318–29.
37. Bhatt DL, Stone GW, Mahaffey KW, et al. Effect of platelet inhibition with cangrelor during PCI on ischemic events. N Engl J Med 2013;368(14):1303–13.
38. Steg PG, Bhatt DL, Hamm CW, et al. Effect of cangrelor on periprocedural outcomes in percutaneous coronary interventions: a pooled analysis of patient-level data. Lancet 2013;382(9909):1981–92.
39. Morrow DA, Braunwald E, Bonaca MP, et al. Vorapaxar in the secondary prevention of atherothrombotic events. N Engl J Med 2012;366(15):1404–13.
40. Cavender MA, Scirica BM, Bonaca MP, et al. Vorapaxar in patients with diabetes mellitus and previous myocardial infarction: findings from the thrombin receptor antagonist in secondary prevention of atherothrombotic ischemic events-TIMI 50 trial. Circulation 2015;131(12):1047–53.

Managing Diabetes and Cardiovascular Risk in Chronic Kidney Disease Patients

 CrossMark

Dragana Lovre, MD[a,b,]*, Sulay Shah, MD[a], Aanu Sihota, MD[a],
Vivian A. Fonseca, MD, FRCP[a,b]

KEYWORDS

- Diabetes mellitus • Chronic kidney disease • Cardiovascular risk factors
- Glycated albumin • Fructosamine • A1C • Dyslipidemia of chronic kidney disease

KEY POINTS

- Treatment of CKD-associated dyslipidemia decreases CVD mortality; statins have a positive effect in mild-moderate CKD; however, statin are less effective in dialysis dependent patients. Addition of Ezetimibe to a statin may be effective in preventing CVD events in patients with CKD.
- Diabetes is the leading cause of CKD; glycemic goals in CKD population are similar to non-CKD patients to prevent microvascular complications, while avoiding hypoglycemia.
- Pharmacologically, the goal in CKD population, should be to focus on treatment that targets multiple risk factors with low risk for side effects.

Disclosure Statement: V.A. Fonseca has served as a paid consultant to Eli Lilly, Takeda, Novo Nordisk, Sanofi- Aventis, Astra- Zeneca, Abbott, Boehringer Ingelheim, and. Tulane University Endocrinology has also received grants and Research Support from Novo- Nordisk, Asahi, Abbott, Sanofi, and Bayer. Dr D. Lovre-has received research grant (to Tulane) from Lexicon. Dr A. Sihota, and Dr S. Shah have nothing to disclose.
Dr V.A. Fonseca is supported in part by the Tullis Tulane Alumni Chair in Diabetes, the Patient Centered Outcomes Research Institute (through Louisiana Clinical Data Research Network [LACDRN]) and grant 1 U54 GM104940 from the National Institute of General Medical Sciences of the National Institutes of Health, which funds the Louisiana Clinical and Translational Science Center. The content is solely the responsibility of the authors and does not necessarily represent the official views of the National Institutes of Health.
Author Contributions: All authors contributed to the literature search and writing of the article. V.F. designed the search strategy, supervised study implementation and reviewed/edited the article.

[a] Section of Endocrinology, Tulane University Health Sciences Center, 1430 Tulane Avenue, #8553, New Orleans, LA 70112, USA; [b] Section of Endocrinology, Southeast Louisiana Veterans Health Care Systems, 2400 Canal Street, New Orleans, LA 70119, USA
* Corresponding author. 1430 Tulane Avenue, #8553, New Orleans, LA 70112.
E-mail address: dlovre@tulane.edu

Endocrinol Metab Clin N Am 47 (2018) 237–257
https://doi.org/10.1016/j.ecl.2017.10.006
0889-8529/18/© 2017 Elsevier Inc. All rights reserved.

INTRODUCTION

Cardiovascular disease (CVD) is a major clinical problem contributing to significant mortality worldwide, especially in populations with chronic kidney disease (CKD) and diabetes.[1,2] According to the US Renal Data System (USRDS) and the adult National Health and Nutrition Examination Survey (NHANES), the prevalence of CVD in patients with CKD is as high as 63% compared with only 5.8% for patients without CKD, and is directly related to the severity of CKD.[3] Because CVD mortality rates are 10 to 30 times higher in patients on dialysis than in the general population,[4] patients with CKD are more likely to die of CVD than reach end-stage renal disease (ESRD).[5–7] USRDS 2016 data showed that 41% of deaths in dialysis patients are due to CVD. A recent systematic review and meta-analysis of global CKD showed mean CKD prevalence of 13.4% for all 5 stages, and 10.6% for stages 3 to 5.[8] According to the World Health Organization, diabetes had an estimated prevalence of 8.5% in 2014, and evidence suggests that CKD may be even more common.[9]

Diabetes mellitus is the leading cause of CKD in the United States, with estimates suggesting that close to 50% of patients with diabetes show evidence of CKD.[10,11] Diabetes is also often difficult to control in the CKD population; several antihyperglycemic agents are contraindicated in patients with CKD, and the pharmacokinetics of others, including insulin, change with declining glomerular filtration rate (GFR).

In this review, we discuss mechanisms of increased CVD in patients with CKD and strategies for managing cardiovascular (CV) risk in patients with CKD. Our focus is mainly on decreasing cardiovascular events (CVEs) and progression of microvascular complications by reducing levels of glucose and lipids. We recognize the importance of blood pressure (BP) control in the management of CKD and prevention of CVD events in this population, but a detailed discussion of blood pressure is beyond the scope of this review. We searched PubMed using the terms "mechanisms of increased CVD in CKD," "CVD and CKD and hyperlipidemia," "CKD and CVD and diabetes," "dyslipidemia and CKD," "ezetimibe and CKD," "statins and CKD/ESRD," "glycemic control and CKD," "glycemic markers," and "glycosylated albumin and fructosamine and CKD" with no limit on the date of the article. All articles were discussed among all authors. We chose pertinent articles, and searched their references in turn for additional relevant publications.

MECHANISMS OF INCREASED CARDIOVASCULAR DISEASE IN CHRONIC KIDNEY DISEASE

The complex relationship between CKD and CVD involves a combination of cardiovascular risk factors, comprising "traditional factors" (eg, advanced age, hypertension, diabetes mellitus, and dyslipidemia) and "nontraditional factors" specific to CKD (eg, anemia, volume overload, mineral metabolism abnormalities, proteinuria, oxidative stress, and inflammation).[12]

An analysis of NHANES data from 2001 to 2010 encompassing (1) the prevalence of CV-related comorbidities and CV risk factors, (2) the utilization of lipid-lowering and BP-lowering agents, and (3) rates of low-density lipoprotein cholesterol (LDL-C) or BP goal attainment in US adults stratified by CKD stage[13] demonstrated that despite a reported increase in lipid and BP treatment, treatment remains suboptimal. Greater efforts are required to improve CVD reduction in the CKD population.[13]

Left Ventricular Dysfunction

The leading cardiac abnormality in patients with CKD and ESRD is left ventricular (LV) dysfunction.[12] One study showed that approximately 74% of patients with ESRD starting dialysis suffer from LV hypertrophy, 32% show LV dilatation, and another

14.8% have systolic dysfunction.[4] A report from the Acute Decompensated Heart Failure National Registry (ADHERE) database on outcomes in 118,465 patients hospitalized with acute decompensated heart failure showed that most have significant renal impairment (27.4% had mild renal dysfunction, 43.5% had moderate renal dysfunction, 13.1% had severe kidney dysfunction, and 7.0% had kidney failure).[14] LV hypertrophy is an adaptive process of the LV in which an increase in cardiac work is induced by an increased afterload (pressure overload), an increased preload (volume overload), or both. Increased afterload may result from arterial hypertension and arterial stiffness, whereas increased preload may be caused by hypervolemia and anemia.[15]

Diabetes Mellitus and Glucose Control

The impact of improved glycemic control in preventing CVD events in patients with diabetes and CKD is controversial. The value of glycemic control in preventing microvascular complications has not been definitively established in advanced CKD, as patients with advanced CKD are often excluded from clinical trials.

In 1 meta-analysis of 7 randomized controlled trials (RCTs) of intensive glycemic control in type 2 diabetes mellitus (T2DM), intensive therapy led to a statistically significant reduction in microalbuminuria and macroalbuminuria; however, data regarding the effect of intensive glycemic control on clinical renal outcomes (doubling of serum creatinine, ESRD, or death from renal disease) were inconclusive.[16] The benefits of intensive glycemic therapy for individuals with diabetes and early-stage CKD have been well established, but there is no consensus on whether intensive therapy slows the progression of established diabetic nephropathy (DN), particularly among individuals who have a reduced GFR.[17,18] In the Action to Control Cardiovascular Risk in Diabetes (ACCORD) trial, despite intensive control of glucose and other risk factors in patients, CKD progressed in a large number of participants and several biomarkers did not adequately identify or predict progression. Additionally, from a safety perspective, intensive glycemic control in advanced CKD may increase the risk of severe hypoglycemia. Nadkarni and colleagues[19] found that patients with T2DM who developed a sustained decrease in renal function also had elevated levels of urinary monocyte chemotactic protein-1/Cr ratio at baseline compared with those who had minimal or no decline in renal function. This may be a useful urinary biomarker to predict renal failure in patients with T2DM.

Hypertension

Hypertension (HTN) and CKD have a unique relationship: each is both a cause and a consequence of the other. Among NHANES (2009) participants with CKD stages 4 to 5, 84% had HTN, compared with just 23% of those without CKD.[3] Furthermore, 80% of NHANES participants with CKD stages 3 to 4 had HTN and only 20% of cases were adequately controlled. In 2010, in the Chronic Renal Insufficiency Cohort (CRIC) of more than 3600 patients with a broad spectrum of renal disease severity, 67% of patients reached their BP goal of lower than 140/90 mm Hg and 46% reached their goal of lower than 130/90 mm Hg,[20] compared with a 50% rate of HTN control for the general population from 2007 to 2008.[21] Even with many well-designed RCTs and observational studies, uncertainty and controversy remain among the guideline committees concerning the optimal BP target required to halt CKD progression.

Dyslipidemia of Chronic Kidney Disease

There are several processes responsible for dyslipidemia of *CKD*, including (1) impaired lipolysis, (2) impaired reverse cholesterol transport, and (3) low and altered High-density lipoproteins (HDL), which are summarized in **Table 1** and discussed in detail as follows.

Table 1	
Dyslipidemia related to chronic kidney disease	
1. Impaired lipolysis	Plasma Apo CIII is higher in patients with CKD with or without diabetes and leads to impaired lipolysis.[40]
	Apo B48 levels are elevated in diabetic and nondiabetic ESRD.[41]
2. Impaired reverse cholesterol transport	Plasma LCAT activity is decreased in chronic uremia,[42] so lower LCAT activity decreases mature HDL production.[44]
	Increased plasma oxidized LDL and IDL result from a decrease in mature HDL.[45]
	Inflammation decreases ABCA1 expression[32] and prevents reverse cholesterol transport.[46]
3. Low and altered HDL	CKD-HDL impairs vascular relaxant properties.[20]

Abbreviations: CKD, chronic kidney disease; ESRD, end-stage renal disease; HDL, high-density lipoprotein; IDL, intermediate-density lipoprotein; LCAT, lecithin-cholesterol acyltransferase; LDL, low-density lipoprotein.

Cardiovascular Calcifications

In patients with CKD, accelerated calcifying atherosclerosis and valvular heart disease is a result of uremic CVD. CV calcifications in CKD are highly prevalent as CKD progresses and are strong predictors of CV mortality in patients with CKD. Vascular calcification manifests as both intimal plaque calcification and medial calcification.[22] Many data sources (including registry data, cross-sectional analyses, experimental and clinical data) have shown that increased calcium phosphate product (Ca x P), caused by hyperphosphatemia and/or hypercalcemia, may be a key determinant of CV mortality and progression factors of undesirable calcifications in uremia.[23–26]

The natural history of disease progression in patients with CKD is being evaluated in the CRIC study, a US multicenter observational cohort study that recruited an ethnically and racially diverse patient population (more specifically, the study oversampled black Americans and individuals with diabetes).[27] The study's goals are to (1) examine risk factors for progression of CKD and CVD, (2) develop models that identify high-risk subgroups, and (3) assist in the development of treatment trials and therapies. The CRIC study will likely be instrumental in revealing controlling factors that contribute to mortality and morbidity in patients with CKD. In the meantime, we can improve our knowledge of currently known worsening factors, and most importantly, focus on prevention and screening for kidney disease in high-risk populations.

IS LIPID-LOWERING THERAPY BENEFICIAL IN CHRONIC KIDNEY DISEASE?

The HMG-CoA reductase inhibitors (statins) have been shown to reduce CVEs by 20% to 25% in clinical trials. However, patients with moderate to severe CKD and dialysis patients were either limited in numbers or excluded in trials.[28] Hence, treating dyslipidemia with statins to reduce CVEs in moderate to severe CKD and dialysis patients lacks a strong evidence basis. Patients with diabetes and CKD are at higher risk of developing CVD compared with either CKD alone or diabetes alone or the general population.[29] Trials, such as the Deutsche Diabetes Dialyze Studie (4D) and A Study to Evaluate Use of Rosuvastatin in subjects on Regular Hemodialysis (AURORA), question the efficacy of statins in moderate to severe CKD and dialysis patients.[30,31]

Several possibilities exist for the lack of benefit of statins in CKD (summarized in **Box 1**). First, CKD-related dyslipidemia is characterized by hypertriglyceridemia and normal cholesterol level.[32,33] Second, in addition to CKD dyslipidemia, hypercoagulability, autonomic dysfunction, electrolyte disturbance, LV hypertrophy, and chronic volume overload

---

Box 1
Possible reasons for lack of benefit of statins in chronic kidney disease (CKD)

1. CKD dyslipidemia is different compared with simple elevation of cholesterol.[32,33]

2. Many cardiovascular deaths in dialysis patients may be due to a combination of chronic volume overload–induced cardiomyopathy or electrolyte disturbance.[34,35]

3. Coronary plaques are prone to destabilization in uremic patients.[36]

4. Increased inflammation, oxidative stress, and pro-atherogenic factors in CKD attenuate effect of statins.[37,38]

5. Chronic hyperglycemia reduces vasodilation and myocardial blood flow in diabetic patients with CKD.[39]

---

collectively increase the risk of cardiovascular deaths.[34,35] Third, uremic patients' coronary intima and media are distinct; coronary plaques are heavily calcified and infiltrated with active macrophages, making them more vulnerable to plaque destabilization than patients with normal renal function.[36] Fourth, increased inflammation, oxidative stress, protein energy malnutrition, sympathetic overactivation, and endothelial dysfunction play critical roles in the development of vascular disease, the combination of which dilutes effects of statins as compared with the presence of only traditional risk factors in the general population.[37,38] Fifth, chronic hyperglycemia impairs endothelial function and potentiates coronary vasoconstriction and thrombosis, ultimately decreasing myocardial blood flow, especially in diabetic patients with CKD.[39] Finally, the optimal LDL-C goal in CKD is unknown and it is unclear whether we should target a lower LDL level in this population.

Dyslipidemia of Chronic Kidney Disease

There are several processes responsible for dyslipidemia of CKD: (1) Impaired lipolysis: Apo CIII levels are higher in patients with CKD with or without diabetes, which leads to impaired lipolysis by chylomicrons, and very low density lipoproteins (VLDL) leads to increased levels of triglyceride (TG) and VLDL (summarized in **Table 1**).[40] Apo B48 levels are elevated in diabetic and nondiabetic ESRD.[41] (2) Impaired reverse cholesterol transport: plasma lecithin-cholesterol acyltransferase (LCAT) activity is decreased in chronic uremia[42] and normalizes after renal transplantation.[43] As a result, decreased LCAT activity, decreased esterification of cholesterol, and maturation of HDL ultimately decreases HDL 2 (mature HDL).[44] HDL 2 carries antioxidant enzymes, and decreased HDL 2 level leads to an increase in oxidized LDL level.[45] Hepatic lipase activities depend on HDL 2, and decreased HDL 2 levels lead to accumulation of IDL. Inflammation in patients with CKD also decreases ABCA1 expression,[32] preventing efflux of cholesterol from lipid-laden macrophages to cholesterol-poor HDL.[46] Dialysis patients have high VLDL and intermediate-density lipoprotein (IDL), high cholesterol/TG ratio, and low HDL and LDL.[47] (3) CKD-HDL anti-atherogenic properties are affected through impaired reverse cholesterol transport. CKD-HDL causes uncoupling of nitric oxide synthase and impairs vascular relaxant properties.[48]

CLINICAL TRIALS OF THE STATINS IN PATIENTS WITH MILD TO SEVERE CHRONIC KIDNEY DISEASE
Statins in Patients with Mild Chronic Kidney Disease

The Scandinavian Simvastatin Survival Study group (4S) trial was conducted to evaluate the effect of simvastatin in CVD for secondary prevention (**Table 2**). In the 4S trial, subgroup analysis in patients with GFR less than 75 mL/min, simvastatin decreased

Table 2
Summary of clinical trials of lipid-lowering therapy in patients with mild to severe chronic kidney disease

Trials and Total Number of Patients	Intervention	Number of Patients with Mild to Moderate CKD	Number of Patients with Severe CKD and Dialysis	Primary Result
4S 4420	Simvastatin vs placebo	2314 patients with GFR <75 Average GFR 65 in these patients with CKD	Excluded	RRR of all-cause mortality decreased by 31%, nonfatal MI and coronary mortality by 35%
4D 1255	Atorvastatin 20 mg vs placebo	None	1255 dialysis patients	No difference in mortality form cardiac causes, nonfatal MI
AURORA 2776	Rosuvastatin 10 mg vs placebo	None	2776 dialysis patients	No difference on major CV events and all-cause mortality
SHARP 9027	Simvastatin 20 mg + ezetimibe 10 mg vs simvastatin 20 mg	88 Patients with GFR >60 mL/min 2155 patients with GFR 30–60 mL/min	2526 patients with GFR 15–30 mL/min 3623 dialysis patients	Decreased major atherosclerotic events by 17%, but not in those on dialysis
VA HIT 2531	Gemfibrozil 1200 mg every 24 h	297 patients with GFR <75 mL/min	Excluded	RRR of 24% of combined outcome of death from nonfatal MI, coronary heart disease, or stroke
ACCORD (Lipid arm) 5000	Simvastatin + fenofibrate vs simvastatin alone	734 patients with GFR 30–50 mL/min	Excluded	No difference in CV outcome
FIELD 9795	Fenofibrate vs placebo	5218 patients with GFR 60–89 mL/min 519 patients with GFR 30–50 mL/min	Excluded	Decrease of CVD events by 14% in patients with low HDL, by 23% in patients with TG >204 mg/dL, and 27% in patients with both
IMPROVE-IT 18,000	Simvastatin 40 mg + ezetimibe 10 mg vs simvastatin 40 mg + placebo	3261 patients with GFR 30–60 mL/min 7026 patients with GFR 60–90 mL/min	Excluded	RRR of 6.4% in nonfatal MI and stroke, hospital admission requiring unstable angina, or coronary revascularization

Abbreviations: 4D, the Deutsche Diabetes Dialyze Studie; 4S, The Scandinavian Simvastatin Survival Study; ACCORD, Action to Control Cardiovascular Risk in Diabetes; AURORA, A Study to Evaluate Use of Rosuvastatin in subjects on Regular Hemodialysis; CKD, chronic kidney disease; CV, cardiovascular; CVD, cardiovascular disease; FIELD, Fenofibrate, Intervention and Event Lowering in Diabetes; GFR, glomerular filtration rate; HDL, high-density lipoprotein; IMPROVE-IT, Vytorin Efficacy International Trial; MI, myocardial infarction; NSS, no statistical significance; RRR, relative risk reduction; SHARP, The Study of Heart and Renal protection; TG, triglyceride; VA HIT, Veterans Affairs High-Density Lipoprotein Cholesterol Intervention Trial Study Group.

relative risk (RR) of all-cause mortality by 31% and reduced nonfatal myocardial infarction (MI) and coronary mortality by 35%. Although subgroup analysis failed to show improvement in all-cause mortality in patients with CKD with GFR less than 60 mL/min, all-cause mortality rate doubled in the diabetic subgroup with GFR less than 75 mL/min compared with the simvastatin group, and the trend was similar for reduction of major coronary events in the simvastatin group. Limitations of subgroup analysis in diabetic patients with CKD include small sample size (95 patients) and post hoc analysis.[49]

In a subgroup analysis of 3 RCTs (West of Scotland Coronary Prevention Study [WOSCPOS], Cholesterol and Recurrent Events trial [CARE], and Long-Term Intervention with Pravastatin in Ischemic Disease study [LIPID]), Tonelli and colleagues[29] studied the effects of pravastatin in patients with mild CKD. In 571 diabetic patients with CKD, pravastatin did not decrease all-cause mortality but decreased RR by 25% of composite outcome (MI, coronary death, or revascularization procedure rate). The Heart Protection Study evaluated the effects of simvastatin on all-cause mortality and fatal and nonfatal vascular events in 20,000 UK patients. Subgroup analysis of 1329 patients with mildly elevated creatinine (>1.24 mg/dL for women and >1.47 mg/dL but <2.26 mg/dL for men) reduced major CVEs by 28% compared with the placebo group, similar to other cohorts.[50]

Statins in Patients with Advanced Chronic Kidney Disease and Dialysis Patients

In the 4D trial, 1255 HD patients with T2DM were randomized to atorvastatin 20 mg or placebo to evaluate possible CV reduction benefit in dialysis patients. Total reduction of LDL-C was similar to that seen in nondialysis patients. Atorvastatin did not significantly decrease mortality from cardiac causes or nonfatal MI, but suggested a downward trend in terms of cardiac death. There was an increased trend of death from cerebrovascular accident (CVA) (confidence interval [CI] 0.81–1.55) and increased incidence of statistically significant fatal stroke (hazard ratio [HR] = 2.03 CI (1.05–3.93), P value 0.04). Lack of benefit of statins is possibly due to dyslipidemia of CKD, delayed treatment with statin, or low dose of statin, as 15% of patients in in placebo group used statins and 25% discontinued atorvastatin in the intervention arm.[30]

In the AURORA trial, 2776 dialysis patients (731 patients with diabetes) were randomized to receive rosuvastatin 10 mg versus placebo. Results showed no benefit of statins on major CVEs and all-cause mortality. The results were similar to the 4D study except there was no increase in the incidence of fatal stroke. The study excluded patients who were previously on statins, so the question remains whether it would show beneficial effects if dialysis patients with previous statin therapy were included in the trial.[31]

The Study of Heart and Renal protection (SHARP) trial was a randomized trial of 9027 patients with advanced CKD and dialysis with primary prevention of CVEs as primary outcome. Results showed that simvastatin 20 mg plus ezetimibe 10 mg reduced major atherosclerotic events by 17% without an increase in side effects.[51] However, the study lacked adequate power to assess separate elements of major atherosclerotic events in patients with CKD. In the study 23% participant had diabetes and there was no evidence of the comparative RR on major atherosclerotic events in patients with or without diabetes with intervention.[51] Subgroup analysis among nondialysis subjects showed relative risk reduction (RRR) of 22% for major atherosclerotic events. The subgroup analysis of 3023 patients on dialysis showed no difference in incidence of major atherosclerotic events or all-cause mortality, despite receiving statin and ezetimibe (of note: one-third of nondialysis patients were started on dialysis during the trial). These encouraging results in the nondialysis subgroup strengthen the possibility of a beneficial effect of intervention in the dialysis group.[51]

CORRECTION OF HYPERTRIGLYCERIDEMIA AND LOW HIGH-DENSITY LIPOPROTEIN

Hypertriglyceridemia and low HDL are common in patients with diabetes.[32,33,40,42] For T2DM-related dyslipidemia, many physicians believe that fibrates are the logical first choice.[52] In the Veterans Affairs High-Density Lipoprotein Cholesterol Intervention Trial Study Group (VA HIT), 2531 patients with similar lipid abnormalities participated.[53] The overall trial showed that treatment with gemfibrozil 1200 mg daily resulted in an RRR of 24% in combined outcome of death from nonfatal MI, coronary heart disease, or stroke, although there was no statically significant change in all-cause mortality. In a post hoc analysis of 297 patients with diabetes and estimated GFR (eGFR) less than 75 mL/min showed 42% RRR in major CVEs. However, the study did not have adequate power for subgroup analysis.[53]

The lipid arm of the ACCORD trial was performed to identify CV benefits of a combination of simvastatin and fenofibrate in 5000 patients with T2DM, low HDL, and high TG. Patients were randomized to receive simvastatin + fenofibrate versus simvastatin alone to assess CV benefits for both primary and secondary prevention. The study did not show a statistically significant difference in CV outcome with simvastatin + fenofibrate, although a statistically nonsignificant downtrend was present after a median follow-up of 4.3 years. There were 734 patients with GFR 30 to 50 mL/min requiring dose adjustment of fenofibrate, and 96 patients with GFR less than 30 mL/min requiring discontinuation of drugs. Subgroup analysis of 734 patients with CKD-3 did not have adequate power to show beneficial effects of the combination. Post hoc analysis showed a subgroup of patients with TG >204 mg/dL and HDL less than 34 mg/dL may have had decreased the rate of CVEs with combination therapy.[54]

In another study, Fenofibrate Intervention and Event Lowering in Diabetes (FIELD), 9795 patients with T2DM and dyslipidemia (5218 patients with eGFR 60–89 mL/min and 519 patients with eGFR 30–59 mL/min[55]) were randomly assigned to fenofibrate or placebo group. Fenofibrate reduced RR of CVEs by 14% in patients with low HDL, by 23% in patients TG >204 mg/dL, and by 27% in patients with combined low HDL and high TG.[56] However, the study was performed in the background of usual care, and patients with moderate to severe CKD were excluded.[52,56] In addition, fibrates increase creatinine and are cleared by the kidneys, so their use in patients with severe CKD and dialysis patients is contraindicated.[57]

WILL LOWERING LOW-DENSITY LIPOPROTEIN TARGET BE BENEFICIAL IN PATIENTS WITH HIGH-RISK AND EXTREMELY HIGH-RISK CHRONIC KIDNEY DISEASE?

Doubling the dose of a statin further reduces plasma LDL by only 6%, but adding another drug to enable combination therapy has a greater effect in lowering LDL.[58] Would lowering LDL target further in high-risk or extremely high-risk individuals be beneficial?[58] This hypothesis has been tested in several clinical trials, including the IMProved Reduction of Outcomes: Vytorin Efficacy International Trial (IMPROVE-IT trial) and the Further Cardiovascular Outcomes Research with proprotein convertase subtilism/kexin type 9 (PCSK 9) Inhibition in Subjects with Elevated Risk (FOURIER) study, and other trials are ongoing.

The IMPROVE-IT trial tested the benefits of lowering LDL by randomizing 18,000 patients with acute coronary syndrome (3261 patients with eGFR 30–60 mL/min, 7026 patients with eGFR 60–90 mL/min, and 40% of patients with diabetes) to determine whether the addition of ezetimibe to statin would provide additional benefits. Nonfatal MI and stroke, hospital admission requiring unstable angina, or coronary revascularization showed RRR of 6.4% (HR 0.936, CI 0.887–0.988, P = .016) in the intervention group, without increasing side effects except for a non–statistically significant increase in event of hemorrhagic stroke. The benefit was particularly pronounced in patients with diabetes (27% of study population) and patients older than 75 years; however, the study excluded patients with severe CKD (GFR <30 mL/min) and dialysis patients at the time of randomization.[59] The FOURIER study was a randomized placebo-controlled trial in 27,500 patients (36% patients with diabetes) on background statin therapy to evaluate the benefits of intensive LDL reduction with evolocumab. Evolocumab reduced LDL cholesterol by 59%: LDL less than 70, less than 40, and less than 25 mg/dL in 87%, 67%, and 40%, respectively. RR of primary endpoint (cardiovascular death, MI, stroke, hospitalization for unstable angina) was reduced by 15% in the evolocumab group, 20% RRR in secondary endpoint (cardiovascular death, MI, and stroke). Results were consistent across major subgroups. Patients with GFR less than 20 mL/min were excluded from the study.[60]

In summary, at present, there is no evidence of nephrotoxicity of statins. Except for Atorvastatin and Fluvastatin, the dose of other statins need to be modified in patients with GFR is <30 mL/min.[57,61] Based on current evidence, early detection and treatment of CKD dyslipidemia is critical to decrease mortality from CVD. Statin is the gold standard treatment for mild-moderate CKD dyslipidemia and early treatment with statins may translate long-term statin benefit in those patients. Patients who are on statin and if they become dialysis dependent, continue statin with dose adjustment. Based on current evidence, dialysis-dependent patients who are not on a statin should not be started on statins.[61,62] In patients with severe CKD and LDL above target, raising statin dose increases the risk of side effects.[61,62] Ezetimibe, which was also tested in the SHARP trial, can be used in combination with statins. Fibrates and PCSK 9 inhibitors should not be used in patients with GFR less than 30. Newer studies (Thrombolysis in Myocardial Infarction [IMPROVE IT trial] and FOURIER) in high-risk or extremely high-risk patients indicate that intensive LDL lowering therapy reduced CVEs; however, patients with severe CKD and dialysis patients were excluded, so further studies are needed to determine the role of intensive lipid-lowering therapy on cardiovascular outcomes (CVOs) in those populations.

DIABETES, GLYCEMIA, AND CHRONIC KIDNEY DISEASE

The management of glycemia is challenging in patients with CKD due to inconclusive data on the value of intensive control, challenges with measurement metrics, such as HbA1c, and changes to the pharmacokinetics and pharmacodynamics of various drugs. Some diabetes medications are contraindicated in advanced CKD. Further, hypoglycemia may be more severe in patients with CKD. As a result, glycemic control is often poor in patients with CKD.

Benefits of Glycemic Control in Patients with Diabetes and CKD

The Diabetes Control and Complications Trial (DCCT) showed that maintaining A1C at less than 7% resulted in decreased microvascular complications, and the UK Prospective Diabetes Study group (UKPDS) confirmed this. However, both DCCT and UKPDS excluded participants with advanced kidney disease. In patients with CKD, not on dialysis, it is not clear whether good glycemic control delays progression of DN and CVEs.[63] The DCCT trial included only participants with early-stage DN and found decreased microvascular complications.[64] In patients with T2DM, both albuminuria and eGFR have been found to be independent risk factors for CVD, renal disease, and mortality.[64–66] Unfortunately, most large studies analyzing the benefits and risks of glycemic control did not include patients with advanced CKD. In a subgroup analysis of CKD in the ACCORD study, 3636 patients met the criteria for CKD stages 1 to 3. These participants had an increase in all-cause mortality (HR 1.3, 95% CI 1.0–1.6) and increased CV mortality (HR 1.4, 95% CI 1.05–1.90).[67] A large retrospective observational study of 23,296 people with T2DM and eGFR less than 60 mL/min/1.73 m^2 found higher mortality with A1C both less than 6.5% and greater than 8.0%.[68] This study did not find more adverse events (AEs) in those with stage 4 CKD and A1C 7% to 9% when compared with A1C <7% in the same population. More studies are needed to evaluate the risks and benefits of strict glycemic control in patients with CKD using additional biomarkers, such as glycated albumin.

A1C as an Indicator of Glycemic Control in Chronic Kidney Disease

Diabetes is the leading cause of CKD, it is therefore crucial to have reliable glycemic markers in this patient population. A1C has been used in clinical practice since 1976[69] as a marker to assess glycemic control in patients with diabetes. American Diabetes Association guidelines from 2017 recommend checking A1C every 3 months in patients with diabetes who have had a change in therapy or are not meeting glycemic goals. Different recommendations do not exist for patients with both diabetes and CKD. Decreased reliability of A1C in CKD may be due in part to the shorter life span of red blood cells (RBCs).[70] Decreased RBC life span includes uremia, which causes increased breakdown. There also may be mechanical damage from the dialysis itself. The mechanical effect of HD is small and transient; it has not been noted to cause a decrease in hemoglobin concentrations.[71] Patients on peritoneal dialysis (PD) do not have the mechanical damage of HD but do have decreased RBC survival due to the uremic environment, although possibly to a lesser extent.[71] In uremia there is increased phosphatidylserine, resulting in increased degradation by erythrocytes.[72] Patients with CKD were noted to have impairment in phospholipid asymmetry; this did not seem to be affected by the presence or absence of dialysis.[72] In fact, uremia is the likely cause of altered phospholipid asymmetry, which can decrease the life span of RBCs.[73] Various studies have looked at the survival of RBCs in dialysis patients, but results vary widely; decrease of RBC life span ranges from 20%[71] to 70%.[74] There are conflicting data regarding whether improvement of the uremic state results in improved RBC survival.[75–77] In addition, some individuals may glycate hemoglobin faster than others, resulting in differences in A1C.[78] In patients with ESRD, differences in acid-base balance and hemoglobin concentration also can affect glycation of RBCs.[79]

Erythropoietin production is decreased in ESRD, and a significant proportion of patients with ESRD receive erythropoietin treatment for normocytic normochromic anemia.[70] Erythropoietin use results in increased production of young RBCs, which are reported to glycate at a slower rate than older cells.[80] Patients with diabetes on dialysis receiving erythropoietin were found to have lower levels of A1C than patients who were not receiving erythropoietin.[70,81,82]

In a uremic environment there is increased production of carboxylate hemoglobin, which may be assayed incorrectly as A1C,[83] resulting in overestimation of A1C levels. Uremia also can suppress bone marrow function.[84,85]

A1C is a result of nonenzymatic glycation of RBCs; therefore, any condition that affects the half-life or metabolism of RBCs can affect A1C values. Several studies have shown a positive correlation coefficient between serum plasma glucose (PG) levels and A1C in patients with stages 3 and 4 CKD,[86] ESRD on HD,[70,84,87–91] and ESRD on PD.[92] In these studies, the correlation coefficient ranged from 0.5 to 0.8; the strongest correlation coefficient was seen in a study conducted by Chen and colleagues[86] that analyzed the glycosylated albumin (GA) and PG in stages 3 and 4 CKD. Poor correlation has been noted between stages 4 and 5 CKD and A1C; this may be secondary to anemia, decreased RBC survival,[70] and use of erythropoietin. Many studies have shown lower than estimated A1C in diabetic patients with ESRD compared with diabetic patients without CKD,[70,86,90,91] suggesting that in this patient population, A1C may underestimate glycemic control. The lower A1C value also may be due to a combination of anemia and erythropoietin injections.[81,93] Inaba and colleagues[70] showed that the regression slope between PG A1C was steeper in patients with diabetes who did not have CKD when compared with patients with diabetes and ESRD.

Glycated Albumin as an Indicator of Glycemic Control in Chronic Kidney Disease

Several studies have suggested that glycated albumin (GA) may be a superior indicator of glycemic control in CKD.[70,89,91] Albumin has a half-life of approximately 2 weeks and therefore is a marker of glycemic control over a shorter duration than A1C.[70,94] GA can be affected by many conditions that lower serum albumin, such as nephrotic syndrome,[95] thyroid function,[96] chronic liver disease,[97] blood loss, and burns.[98] There also may be increased protein loss during dialysis.[99,100] In addition, GA is lower than expected in Cushing syndrome,[101] and thyroid hormone levels were found to be inversely related to GA. GA also has been found to be lower in obese patients with diabetes compared with nonobese patients with diabetes,[51,98,102] likely due to the increased microinflammation in obese patients.[51] High serum albumin has been associated with less glycation, and low albumin levels are associated with increased glycation,[103] as CKD worsens the rate of proteinuria and albuminuria increases and the serum albumin levels decrease. Of note, no significant correlation has been found between GA and PG when serum albumin was less than 3.5 g/dL.[51,96–98,104,105]

Comparison of A1C with Glycated Albumin

Some studies have shown that GA may be a better marker than A1C for glycemic control,[70,89,91] whereas others show that A1C correlated more closely with PG.[84] Chronic liver disease can affect both A1C and GA due to increased turnover of RBCs and decreased levels of serum albumin.[97] Likely due to increased RBC turnover, A1C values in patients with chronic liver disease were lower than the estimated A1C based on PG values, and GA levels were increased when compared with PG.[97] Inaba and colleagues[70] found a significant and positive correlation between A1C and GA in patients with diabetes with both ESRD and diabetic patients without CKD. Vos and colleagues[94] found a poor and nonsignificant correlation between A1C and PG in patients with stages 4 and 5 CKD, whereas GA showed significant and positive ($r = 0.54$) correlation in patients with and without CKD stages 4 and 5. Two observational studies have shown that in patients with diabetes on HD, GA but not A1C was a good predictor of all-cause mortality and CV mortality.[106,107] Harada and colleagues[104] found a positive correlation between PG and GA when eGFR was greater than 30 mL/min/1.73 m^2; they did not find a significant correlation if the eGFR was less than 30 mL/min/1.73 m^2.

Fructosamine as an Indicator of Glycemic Control in Chronic Kidney Disease

Fructosamine is composed of glycated serum proteins that have become stable ketoamines though nonenzymatic glycation. Albumin makes up approximately 90% of fructosamine.[94] The different proteins that make up fructosamine have different half-lives and react differently with glucose. In addition, serum urea and uric acid can influence fructosamine levels.[108] Several studies have suggested that fructosamine should be corrected for serum albumin or protein levels.[109,110]

Self-Blood Glucose Monitoring and Continuous Glucose Monitoring in Chronic Kidney Disease

Regardless of which glycemic marker is chosen, self-monitoring blood glucose (SMBG) and/or continuous glucose monitoring (CGM) is essential in patients with end-stage DN given the high degree of glycemic variability. Jin and colleagues[111] found lower blood glucose levels in patients with diabetes on dialysis days, with increased mean amplitude of glycemic excursions compared with nondialysis days. Hypoglycemia has also been noted on CGM without symptoms in patients with end-stage DN.[111] SMBG or CGM is essential in this patient population given the chance of asymptomatic hypoglycemia. In addition, studies suggest that glucose fluctuation is an independent risk factor for diabetes complications.[112]

Glycemic Markers in Summary

In summary, some recent studies have suggested that GA may be a better glycemic indicator in patients with diabetes with CKD.[70,89,91] It should be noted that a significant correlation has not been found between GA and PG when the serum albumin was less than 3.5 g/dL.[51,96–98,104,105] Several of these studies looked at a limited number of blood glucose values to determine the average blood glucose, but these values may be more dynamic in patients on dialysis. In addition, further studies directly comparing A1C, GA, and serum albumin levels are warranted. In our review, when choosing a glycemic marker in patients with eGFR less than 30 mL/min/1.73 m^2 who also have serum albumin $\geq$3.5 g/d, GA appears to be superior to A1C.

Treatment of Diabetes in Chronic Kidney Disease

Diabetic kidney disease carries an increased risk of hypoglycemia. In a fasting state, an estimated 20% to 25% of glucose released into circulation originates from renal gluconeogenesis.[113,114] In addition, renal gluconeogenesis increases following a meal, which in turn may contribute to hepatic glycogen stores.[113,114] Renal impairment leads to decreased renal gluconeogenesis, and there is also decreased sympathetic response due to autonomic neuropathy.[115] Renal insulin clearance is decreased and uremic toxins decrease insulin metabolism in the liver.[116] Prevention of hypoglycemia is crucial in this patient population. Summarized in **Table 3** are various antihyperglycemic treatment options with recommended dose adjustments for the CKD population.

STRATEGIES TO IMPROVE OVERALL METABOLIC CONTROL

Owing to CKD association with high CV risk, morbidity, and mortality, in addition to a lack of studies demonstrating methods to decrease CV risk as compared with populations without CKD, for many treatments we must resort to applying data results obtained from non-CKD population studies. To improve overall metabolic control, health care providers should pay close attention to what we commonly think of as the "traditional factors" (eg, advanced age, hypertension, diabetes mellitus, and dyslipidemia), as well as the "nontraditional factors" specific to CKD (eg, anemia, volume status, mineral metabolism abnormalities, and proteinuria).

As covered previously, treatment of CKD-associated dyslipidemia is important to decrease mortality from cardiovascular disease. Most studies showed a positive effect of statins in mild to moderate CKD; however, risks and benefits should be

Table 3
Recommended dose adjustments in CKD for antihyperglycemic drugs

Drug Class/Drug	Recommended Dose Adjustments with Impaired GFR	Rationale
Insulin	Decrease dose	Prolonged half-life due to decreased renal metabolism of exogenous insulin
Biguanides		
Metformin	eGFR >45: dose adjustment not required eGFR 30–45: do not start treatment; if patient is already on it, monitor renal function changes carefully eGFR<30: do not use	Concern for lactic acid accumulation in kidney disease
Thiazolidinediones		
Pioglitazone and rosiglitazone	Dose adjustment not required, avoid use in advanced CKD	Causes fluid retention; therefore, avoid use in advanced CKD; does not cause hypoglycemia, metabolized by the liver
Sulfonylureas		
Glyburide	Avoid use	Accumulation of active metabolites can result in hypoglycemia
Glimepiride	Start at 1 mg daily	Causes less hypoglycemia than glyburide
Glipizide	Dose adjustment not required	Metabolized by the liver to inactive metabolites
Meglitinides		
Repaglinide Nateglinide	eGFR <30: start 0.5 mg with meals eGFR<30: start 60 mg with meals	Decreased renal clearance; increased risk of hypoglycemia[79] Lower dose recommended in CKD
α-Glucosidase inhibitors		
Acarbose and miglitol	Use with caution if eGFR <30	Plasma levels can increase in CKD[117]
Dipeptidyl peptidase-4 inhibitors		
Linagliptin	Dose adjustment not required	Mainly excreted by enterohepatic circulation
Sitagliptin	eGFR >50: 100 mg daily eGFR 30–50: 50 mg daily eGFR <30: 25 mg daily	Varying renal excretion ranging from 12% to 80% SGLT2 may have decreased function in renal impairment
Saxagliptin	eGFR >50: 5 mg daily eGFR ≤50: 2.5 mg daily	
Alogliptin	eGFR >60: 25 mg daily eGFR 30–60: 12.5 mg daily eGFR <30: 6.25 mg daily	
Glucagonlike peptide 1 receptor agonists		
Exenatide	eGFR<30: not recommended	Renally excreted, clearance decreased by 64% if eGFR is <30[118] May be associated with acute kidney injury and worsening kidney function[119,120]

(*continued on next page*)

Table 3
(*continued*)

Drug Class/Drug	Recommended Dose Adjustments with Impaired GFR	Rationale
Liraglutide	Dose adjustment not required as per manufacturer	Kidneys are not the main organ of elimination[121] More GI adverse effects may occur in CKD[122]
Lixisenatide	eGFR 30–59 dosage adjustment not required, close monitoring recommended eGFR 15–29, limited clinical experience, monitor kidney function eGFR <15: avoid use	
Albiglutide	eGFR >15, dosage adjustment not required	
Dulaglutide	Dose adjustment not required per manufacturer	
Amylinomimetic		
Pramlintide	Avoid use in stage 4 CKD	Primarily metabolized and excreted by kidneys
Sodium glucose cotransporter 2 inhibitors		
Canagliflozin	eGFR >60: no dose adjustments eGFR 45–59: 100 mg daily eGFR <45: avoid use	SGLT 2 inhibitors may be less effective in lowering blood glucose in presence of renal impairment
Dapagliflozin	eGFR <60: avoid starting eGFR <30: contraindicated	
Empagliflozin	eGFR ≥45: dose adjustment not required eGFR <30: contraindicated eGFR 30-44 avoid use	

Abbreviations: CKD, chronic kidney disease; eGFR, estimated glomerular filtration rate; GI, gastrointestinal; SGLT2, sodium glucose cotransporter 2.

closely evaluated, and statin doses should be adjusted once the patient is dialysis dependent. Because diabetes is the leading cause of CKD, and as the incidence of diabetes continues to rise, more studies are needed to evaluate and identify a glycemic threshold to slow the progression of CKD. For now, due to lack of such data, goals similar to those for patients without CKD are used to prevent microvascular complications, paying special attention to avoid hypoglycemia. Another difficult part of diabetes control in CKD is the lack of one ideal marker to assess and follow glycemic control. Again, most large studies analyzing the benefits and risks of glycemic control did not include patients with advanced CKD.

Exercise, smoking cessation, optimal protein intake, and treatment of anemia and deficiency of active vitamin D are other factors that should be monitored in patients with CKD. In addition to specific data reviews on lipids and diabetes in this article, and BP control addressed in the article by Farheen K. Dojki and George L. Bakris, "Blood Pressure Control and Cardiovascular/Renal Outcomes," elsewhere in this issue, optimizing volume status, correcting anemia, and ensuring the patient is on appropriate treatment to decrease proteinuria are essential. Pharmacologically, focusing on treatment that targets multiple risk factors with low risk for side effects is optimal for patients with CKD. Evidence from clinical trials indicates that mild to moderate CKD is also much easier to treat, and we assume similar benefits to patients without CKD with slight medication dose adjustment. Further studies are needed on patients with severe CKD and dialysis patients to determine the effects of controlling traditional and nontraditional cardiovascular factors.

SUMMARY

Diabetes is the leading cause of CKD, and the incidence of diabetes continues to rise. Treatment and control of CVD risk factors among people with CKD and diabetes remains poorly understood, mostly due to a lack of studies on CVD risk in patients with CKD. Therefore, for many treatments, we resort to applying results obtained from non-CKD population studies to decrease CV risk in patients with CKD. Due to a lack of studies, including advanced CKD populations, combined with the lack of a reliable marker of glycemic control in patients with CKD and high risk of hypoglycemia, the benefits of good glycemic control on CV risk has not been clearly shown in patients with advanced CKD. Conversely, most studies show that statins benefit mild to moderate CKD, although statin doses may need to be adjusted once the patient is dialysis dependent. Further research on screening, preventive methods, and the development of medications targeting these specific patients is necessary to improve CKD treatment and prevent cardiovascular mortality.

REFERENCES

1. WHO. Cardiovascular diseases. 2016; WHO fact sheet on cardiovascular disease. Available at: http://www.who.int/mediacentre/factsheets/fs317/en/. Accessed March 11, 2017.
2. K/DOQI clinical practice guidelines for chronic kidney disease: evaluation, classification, and stratification. Am J Kidney Dis 2002;39(2 Suppl 1):S1–266.
3. USRDS. Chronic kidney disease in the adult NHANES population 2009. In. USRDS Annual Report Data. Available at: https://www.usrds.org/2009/pdf/V1_01_09.PDF.
4. Foley RN, Parfrey PS, Sarnak MJ. Clinical epidemiology of cardiovascular disease in chronic renal disease. Am J Kidney Dis 1998;32(5 Suppl 3):S112–9.
5. Collins AJ, Li S, Gilbertson DT, et al. Chronic kidney disease and cardiovascular disease in the Medicare population. Kidney Int Suppl 2003;87:S24–31.
6. Dalrymple LS, Katz R, Kestenbaum B, et al. Chronic kidney disease and the risk of end-stage renal disease versus death. J Gen Intern Med 2011;26(4):379–85.
7. Go AS, Chertow GM, Fan D, et al. Chronic kidney disease and the risks of death, cardiovascular events, and hospitalization. New Engl J Med 2004;351(13): 1296–305.
8. Hill NR, Fatoba ST, Oke JL, et al. Global prevalence of chronic kidney disease–a systematic review and meta-analysis. PLoS One 2016;11(7):e0158765.
9. World Health Organization. Global report on diabetes. WHO; 2016. Available at: http://www.who.int/diabetes/global-report/en/.
10. Koro CE, Lee BH, Bowlin SJ. Antidiabetic medication use and prevalence of chronic kidney disease among patients with type 2 diabetes mellitus in the United States. Clin Ther 2009;31(11):2608–17.
11. Tuttle KR, Bakris GL, Bilous RW, et al. Diabetic kidney disease: a report from an ADA consensus conference. Diabetes Care 2014;37(10):2864.

12. Segall L, Nistor I, Covic A. Heart failure in patients with chronic kidney disease: a systematic integrative review. Biomed Res Int 2014;2014:937398.

13. Kuznik A, Mardekian J, Tarasenko L. Evaluation of cardiovascular disease burden and therapeutic goal attainment in US adults with chronic kidney disease: an analysis of National Health and Nutritional Examination Survey data, 2001-2010. BMC Nephrol 2013;14:132.

14. Heywood JT, Fonarow GC, Costanzo MR, et al. High prevalence of renal dysfunction and its impact on outcome in 118,465 patients hospitalized with acute decompensated heart failure: a report from the ADHERE database. J Card Fail 2007;13(6):422–30.

15. Middleton RJ, Parfrey PS, Foley RN. Left ventricular hypertrophy in the renal patient. J Am Soc Nephrol 2001;12(5):1079–84.

16. Coca SG, Ismail-Beigi F, Haq N, et al. Role of intensive glucose control in development of renal endpoints in type 2 diabetes: systematic review and meta-analysis. Arch Intern Med 2012;172(10):761–9.

17. Jun M, Perkovic V, Cass A. Intensive glycemic control and renal outcome. Contrib Nephrol 2011;170:196–208.

18. Ruospo M, Saglimbene VM, Palmer SC, et al. Glucose targets for preventing diabetic kidney disease and its progression. Cochrane Database Syst Rev 2017;(6):CD010137.

19. Nadkarni GN, Rao V, Ismail-Beigi F, et al. Association of urinary biomarkers of inflammation, injury, and fibrosis with renal function decline: the ACCORD trial. Clin J Am Soc Nephrol 2016;11(8):1343–52.

20. Muntner P, Anderson A, Charleston J, et al. Hypertension awareness, treatment, and control in adults with CKD: results from the Chronic Renal Insufficiency Cohort (CRIC) Study. Am J Kidney Dis 2010;55(3):441–51.

21. Egan BM, Zhao Y, Axon RN. US trends in prevalence, awareness, treatment, and control of hypertension, 1988-2008. Jama 2010;303(20):2043–50.

22. Ketteler M, Schlieper G, Floege J. Calcification and cardiovascular health: new insights into an old phenomenon. Hypertension 2006;47(6):1027–34.

23. Block GA, Klassen PS, Lazarus JM, et al. Mineral metabolism, mortality, and morbidity in maintenance hemodialysis. J Am Soc Nephrol 2004;15(8):2208–18.

24. Ganesh SK, Stack AG, Levin NW, et al. Association of elevated serum PO(4), Ca x PO(4) product, and parathyroid hormone with cardiac mortality risk in chronic hemodialysis patients. J Am Soc Nephrol 2001;12(10):2131–8.

25. Stevens LA, Djurdjev O, Cardew S, et al. Calcium, phosphate, and parathyroid hormone levels in combination and as a function of dialysis duration predict mortality: evidence for the complexity of the association between mineral metabolism and outcomes. J Am Soc Nephrol 2004;15(3):770–9.

26. Block GA, Hulbert-Shearon TE, Levin NW, et al. Association of serum phosphorus and calcium x phosphate product with mortality risk in chronic hemodialysis patients: a national study. Am J Kidney Dis 1998;31(4):607–17.

27. Denker M, Boyle S, Anderson AH, et al. Chronic Renal Insufficiency Cohort Study (CRIC): Overview and summary of selected findings. Clin J Am Soc Nephrol 2015;10(11):2073–83.

28. Navaneethan SD, Pansini F, Perkovic V, et al. HMG CoA reductase inhibitors (statins) for people with chronic kidney disease not requiring dialysis. Cochrane Database Syst Rev 2009;(2):CD007784.

29. Tonelli M, Keech A, Shepherd J, et al. Effect of pravastatin in people with diabetes and chronic kidney disease. J Am Soc Nephrol 2005;16(12):3748–54.

30. Wanner C, Krane V, Marz W, et al. Atorvastatin in patients with type 2 diabetes mellitus undergoing hemodialysis. N Engl J Med 2005;353(3):238–48.
31. Fellstrom BC, Jardine AG, Schmieder RE, et al. Rosuvastatin and cardiovascular events in patients undergoing hemodialysis. N Engl J Med 2009;360(14):1395–407.
32. Kaysen GA. Lipid and lipoprotein metabolism in chronic kidney disease. J Ren Nu 2009;19(1):73–7.
33. Ananthakrishnan S, Kaysen GA. Treatment of hyperlipidemia changes with level of kidney function—rationale. Adv Chronic Kidney Dis 2016;23(4):247–54.
34. Karnik JA, Young BS, Lew NL, et al. Cardiac arrest and sudden death in dialysis units. Kidney Int 2001;60(1):350–7.
35. Herzog CA. How to manage the renal patient with coronary heart disease: the agony and the ecstasy of opinion-based medicine. J Am Soc Nephrol 2003; 14(10):2556–72.
36. Schwarz U, Amann K, Ritz E. Why are coronary plaques more malignant in the uraemic patient? Nephrol Dial Transpl 1999;14(1):224–5.
37. Kalantar-Zadeh K, Block G, Humphreys MH, et al. Reverse epidemiology of cardiovascular risk factors in maintenance dialysis patients. Kidney Int 2003;63(3): 793–808.
38. Stenvinkel P, Carrero JJ, Axelsson J, et al. Emerging biomarkers for evaluating cardiovascular risk in the chronic kidney disease patient: how do new pieces fit into the uremic puzzle? Clin J Am Soc Nephrol 2008;3(2):505–21.
39. Di Carli MF, Janisse J, Grunberger G, et al. Role of chronic hyperglycemia in the pathogenesis of coronary microvascular dysfunction in diabetes. J Am Coll Cardiol 2003;41(8):1387–93.
40. Hirano T, Sakaue T, Misaki A, et al. Very low-density lipoprotein-apoprotein CI is increased in diabetic nephropathy: comparison with apoprotein CIII. Kidney Int 2003;63(6):2171–7.
41. Hayashi T, Hirano T, Taira T, et al. Remarkable increase of apolipoprotein B48 level in diabetic patients with end-stage renal disease. Atherosclerosis 2008; 197(1):154–8.
42. Guarnieri GF, Moracchiello M, Campanacci L, et al. Lecithin-cholesterol acyltransferase (LCAT) activity in chronic uremia. Kidney Int Suppl 1978;(8):S26–30.
43. Chan MK, Ramdial L, Varghese Z, et al. Plasma LCAT activities in renal allograft recipients. Clin Chim Acta 1982;124(2):187–93.
44. Miida T, Miyazaki O, Hanyu O, et al. LCAT-dependent conversion of prebeta1-HDL into alpha-migrating HDL is severely delayed in hemodialysis patients. J Am Soc Nephrol 2003;14(3):732–8.
45. Dantoine TF, Debord J, Charmes JP, et al. Decrease of serum paraoxonase activity in chronic renal failure. J Am Soc Nephrol 1998;9(11):2082–8.
46. Oram JF, Lawn RM, Garvin MR, et al. ABCA1 is the cAMP-inducible apolipoprotein receptor that mediates cholesterol secretion from macrophages. J Biol Chem 2000;275(44):34508–11.
47. Shoji T, Nishizawa Y, Kawagishi T, et al. Atherogenic lipoprotein changes in the absence of hyperlipidemia in patients with chronic renal failure treated by hemodialysis. Atherosclerosis 1997;131(2):229–36.
48. Shroff R, Speer T, Colin S, et al. HDL in children with CKD promotes endothelial dysfunction and an abnormal vascular phenotype. J Am Soc Nephrol 2014; 25(11):2658–68.
49. Chonchol M, Cook T, Kjekshus J, et al. Simvastatin for secondary prevention of all-cause mortality and major coronary events in patients with mild chronic renal insufficiency. Am J Kidney Dis 2007;49(3):373–82.

50. MRC/BHF heart protection study of cholesterol lowering with simvastatin in 20,536 high-risk individuals: a randomised placebo-controlled trial. Lancet 2002;360(9326):7–22.

51. Baigent C, Landray MJ, Reith C, et al. The effects of lowering LDL cholesterol with simvastatin plus ezetimibe in patients with chronic kidney disease (study of heart and renal protection): a randomised placebo-controlled trial. Lancet 2011;377(9784):2181–92.

52. The need for a large-scale trial of fibrate therapy in diabetes: the rationale and design of the Fenofibrate Intervention and Event Lowering in Diabetes (FIELD) study [ISRCTN64783481]. Cardiovasc Diabetol 2004;3:9.

53. Rubins HB, Robins SJ, Collins D, et al. Gemfibrozil for the secondary prevention of coronary heart disease in men with low levels of high-density lipoprotein cholesterol. Veterans Affairs High-Density Lipoprotein Cholesterol Intervention Trial study group. N Engl J Med 1999;341(6):410–8.

54. Ginsberg HN, Elam MB, Lovato LC, et al. Effects of combination lipid therapy in type 2 diabetes mellitus. N Engl J Med 2010;362(17):1563–74.

55. Drury PL, Ting R, Zannino D, et al. Estimated glomerular filtration rate and albuminuria are independent predictors of cardiovascular events and death in type 2 diabetes mellitus: the Fenofibrate Intervention and Event Lowering in Diabetes (FIELD) study. Diabetologia 2011;54(1):32–43.

56. Scott R, O'Brien R, Fulcher G, et al. Effects of fenofibrate treatment on cardiovascular disease risk in 9,795 individuals with type 2 diabetes and various components of the metabolic syndrome: the Fenofibrate Intervention and Event Lowering in Diabetes (FIELD) study. Diabetes Care 2009;32(3):493–8.

57. Hager MR, Narla AD, Tannock LR. Dyslipidemia in patients with chronic kidney disease. Rev Endocr Metab Disord 2017;18(1):29–40.

58. Feingold KR, Grunfeld C. Cholesterol lowering drugs. In: De Groot LJ, Chrousos G, Dungan K, et al, editors. Endotext. South Dartmouth (MA): MDText.com, Inc; 2000.

59. Cannon CP, Blazing MA, Giugliano RP, et al. Ezetimibe added to statin therapy after acute coronary syndromes. N Engl J Med 2015;372(25):2387–97.

60. Sabatine MS, Giugliano RP, Keech AC, et al. Evolocumab and clinical outcomes in patients with cardiovascular disease. N Engl J Med 2017;376(18):1713–22.

61. KDOQI clinical practice guideline for diabetes and CKD: 2012 update. Am J Kidney Dis 2012;60(5):850–86.

62. Wanner C, Tonelli M. KDIGO clinical practice guideline for lipid management in CKD: summary of recommendation statements and clinical approach to the patient. Kidney Int 2014;85(6):1303–9.

63. Fukami K, Shibata R, Nakayama H, et al. Serum albumin-adjusted glycated albumin reflects glycemic excursion in diabetic patients with severe chronic kidney disease not treated with dialysis. J Diabetes Complications 2015;29(7):913–7.

64. The effect of intensive treatment of diabetes on the development and progression of long-term complications in insulin-dependent diabetes mellitus. The diabetes control and complications trial research group. N Engl J Med 1993; 329(14):977–86.

65. Ninomiya T, Perkovic V, de Galan BE, et al. Albuminuria and kidney function independently predict cardiovascular and renal outcomes in diabetes. J Am Soc Nephrol 2009;20(8):1813–21.

66. Vigil L, Lopez M, Condés E, et al. Cystatin C is associated with the metabolic syndrome and other cardiovascular risk factors in a hypertensive population. J Am Soc Hypertens 2009;3(3):201–9.

67. Papademetriou V, Lovato L, Doumas M, et al. Chronic kidney disease and intensive glycemic control increase cardiovascular risk in patients with type 2 diabetes. Kidney Int 2015;87(3):649–59.
68. Shurraw S, Hemmelgarn B, Lin M, et al. Association between glycemic control and adverse outcomes in people with diabetes mellitus and chronic kidney disease: a population-based cohort study. Arch Intern Med 2011;171(21):1920–7.
69. Koenig RJ, Peterson CM, Jones RL, et al. Correlation of glucose regulation and hemoglobin Alc in diabetes mellitus. N Engl J Med 1976;295(8):417–20.
70. Inaba M, Okuno S, Kumeda Y, et al. Glycated albumin is a better glycemic indicator than glycated hemoglobin values in hemodialysis patients with diabetes: effect of anemia and erythropoietin injection. J Am Soc Nephrol 2007;18(3): 896–903.
71. Viazzi F, Bonino B, Ratto E, et al. Early renal abnormalities as an indicator of cardiovascular risk in type 2 diabetes. High Blood Press Cardiovasc Prev 2014; 21(4):257–60.
72. Bonomini M, Sirolli V, Settefrati N, et al. Increased erythrocyte phosphatidylserine exposure in chronic renal failure. J Am Soc Nephrol 1999;10(9):1982–90.
73. Palsson R, Patel UD. Cardiovascular complications of diabetic kidney disease. Adv Chronic Kidney Dis 2014;21(3):273–80.
74. Halimi JM. The emerging concept of chronic kidney disease without clinical proteinuria in diabetic patients. Diabetes Metab 2012;38(4):291–7.
75. Gajjala PR, Sanati M, Jankowski J. Cellular and molecular mechanisms of chronic kidney disease with diabetes mellitus and cardiovascular diseases as its comorbidities. Front Immunol 2015;6:340.
76. Maurin N. The role of platelets in atherosclerosis, diabetes mellitus, and chronic kidney disease. An attempt at explaining the TREAT study results. Med Klin (munich) 2010;105(5):339–44 [in German].
77. Kovesdy CP, Park JC, Kalantar-Zadeh K. Glycemic control and burnt-out diabetes in ESRD. Semin Dial 2010;23(2):148–56.
78. Modan M, Meytes D, Rozeman P, et al. Significance of high HbA1 levels in normal glucose tolerance. Diabetes Care 1988;11(5):422–8.
79. Tuttle KR, Bakris GL, Bilous RW, et al. Diabetic kidney disease: a report from an ADA consensus conference. Am J Kidney Dis 2014;64(4):510–33.
80. Fitzgibbons JF, Koler RD, Jones RT. Red cell age-related changes of hemoglobins Ala+b and Alc in normal and diabetic subjects. J Clin Invest 1976;58(4): 820–4.
81. Ioannidis I. Diabetes treatment in patients with renal disease: is the landscape clear enough? World J Diabetes 2014;5(5):651–8.
82. Patel T, Charytan DM. Cardiovascular complications in diabetic kidney disease. Semin Dial 2010;23(2):169–77.
83. Lytvyn Y, Perkins BA, Cherney DZ. Uric acid as a biomarker and a therapeutic target in diabetes. Can J Diabetes 2015;39(3):239–46.
84. Ichikawa H, Nagake Y, Takahashi M, et al. What is the best index of glycemic control in patients with diabetes mellitus on hemodialysis? Nihon Jinzo Gakkai Shi 1996;38(7):305–8.
85. Eschbach JW, Adamson JW. Modern aspects of the pathophysiology of renal anemia. Contrib Nephrol 1988;66:63–70.
86. Chen HS, Wu TE, Lin HD, et al. Hemoglobin A(1c) and fructosamine for assessing glycemic control in diabetic patients with CKD stages 3 and 4. Am J Kidney Dis 2010;55(5):867–74.

87. Nunoi K, Kodama T, Sato Y, et al. Comparison of reliability of plasma fructos-amine and glycosylated hemoglobin assays for assessing glycemic control in diabetic patients on hemodialysis. Metabolism 1991;40(9):986–9.

88. Joy MS, Cefalu WT, Hogan SL, et al. Long-term glycemic control measurements in diabetic patients receiving hemodialysis. Am J Kidney Dis 2002;39(2): 297–307.

89. Nagayama H, Inaba M, Okabe R, et al. Glycated albumin as an improved indi-cator of glycemic control in hemodialysis patients with type 2 diabetes based on fasting plasma glucose and oral glucose tolerance test. Biomed Pharmacother 2009;63(3):236–40.

90. Riveline JP, Teynie J, Belmouaz S, et al. Glycaemic control in type 2 diabetic pa-tients on chronic haemodialysis: use of a continuous glucose monitoring system. Nephrol Dial Transpl 2009;24(9):2866–71.

91. Vos FE, Schollum JB, Coulter CV, et al. Assessment of markers of glycaemic control in diabetic patients with chronic kidney disease using continuous glucose monitoring. Nephrology (Carlton) 2012;17(2):182–8.

92. Bilo HJ, Struijk DG, Boeschoten EW, et al. A comparison of three methods to assess metabolic control in diabetic patients on CAPD treatment. Neth J Med 1988;33(5–6):217–24.

93. Suzuki H, Kikuta T, Inoue T, et al. Time to re-evaluate effects of renin-angiotensin system inhibitors on renal and cardiovascular outcomes in diabetic nephropa-thy. World J Nephrol 2015;4(1):118–26.

94. Vos FE, Schollum JB, Walker RJ. Glycated albumin is the preferred marker for assessing glycaemic control in advanced chronic kidney disease. NDT Plus 2011;4(6):368–75.

95. Okada T, Nakao T, Matsumoto H, et al. Influence of proteinuria on glycated al-bumin values in diabetic patients with chronic kidney disease. Intern Med 2011;50(1):23–9.

96. Koga M, Murai J, Saito H, et al. Effects of thyroid hormone on serum glycated albumin levels: study on non-diabetic subjects. Diabetes Res Clin Pract 2009; 84(2):163–7.

97. Koga M, Kasayama S, Kanehara H, et al. CLD (chronic liver diseases)-HbA1C as a suitable indicator for estimation of mean plasma glucose in patients with chronic liver diseases. Diabetes Res Clin Pract 2008;81(2):258–62.

98. Jindal A, Garcia-Touza M, Jindal N, et al. Diabetic kidney disease and the car-diorenal syndrome: old disease, new perspectives. Endocrinol Metab Clin North Am 2013;42(4):789–808.

99. Ikizler TA, Pupim LB, Brouillette JR, et al. Hemodialysis stimulates muscle and whole body protein loss and alters substrate oxidation. Am J Physiol Endocrinol Metab 2002;282(1):E107–16.

100. Cooper S, Iliescu EA, Morton AR. The relationship between dialysate protein loss and membrane transport status in peritoneal dialysis patients. Adv Perit Dial 2001;17:244–7.

101. Kitamura T, Otsuki M, Tamada D, et al. Glycated albumin is set lower in relation to plasma glucose levels in patients with Cushing's syndrome. Clin Chim Acta 2013;424:164–7.

102. Domingueti CP, Dusse LM, Carvalho M, et al. Hypercoagulability and car-diovascular disease in diabetic nephropathy. Clin Chim Acta 2013;415: 279–85.

103. Schleicher ED, Olgemöller B, Wiedenmann E, et al. Specific glycation of albu-min depends on its half-life. Clin Chem 1993;39(4):625–8.

104. Harada K, Sumida K, Yamaguchi Y, et al. Relationship between the accuracy of glycemic markers and the chronic kidney disease stage in patients with type 2 diabetes mellitus. Clin Nephrol 2014;82(2):107–14.

105. Okada T, Nakao T, Matsumoto H, et al. Influence of age and nutritional status on glycated albumin values in hemodialysis patients. Intern Med 2009;48(17):1495–9.

106. Isshiki K, Nishio T, Isono M, et al. Glycated albumin predicts the risk of mortality in type 2 diabetic patients on hemodialysis: evaluation of a target level for improving survival. Ther Apher Dial 2014;18(5):434–42.

107. Freedman BI, Andries L, Shihabi ZK, et al. Glycated albumin and risk of death and hospitalizations in diabetic dialysis patients. Clin J Am Soc Nephrol 2011; 6(7):1635–43.

108. Goldstein DE, Little RR, Lorenz RA, et al. Tests of glycemia in diabetes. Diabetes Care 2004;27(7):1761–73.

109. Hindle EJ, Rostron GM, Gatt JA. The estimation of serum fructosamine: an alternative measurement to glycated haemoglobin. Ann Clin Biochem 1985;22(Pt 1):84–9.

110. Van Dieijen-Visser MP, Seynaeve C, Brombacher PJ. Influence of variations in albumin or total-protein concentration on serum fructosamine concentration. Clin Chem 1986;32(8):1610.

111. Jin YP, Su XF, Yin GP, et al. Blood glucose fluctuations in hemodialysis patients with end stage diabetic nephropathy. J Diabetes Complications 2015;29(3): 395–9.

112. Home P. Contributions of basal and post-prandial hyperglycaemia to micro- and macrovascular complications in people with type 2 diabetes. Curr Med Res Opin 2005;21(7):989–98.

113. Gerich JE. Role of the kidney in normal glucose homeostasis and in the hyperglycaemia of diabetes mellitus: therapeutic implications. Diabet Med 2010; 27(2):136–42.

114. Wilding JP. The role of the kidneys in glucose homeostasis in type 2 diabetes: clinical implications and therapeutic significance through sodium glucose co-transporter 2 inhibitors. Metabolism 2014;63(10):1228–37.

115. Adrogué HJ. Glucose homeostasis and the kidney. Kidney Int 1992;42(5): 1266–82.

116. DeFronzo RA, Alvestrand A. Glucose intolerance in uremia: site and mechanism. Am J Clin Nutr 1980;33(7):1438–45.

117. Charpentier G, Riveline JP, Varroud-Vial M. Management of drugs affecting blood glucose in diabetic patients with renal failure. Diabetes Metab 2000; 26(Suppl 4):73–85.

118. Snyder RW, Berns JS. Use of insulin and oral hypoglycemic medications in patients with diabetes mellitus and advanced kidney disease. Semin Dial 2004; 17(5):365–70.

119. Weise WJ, Sivanandy MS, Block CA, et al. Exenatide-associated ischemic renal failure. Diabetes Care 2009;32(2):e22–3.

120. Johansen OE, Whitfield R. Exenatide may aggravate moderate diabetic renal impairment: a case report. Br J Clin Pharmacol 2008;66(4):568–9.

121. Jacobsen LV, Hindsberger C, Robson R, et al. Effect of renal impairment on the pharmacokinetics of the GLP-1 analogue liraglutide. Br J Clin Pharmacol 2009; 68(6):898–905.

122. Davies MJ, Bain SC, Atkin SL, et al. Efficacy and safety of liraglutide versus placebo as add-on to glucose-lowering therapy in patients with type 2 diabetes and moderate renal impairment (LIRA-RENAL): a randomized clinical trial. Diabetes Care 2016;39(2):222–30.

Moving?

Make sure your subscription moves with you!

To notify us of your new address, find your **Clinics Account Number** (located on your mailing label above your name), and contact customer service at:

Email: journalscustomerservice-usa@elsevier.com

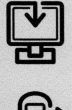

800-654-2452 (subscribers in the U.S. & Canada)
314-447-8871 (subscribers outside of the U.S. & Canada)

Fax number: 314-447-8029

Elsevier Health Sciences Division
Subscription Customer Service
3251 Riverport Lane
Maryland Heights, MO 63043